Biosignal Processing

Edited by Vahid Asadpour and Selcan Karakuş

Published in London, United Kingdom

Biosignal Processing
http://dx.doi.org/10.5772/intechopen.97943
Edited by Vahid Asadpour and Selcan Karakuş

Contributors
Vandana Roy, Fatima M. Baqer, Salah Albermany, Umamaheswari K, Shrichandran G.V., Jeba Derwin D., Marwa Fradi, Kais Bouallegue, Philippe Lasaygues, Mohsen Machhout, Hideaki Nakamura, Anton Yudhana, Liya Yusrina Sabila, Arsyad Cahya Subrata, Hendriana Helda Pratama, Muhammad Syahrul Akbar, Saptarshi Biswas, Sumagna Dey, Rohan Pal, Toshikazu Shinba, Kristin S. S. Williams, Taouli Sidi Ahmed, Alma T. Banigo, Chigozie A. Nnadiekwe, Emmanuel M. Beasi, David Marcarian, Anielle Almeida C.A. Silva, Eliete A. Alvin, Lais S. de Jesus, Caio C.L. de França, Marílya P.G. da Silva, Samaysa L. Lins, Diógenes Meneses, Marcela R. Lemes, Rhanoica O. Guerra, Marcos V. da Silva, Carlo J.F. de Oliveira, Virmondes Rodrigues Junior, Renata M. Etchebehere, Bruno G. Lucca, Fabiane C. de Abreu, Sanívia A.L. Pereira, Rodrigo C. Rosa, Noelio Oliveira O. Dantas, Hiroaki Matsui, Marlon S. Sheldon Thomas, Selcan Karakuş, Nuray Beköz Üllen, Gizem Karabulut

First published in London, United Kingdom, 2022 by IntechOpen
IntechOpen is the global imprint of INTECHOPEN LIMITED, registered in England and Wales, registration number: 11086078, 5 Princes Gate Court, London, SW7 2QJ, United Kingdom
Printed in Croatia

British Library Cataloguing-in-Publication Data
A catalogue record for this book is available from the British Library

Additional hard and PDF copies can be obtained from orders@intechopen.com

Biosignal Processing
Edited by Vahid Asadpour and Selcan Karakuş
p. cm.

This title is part of the Biomedical Engineering Book Series, Volume 14
Topic: Bioinformatics and Medical Informatics
Series Editor: Robert Koprowski
Topic Editor: Slawomir Wilczynski

Print ISBN 978-1-80355-561-4
Online ISBN 978-1-80355-562-1
eBook (PDF) ISBN 978-1-80355-563-8
ISSN 2631-5343

For EU product safety concerns:
IN TECH d.o.o., Prolaz Marije Krucifikse Kozulić 3, 51000 Rijeka, Croatia,
info@intechopen.com or visit our website at intechopen.com.

IntechOpen Book Series

Biomedical Engineering

Volume 14

Aims and Scope of the Series

Biomedical Engineering is one of the fastest-growing interdisciplinary branches of science and industry. The combination of electronics and computer science with biology and medicine has improved patient diagnosis, reduced rehabilitation time, and helped to facilitate a better quality of life. Nowadays, all medical imaging devices, medical instruments, or new laboratory techniques result from the cooperation of specialists in various fields. The series of Biomedical Engineering books covers such areas of knowledge as chemistry, physics, electronics, medicine, and biology. This series is intended for doctors, engineers, and scientists involved in biomedical engineering or those wanting to start working in this field.

Meet the Series Editor

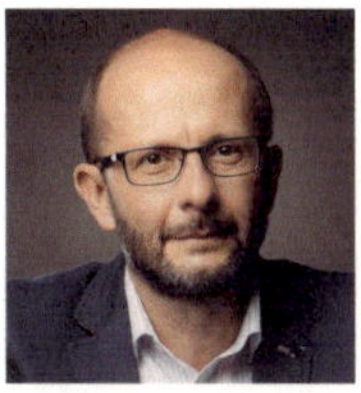

Robert Koprowski, MD (1997), Ph.D. (2003), Habilitation (2015), is an employee of the University of Silesia, Poland, Institute of Computer Science, Department of Biomedical Computer Systems. For 20 years, he has studied the analysis and processing of biomedical images, emphasizing the full automation of measurement for a large inter-individual variability of patients. Dr. Koprowski has authored more than a hundred research papers with dozens in impact factor (IF) journals and has authored or co-authored six books. Additionally, he is the author of several national and international patents in the field of biomedical devices and imaging. Since 2011, he has been a reviewer of grants and projects (including EU projects) in biomedical engineering.

Meet the Volume Editors

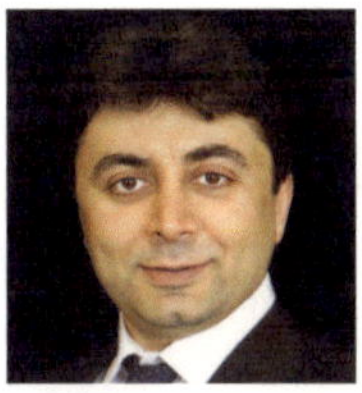

Vahid Asadpour is currently with Kaiser Permanente Southern California at the Department of Research and Evaluation. He graduated with an MS and Ph.D. in Biomedical Engineering. He was a research scientist at the University of California Los Angeles (UCLA) and visiting professor and researcher at the University of North Dakota. He works in artificial intelligence and its applications in medical signal processing. In addition, he is using digital signal processing in medical imaging and speech processing. Dr. Asadpour developed brain computer interfacing algorithms and published multiple books, book chapters, and several journal and conference papers in this field and other areas of intelligent signal processing. He has also designed medical devices, including a laser Doppler monitoring system.

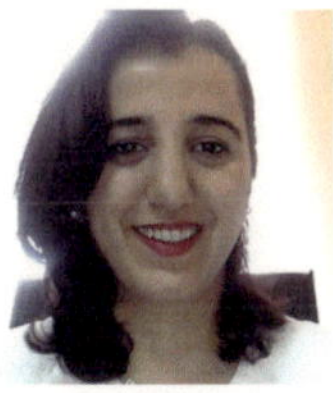

Selcan Karakuş is currently an Associate Professor in the Department of Chemistry, at Istanbul University-Cerrahpasa (IUC), Turkey. She received her Master of Science degree in physical chemistry from Istanbul University (IU) in 2006, and her Ph.D. in physical chemistry from IU in 2011. She has been a visiting researcher at the University of Massachusetts, Department of Polymer Science and Engineering. She has research experience in drug carrier systems, nanoparticles, nanocomposites, nano-emulsion self-assembled polymeric nanostructures, and copolymer blends. She has worked on a variety of projects funded by IUC and has published several research articles and book chapters.

Contents

Preface XV

Section 1
Biosignals Theory 1

Chapter 1 3
Characteristic Profiles of Heart Rate Variability in Depression and Anxiety
by Toshikazu Shinba

Chapter 2 13
Mathematical Morphology and the Heart Signals
by Taouli Sidi Ahmed

Chapter 3 33
Applications of Quantum Mechanics, Laws of Classical Physics, and Differential Calculus to Evaluate Source Localization According to the Electroencephalogram
by Kristin S. Williams

Chapter 4 43
Protecting Bioelectric Signals from Electromagnetic Interference in a Wireless World
by David Marcarian

Section 2
Biosignal Processing Algorithms and Applications 53

Chapter 5 55
Non-Invasive Approach for Glucose Detection in Urine Quality Using Its Image Analysis
by Anton Yudhana, Liya Yusrina Sabila, Arsyad Cahya Subrata, Hendriana Helda Pratama and Muhammad Syahrul Akbar

Chapter 6 73
Deep Learning Algorithms for Efficient Analysis of ECG Signals to Detect Heart Disorders
by Sumagna Dey, Rohan Pal and Saptarshi Biswas

Chapter 7 97
EEG Authentication System Using Fuzzy Vault Scheme
by Fatima M. Baqer and Salah Albermany

Chapter 8 113
Automatic Noise Reduction in Ultrasonic Computed Tomography Image for Adult Bone Fracture Detection
by Marwa Fradi, Kais Bouallegue, Philippe Lasaygues and Mohsen Machhout

Chapter 9 131
Soft Tissue Image Reconstruction Using Diffuse Optical Tomography
by Umamaheswari K, Shrichandran G.V. and Jeba Derwin D.

Chapter 10 143
Effective EEG Artifact Removal from EEG Signal
by Vandana Roy

Section 3
Biosignal Sensors 161

Chapter 11 163
Developmental Studies on Practical Enzymatic Phosphate Ion Biosensors and Microbial BOD Biosensors, and New Insights into the Future Perspectives of These Biosensor Fields
by Hideaki Nakamura

Chapter 12 189
Nanostructures in Biosensors: Development and Applications
by Gizem Karabulut, Nuray Beköz Üllen and Selcan Karakuş

Chapter 13 209
Biological Sensing Using Infrared SPR Devices Based on ZnO
by Hiroaki Matsui

Chapter 14 227
Development of Simple and Portable Surface Acoustic Wave Biosensors for Applications in Biology and Medicine
by Marlon S. Thomas

Chapter 15 241
Recent Advances in Biosensing in Tissue Engineering and Regenerative Medicine
by Alma T. Banigo, Chigozie A. Nnadiekwe and Emmanuel M. Beasi

Chapter 16 275
NanoBioSensors: From Electrochemical Sensors Improvement to Theranostic Applications
by Anielle C.A. Silva, Eliete A. Alvin, Lais S. de Jesus, Caio C.L. de França, Marílya P.G. da Silva, Samaysa L. Lins, Diógenes Meneses, Marcela R. Lemes, Rhanoica O. Guerra, Marcos V. da Silva, Carlo J.F. de Oliveira, Virmondes Rodrigues Junior, Renata M. Etchebehere, Fabiane C. de Abreu, Bruno G. Lucca, Sanívia A.L. Pereira, Rodrigo C. Rosa and Noelio O. Dantas

Preface

Advances in biosignal processing have made it one of the most important interpretations and therapeutic tools in medicine. The use of advanced instruments and processing techniques in modern signal processing has improved the accuracy and reliability of medical diagnoses. This book presents a wide range of new methods that play an important role in the state-of-the-art improvement of biosignal processing.

Chapters discuss biosignal theory, biosignal processing algorithms and applications, and biosignal sensors. They examine such topics as glucose detection, tissue engineering, fuzzy electroencephalogram analysis, deep learning electrocardiogram analysis, protein bioelectric signal, soft tissue optical tomography, heart rate variability, nano biosensors, ultrasonic bone fractures detection, source localization and enzymic biosensors, and more. The book also gives an understanding of how to apply artificial intelligence and machine learning to biosignal techniques. It provides a forum for researchers, engineers, and graduate students who are seeking advanced approaches to biomedical signal analysis, algorithms, and applications. This book is a useful resource for advanced research scholars in the field of brain signal processing and biomedical engineering.

Dr. Vahid Asadpour
Department of Research and Evaluation,
Kaiser Permanente Southern California,
Pasadena, USA

Selcan Karakuş
Faculty of Engineering,
Department of Chemistry,
Istanbul University-Cerrahpasa,
Istanbul, Turkey

Section 1

Biosignals Theory

Chapter 1

Characteristic Profiles of Heart Rate Variability in Depression and Anxiety

Toshikazu Shinba

Abstract

This chapter on heart rate variability (HRV) presents a view based on our published data that HRV profiles in depression and anxiety show differences and can be used for the differentiation of these two disorders in clinical practices. Characteristic HRV profiles in depression and anxiety are revealed by measurements incorporating task load. Analysis of two frequency-domain HRV parameters, low frequency (LF) and high frequency (HF), together with heart rate (HR) itself measured at rest (Rest), during the task load (Task), and at rest after the task (After) enables the evaluation of the autonomic regulation in response to behavioral changes with different stress levels. LF is the heart rate modulation related to blood pressure changes to stabilize circulation. HF is related to breathing rhythm and reflects parasympathetic activity. It has been indicated that LF, HF, their ratio LF/HF and HR in depression and anxiety show characteristic dysregulations during Rest, Task and After. These HRV profiles are useful for understanding the pathophysiology of the disorders.

Keywords: heart rate variability, baseline and reactivity, autonomic dysregulation, depression, anxiety

1. Introduction

Depression and anxiety are frequent mental disturbances that seriously affect human life. They are commonly encountered in clinical practices, but comorbidity is often and differentiation of depressive and anxiety states is important with respect to therapeutic processes [1]. Psychiatric diagnosis at present is mostly based on psychological and behavioral assessments [2]. Additional use of objective measures as biomarkers to evaluate the symptoms and to make the differential diagnosis will be useful for the adequate treatment of depression and anxiety. A biomarker is defined as an indicator of biological and pathogenic processes or responses to exposure and intervention and is classified as molecular, histological, radiographical, or physiological index [3]. Various types of biomarkers for depression and anxiety have been studied, including genetic, biochemical, hormonal, imaging, and electrophysiological measurers, and some studies tried to use them to differentiate depression and anxiety [4]. Among physiological measures, the present chapter focuses on heart rate variability (HRV) that has been utilized for analyzing autonomic activities to characterize and differentiate depression and anxiety.

2. Autonomic biomarkers of psychiatric disorders

Autonomic measures are interesting because some of the clinical symptoms of depression and anxiety are related to autonomic disturbances. In depression, appetite decreases, and weight loss is frequent. Bowel movement is also unstable. In anxiety, the patients report palpitation and cardiac discomfort without electrocardiographic abnormalities. Perspiration also increases. These somatic symptoms of depression and anxiety can be generated by autonomic dysregulations, supporting the feasibility of autonomic measures as biomarkers for depression and anxiety.

Although autonomic dysregulations are frequent in depression and anxiety, the methods for objective evaluation of autonomic symptoms are limited. Physiological indices of autonomic activity include pupil size, salivary amylase, gut movement, skin conductance, heart rate, and HRV. Among them, HRV has been intensively utilized in the analysis of autonomic function in depression and anxiety [5, 6]. HRV is easily measured by analyzing the electrocardiogram or pulse oximetric plethysmogram. A measurement takes only a few minutes and is less stressful for the patients. The measurement devices are small and portable and can be installed in regular clinical offices or in non-medical places. HRV is useful and convenient to characterize the autonomic dysregulations found in depression and anxiety.

3. Heart rate variability (HRV) measurement for evaluation of autonomic activity

HRV is a variation of inter-heartbeat intervals (**Figure 1**). The heart beats constantly but the rhythm is not regular. The heartbeat slows and accelerates, and the inter-heartbeat interval varies. It has been known that the heartbeat rhythm is composed of multiple components with different frequency ranges [7].

In HRV analysis, heartbeats or pulse beats are first identified conventionally by peak detection (**Figure 2**). The inter-beat interval trend made of the sequence of peak-to-peak intervals is processed by frequency analysis to yield the power spectrum of HRV. The power spectrum can reveal the presence of multiple heart rate rhythms with different frequencies ranges; high frequency (HF), low frequency (LF), very low frequency (VLF), and ultra-very low frequency (UVLF). HF and LF components are often used for the evaluation of autonomic activities in mental disorders, and

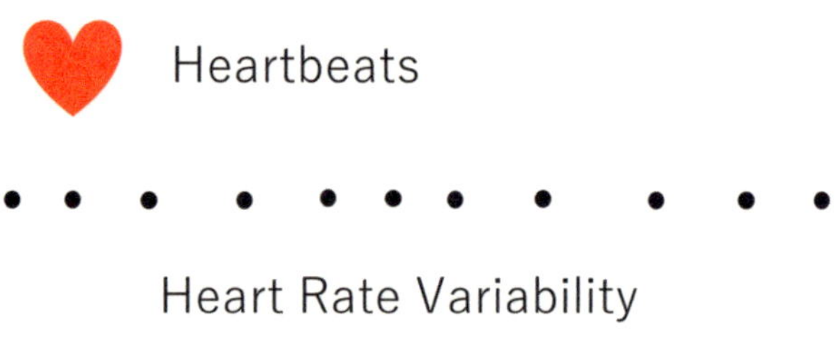

Figure 1.
Inter-heartbeat intervals increase and decrease presenting the heart rate variability (HRV).

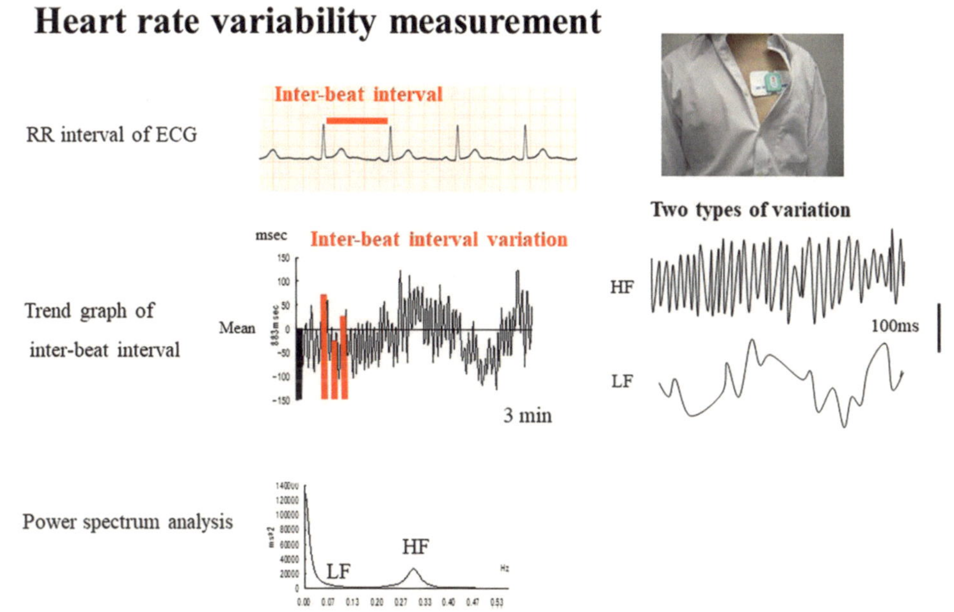

Figure 2.
The methods for heart rate variability (HRV) measurement. RR intervals of electrocardiogram (ECG) are used for creating the RR interval trend graph, which contains both low and high-frequency components (LF and HF). The power spectrum of the trend graph is used to calculate LF and HF by integrating the power in the range designated for LF and HF (0.04–0.15 Hz, 0.15–0.4 Hz, respectively).

their physiological bases have been clarified. The frequency ranges of HF and LF are usually set at 0.15–0.4 Hz and 0.04–0.15 Hz, respectively.

The rhythm of the HF component is related to breathing. Inspiration is accompanied by an increase in heart rate, and expiration by a decrease (**Figure 3**). This modulation is inhibited by the administration of anticholinergic agents such as atropine and is considered to be dependent on parasympathetic activity [8]. The physiological significance for the coupling of breathing rhythm and heart rhythm is not clarified but would be related to the maintenance of constant blood flow under the fluctuation of intrathoracic pressure during breathing activity.

LF component of HRV is generated under the control of baroreceptor [9], and is intimately related to blood pressure fluctuation. When the blood pressure is recorded continuously, the systolic peak fluctuates with an interval of about 10 to 20 seconds. This fluctuation is known as Mayer wave (**Figure 4**). Accompanying this blood pressure fluctuation, heartbeats also vary. When the systolic blood pressure is high, the inter-beat interval is long. When the blood pressure is low, the interval is short (**Figure 4**). It is a homeostatic control to stabilize the blood flow by adjusting the heart rate in response to the changes in blood pressure. Both sympathetic and parasympathetic systems are involved in generating the LF variation.

These observations indicate that HF variation controls the blood flow during various breathing rhythms. LF variation on the other hand stabilizes the blood flow during various activities that accompany changes in blood pressure. Both HF and LF variations serve as safety systems to avoid abrupt changes in blood flow in response to alterations of breathing and somatic condition, respectively. Blood pressure is adjusted automatically, but breathing is modified both unconsciously and consciously. Conscious control of breathing is observed not only during respiration

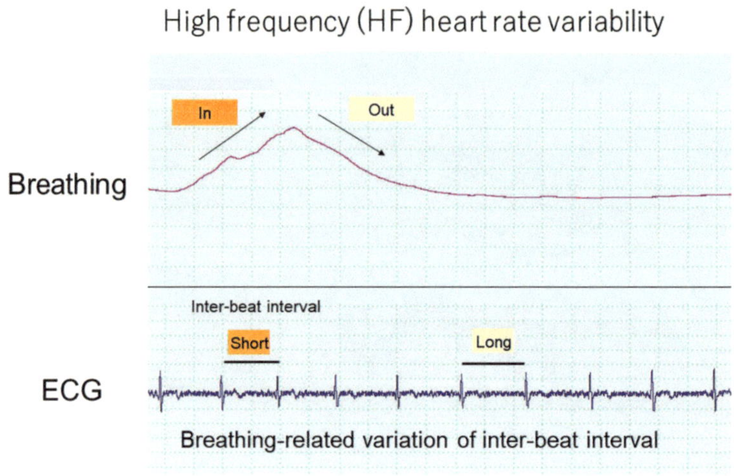

Figure 3.
High frequency (HF) heart rate variability related to breathing. Inspiration (In) is accompanied by shortening of inter-beat interval measured with R-R interval of electrocardiogram (ECG). Expiration (Out) is accompanied by its elongation.

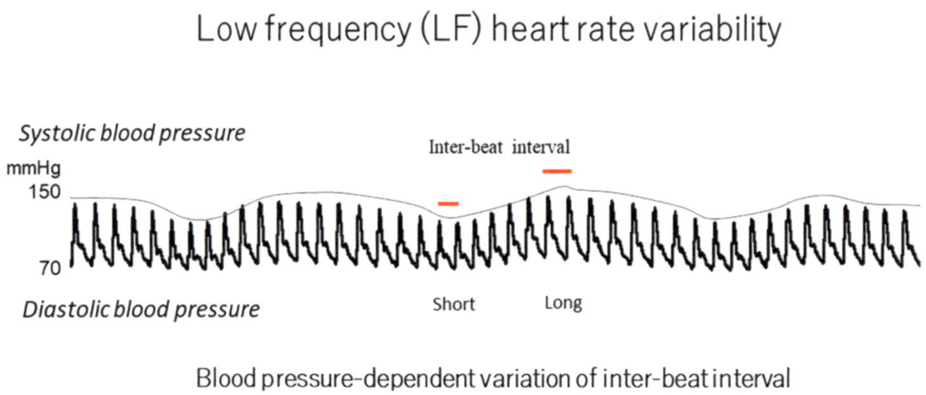

Figure 4.
Low frequency (LF) heart rate variability is dependent on blood pressure. Continuous measurement of blood pressure indicates systolic peaks fluctuate, generating Mayer wave. In response to Mayer wave, inter-heartbeat intervals vary. When the blood pressure is high, the inter-beat interval is long. When the blood pressure is low, it is short.

but during various activities including speaking, singing, and shouting. In various conditions, the HF and LF safeties will be switched on or off to adjust the blood flow and to meet the physiological demand.

HRV is controlled by the autonomic nervous system; sympathetic and parasympathetic. HF variation is large when the parasympathetic system is activated. Interpretation of LF changes in terms of sympathetic or parasympathetic changes is complex because LF variation is controlled by both sympathetic and parasympathetic systems. LF/HF ratio is sometimes used as a parameter representing sympathetic activity, although it is not recommended in some studies [9]. LF/HF can be used to evaluate the balance between breathing-related autonomic activity and blood pressure-dependent autonomic activity.

4. Measurements at rest and during the task load

In the studies on HRV in depression and anxiety, the data at rest condition have been frequently used to analyze the autonomic activity. And in some studies, the data were also recorded during task load or stress. An introduction of task load or stress enables the evaluation of autonomic responsiveness to the load. Random number generation task has been used for the task load in our studies. Random number generation is related to frontal cortical function. In the task, the subject makes a series of digit numbers (0–9) in random order at the speed of 1 Hz [10].

We propose to record HRV at rest (Rest), during task load (Task), and at rest after the task (After) (**Figure 5**). **Figure 5** shows sample data of a normal healthy subject. HF decreases, and LF/HF and HR increase during the task load. These changes of HRV are possibly related to the autonomic modulation in response to the task load and reflect both physical and mental adjustment to stress. Introduction of task load to the assessment of HRV has been found informative on analyzing the autonomic dysfunction of mental disorders [11]. The present chapter is intended to summarize that the Rest, Task, and After scores of HRV are differently altered in depression and anxiety.

Our previous study [12] has indicated the importance of analyzing the change from the rest data to that during the task load. Task/Rest ratio of the HRV indices is

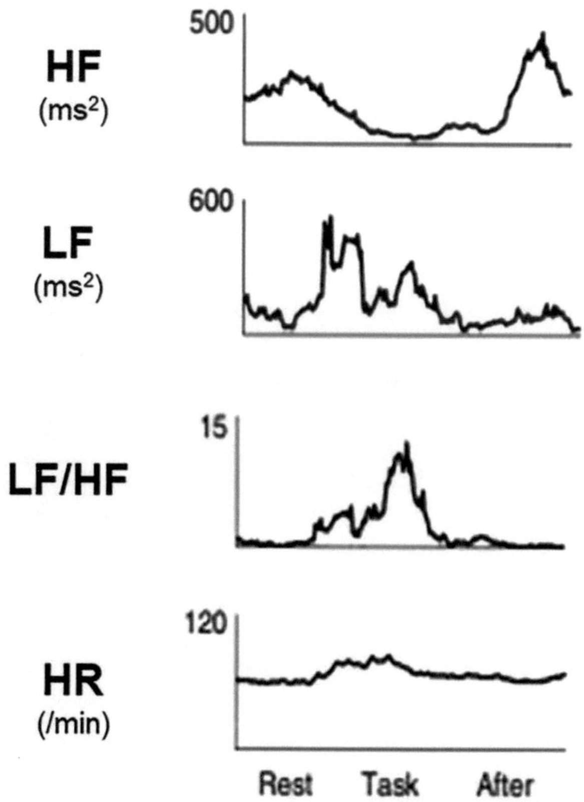

Figure 5.
A sample data of heart rate variability indices at the initial rest period (Rest), during the task load (Task), and during the rest period after the task (After).

used for this purpose, especially for evaluating depressiveness and anxiety. In this study on normal subjects, subjective depressiveness and anxiety were scored by questionnaires; Self-rating Depression Scale (SDS) and State-Trait Anxiety Inventory (STAI) [12]. It has been revealed that the Task/Rest ratio of HF index is significantly correlated with both SDS and STAI scores, confirming the importance of Task/Rest ratio in evaluating depression and anxiety. Below are the HRV profiles of depression and anxiety showing different patterns in the Rest-Task-After paradigm.

5. Characteristic HRV profiles in depression

Figure 6 presents the characteristic HRV profiles at the baseline rest condition (Rest), during the task load (Task) and during the rest condition after the task (After) in the control healthy subjects, in the patients with major depressive disorder (MDD) and in the patients with a general anxiety disorder (GAD). The HRV profiles of MDD and GAD were used in the present chapter to represent that in depression and anxiety. The schematic diagrams are made based on our published data [13]. The data in each measurement condition are connected by lines to clarify the characteristic profiles. LF data are connected by dashed lines to indicate that the inter-subject differences are large not only in the healthy subjects but in the patients with MDD and GAD.

The healthy HF pattern takes the form of a V shape and the healthy LF/HF and HR patterns have inverted V shapes. HF decreases, and LF/HF and HR increase during Task, and they return to the original level at After. This indicates that the breathing-related control of heart rate reflecting parasympathetic activity decreases during Tasks in healthy subjects. It is interesting that inhibition of parasympathetic activity during task load is observed in this paradigm. The parasympathetic inhibition during task load should be a healthy response of the autonomic system to stressful events. LF responses are not consistent. HF and LF react to stressful events differently. HR behaves similar to LF/HF.

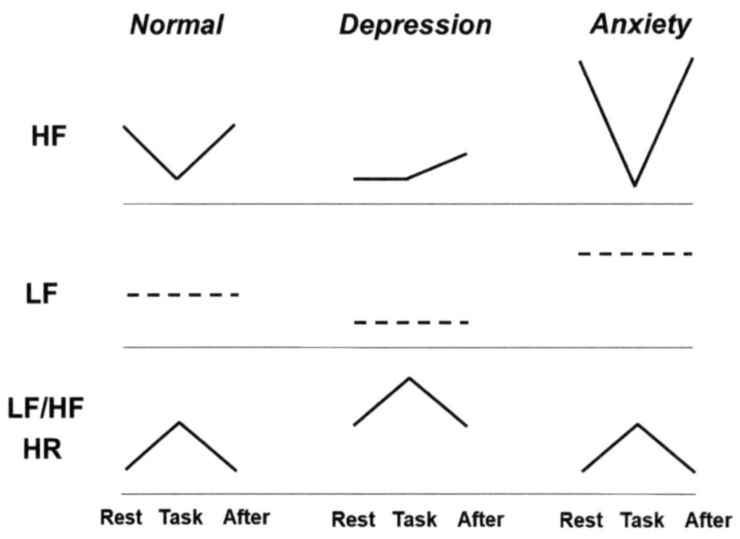

Figure 6.
Schematic diagrams of heart rate variability profiles in major depressive disorder (MDD) and generalized anxiety disorder (GAD). Detailed descriptions are found in the text.

In depression, HF at the resting state is low, indicating the underactivity of parasympathetic system. Parasympathetic underactivity is found not only in depression but in cardiovascular, neurological, and other psychiatric disturbances. In ischemic heart disorder and diabetic neuropathy, the peripheral autonomic nerve function is disturbed. In dementia and epilepsy, organic changes of the brain lead to autonomic alteration. In depression, functional changes of the responsible brain areas should involve the central autonomic system to generate HRV changes.

In addition to baseline change of the parasympathetic activity reflected in low HF, response of HF to the task load is disturbed in depression, making Task/Rest ratio high. Parasympathetic activity cannot be switched off during the task indicating the difficulty in modifying the autonomic activity in response to alteration of arousal level or attention. Unresponsiveness of HF is found not only in MDD [11] but in normal subjects with high depressiveness and anxiety [12]. Subjective scores for depressiveness and anxiety were correlated with Task/Rest ratio of HF in normal controls. Depressiveness and anxiety may be related to parasympathetic unresponsiveness to stress.

Depression is also accompanied by an increase of HF during the rest period after the task load. The rebound-like increase starts after the end of the task and lasts for several tens of seconds. The functional significance of this transient change of HF may be related to excessive excitation of the parasympathetic system after suppression during the task load. Overall, depression is accompanied by continuous suppression together with the uncontrollability of the parasympathetic system.

As for LF, a reduction in the baseline level is observed in depression. But the rebound-like increase is present at the resting state after the task load possibly because LF reflects both sympathetic and parasympathetic activity. LF/HF and HR are higher in depression than in control. Parasympathetic underactivity is also responsible for these changes. It is interesting to observe that LF/HF and HR increase in response to task load although HF and LF are unchanged during the task load. Individual differences during the task load may account for this discrepancy.

6. Characteristic HRV profiles in anxiety

On the other hand, the patients with GAD show an elevation of both HF and LF when they are free of a panic attack or severe phobic symptoms. In contrast to the HRV profile in depression, the parasympathetic system is activated, and breathing-related and blood pressure-dependent modulation of heart rate is enhanced. The elevation of HF and LF at the resting state may be considered as a regulation of autonomic activity to cope with anxiety-related changes. When the regulation does not work, panic attack may occur. During panic attacks and exacerbation of anxiety symptoms, HF decreases and LF/HF increases, reflecting parasympathetic inhibition [6]. But when the anxious state is ameliorated, HRV indices return to the original level [13].

The elevated HF in GAD reacts to the task load by decreasing as in the normal control. Reactivity of parasympathetic activity is maintained in anxiety patients. The elevated LF can contribute to the stabilization of blood flow when the fluctuation of blood flow is large. Such fluctuation would be present during the time of stress. LF elevation may be the sign of an increased control of stress-induced circulatory changes. HRV profiles in GAD can be the result of autonomic accommodation to the anxious state.

7. Conclusions

The present chapter described the different profiles of HRV found in MDD and GAD, and tried to delineate the functional significance of the findings in terms of autonomic activity. It is interesting to use HF and LF indices to evaluate the pathophysiology of mental disorders based on the physiological mechanisms underlying HRV.

Although depression and anxiety coexist frequently, the patterns of autonomic dysregulation show differences when viewed from HRV analyses. Depression is mainly accompanied by parasympathetic inhibition and unresponsiveness. In anxiety, augmentation of parasympathetic activity is present during the condition when the symptoms are controlled. When phobic symptoms appear, parasympathetic activity lowers and the autonomic balance is lost. Then the autonomic dysregulation in anxiety becomes similar to that of depression.

It should be important to understand the differences and similarities to evaluate the pathophysiology of depression and anxiety in clinical practices. Differentiation of depressive and anxious conditions using HRV measures can be useful for adequate pharmacological, psychological, and behavioral therapies [14].

Conflict of interest

The author declares no conflict of interest.

Author details

Toshikazu Shinba
Autonomic Nervous System Consulting, Department of Psychiatry, Shizuoka Saiseikai General Hospital, Shizuoka, Japan

*Address all correspondence to: t156591@siz.saiseikai.or.jp

References

[1] Gorman JM. Comorbid depression and anxiety spectrum disorders. Depression and Anxiety. 1996-1997;**4**:160-168

[2] American Psychiatric Association, editor. Diagnostic and Statistical Manual of Mental Disorders: DSM-5. 5th ed. American Psychiatric Association: Washington, DC, USA; 2013

[3] Kozlowski S. FDA Perspectives on Biomarkers. Maryland, USA: US Food & Drug Administration; 2022. Available from: https://sitc.sitcancer.org/meetings/am09/workshop09/presentations/Kozlowski_800am.pdf

[4] Lai CH. The regional homogeneity of cingulate-precuneus regions: The putative biomarker for depression and anxiety. Journal of Affective Disorders. 2018;**229**:171-176

[5] Kemp AH, Quintana DS, Gray MA, Felmingham KL, Brown K, Gatt JM. Impact of depression and antidepressant treatment on heart rate variability: A review and meta-analysis. Biological Psychiatry. 2010;**67**:1067-1074

[6] Chalmers JA, Quintana DS, Abbott MJA, Kemp AH. Anxiety disorders are associated with reduced heart rate variability: A meta-analysis. Frontiers in Psychiatry. 2014;**5**:80. DOI: 10.3389/fpsyt.2014.00080

[7] Malik M. Heart rate variability: Standards of measurement, physiological interpretation, and clinical use. Circulation. 1996;**93**:1043-1065

[8] Akselrod S, Gordon D, Madwed JB, Snidman NC, Shannon DC, Cohen RJ. Hemodynamic regulation: Investigation by spectral analysis. American Journal of Physiology. 1985;**249**:H867-H875

[9] Goldstein DS, Bentho O, Park MY, Sharabi Y. Low-frequency power of heart rate variability is not a measure of cardiac sympathetic tone but may be a measure of modulation of cardiac autonomic outflows by baroreflexes. Experimental Physiology. 2011;**96**:1255-1261

[10] Shinba T, Shinozaki T, Kariya N, Ebata K. Random number generation deficit in schizophrenia characterized by oral vs written response modes. Perceptual and Motor Skills. 2000;**91**:1091-1105

[11] Shinba T. Altered autonomic activity and reactivity in depression revealed by heart-rate variability measurement during rest and task conditions. Psychiatry and Clinical Neurosciences. 2014;**68**:225-233

[12] Shinba T, Kariya N, Matsui Y, Ozawa N, Matsuda Y, Yamamoto K. Decrease in heart rate variability response to task is related to anxiety and depressiveness in normal subjects. Psychiatry and Clinical Neurosciences. 2008;**62**:603-609

[13] Shinba T. Major depressive disorder and generalized anxiety disorder show different autonomic dysregulations revealed by heart-rate variability analysis in first-onset drug-naïve patients without comorbidity. Psychiatry and Clinical Neurosciences. 2017;**71**:135-145

[14] Shinba T, Murotsu K, Usui Y, Andow Y, Terada H, Kariya N, et al. Return-to-work screening by linear discriminant analysis of heart rate variability indices in depressed subjects. Sensors (Basel). 2021;**21**:5177. DOI: 10.3390/s21155177

Chapter 2

Mathematical Morphology and the Heart Signals

Taouli Sidi Ahmed

Abstract

Nowadays, signal processing is integrated into most systems for analyzing and interpreting ECG and PCG signals. Its objectives are multiple and mainly include compensating for the addition of artifacts to the signals of interest, and extracting information that is not visible by direct visual analysis. Considering that useful clinical information is found in the characteristic waves of the ECG, in particular, the P wave, the QRS complex, the T wave and the heart sounds of the PCG signal. These signals provide important indicators for the diagnosis of heart disease because they reflect physiological processes. These are non-stationary signals that are very sensitive to noise, hence the need to have optimal conditions to record them. It is necessary to use appropriate signal processing tools for noise suppression and wave detection of the ECG signal. Our method uses Morphological filtering, multi-scale morphological and the other by top-hat transform, which are based on mathematical morphology. The latter is based on mathematical operators called opening and closing morphology operators. These methods are also tested, with the aim of removing the noise and detection of the waves of the ECG signal and of the pathological sounds of the PCG signal.

Keywords: ECG signal, PCG signal, morphological filtering, multi-scale morphological, top-hat transform

1. Introduction

In the Western world, the leading cause of death is cardiovascular diseases. Even if the knowledge acquired in cardiology is great, the heart has not yet revealed all its secrets. However, doctors have many ways to study and verify its proper functioning. In particular, they use cardiac signals, the electrocardiogram (ECG) and the phonocardiogram (PCG) which are an important tools in the diagnosis of cardiac pathologies.

The ECG is the signal reflecting the recording of the bioelectrical activities of the cardiac system. It is rich in information on the functional aspects of the heart and the cardiovascular system.

The electrocardiogram includes three important waves called the P wave, complex QRS and T wave which translate respectively the atrial activity, the ventricular activity and ventricular repolarization. From these waves are determined intervals known by the PR interval which defines the atrioventricular conduction time, the ST segment which corresponds to the ventricular repolarization phase, a phase during which the ventricular cells are all depolarized, and the RR interval which indicates the cardiac period, i.e. the time between two successive beats. Inverting it, we get then the heart rate commonly expressed in beats per minute.

The QT interval reflects all ventricular activity, i.e. phases of depolarization and repolarization. The time intervals between these different ECG waves provide important indicators for the diagnosis of heart disease because they reflect physiological processes of the heart and autonomic nervous system [1–3].

The analysis of these different intervals often involves the study of their variability.

At the level of the PCG signal, this signal produces two noises (S1 and S2) during the opening and closing of the valves under normal conditions. Two other noises (S3 and S4) with significantly lower amplitudes than the first two sometimes appear at the level of the cardiac cycle due to the effect of pathology or age [4].

The S1 sound occurs just after the onset of systole and is preferentially due to the closure of the atrioventricular valves. The S2 sound is produced at the beginning of diastole and is due to the closure of the aortic and pulmonary valves. However, doctors use heart auscultation to hear two normal sounds S1 and S2 using a medical instrument called a stethoscope. Also, cardiac synchronization can simultaneously gives the two physiological signals ECG and PCG, such that the S1 noise appears at the end of the R peak and the S2 noise at the end of the ECG segment, as for the S3 and S4 noises, they originate respectively at the end of the P wave and in the middle of the diastolic phase of the electrocardiogram (**Figure 1**).

Generally, the recording conditions of the ECG and PCG make that the signals are necessarily noisy by processes other than cardiac. These artifacts can be of physiological origin (skin, muscle, breathing ...) or environmental (mains current, electromagnetic artifacts, placement of the electrode ...).

The practitioner who analyses the ECG can then be discomfort by the presence of noise: in the case where, for example, he looks for the existence of a normal sinus rhythm and he is looking for the presence of the P wave preceding the R wave, the P wave, which is of low amplitude, can be drowned in noise. In the same way, a strong variation of the base line can prevent discerning an anomaly of the over- or under-shift type of the S-T segment, for example. To be able effectively segment heartbeats without altering clinical information, a certain number of pre-treatments are necessary. The purpose of this step is attenuate, or at by eliminates noises present in the raw ECG signal such as baseline variations or sector the interference at 50 Hz. Also, the

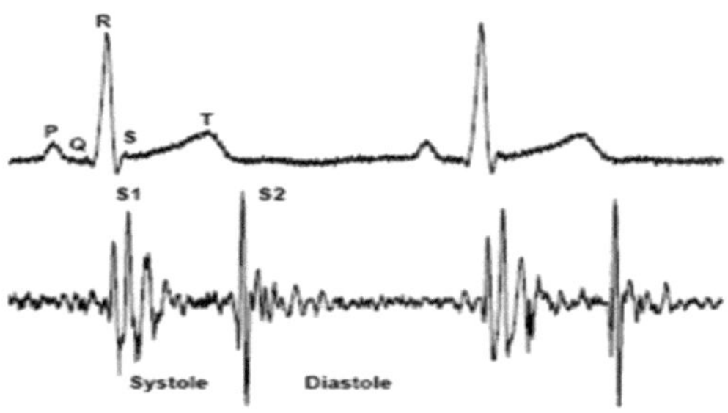

Figure 1.
Synchronization between ECG and PCG signal.

doctor finds it difficult to listen to the S1 and S2 heart sounds due to the presence of heart murmurs and this prevents the doctor from diagnosing the patient.

These heart murmurs are an additional noise; it was produced by a turbulent circulation of blood toward the heart. In fact the objective is to filter the non-stationary ECG and PCG signals and the extraction useful clinical information is found in the time intervals defined by the ECG waves characteristic, including the P wave, QRS complex, T wave, PR interval, ST segment, and interval QT, the defined time intervals between two characteristics ECG waves provide important indicators for the diagnosis of heart disease because they reflect physiological processes.

However, it is clear that to achieve this study, it is essential to perform a pre-processing of the ECG and PCG signals in order to then detect the different waves of the ECG signal.

In this article the morphological transform is used to remove noise and to detect the characteristics of the ECG and PCG signal.

This transformation uses mathematical morphology to realize, in particular the morphological filtering and the top hat transform. Mathematical morphology, based on set operations, provides an approach to developing nonlinear signal processing methods in which the shape of a signal's information is incorporated [5]. In these operations, the result of one set of data transformed by another set depends on the shapes of the two sets involved. A structuring element must be designed according to the shape characteristics of the signal that must be extracted. There are two basic morphological operators: erosion and dilation. Opening and closing are derived operators defined in terms of erosion and dilation [6].

Dilation reduces the peaks in a signal and to widen the valleys, erosion fills in the valleys and thickens the peaks in the signal; opening removes the peaks but preserves the valleys, and closing fills in the valleys, removes the wells (or valleys). The "closing" and "opening" operators behave like filters; we will speak of "Morphological Filter" [7].

An important number of researches work using different tools and methods of noise filtering have been presented in the literature. The methods often based on classical linear high-pass filtering, low-pass or band-pass [8–10], linear adaptive filtering [11], filtering based on neural networks [12–15], have been proposed to eliminate noise affecting the line of basis of the ECG signal. The major disadvantage of these methods is the distortion of the signal due to the overlapping of the spectra of the ECG, PCG and their noises. On the other hand, a large number of methods have been proposed for the detection of ECG signal waves [12–20]. The majority of these methods are based on adaptive filtering or thresholding, which shows the limitation of the application. The emergence of treatment method in the non-stationary case has helped the researchers to develop new tools better suited to filtering. Techniques based on the wavelet theory have already proved their worth for the filtering of noise from the ECG signal. Donoho and Johnston proposed a denoising method by thresholding of wavelet [21, 22]. The denoising method by wavelet thresholding was treated the wavelet coefficients by a threshold which must be chosen in advance. Approaches for estimate the value of this threshold can be found in [23, 24].

In this chapter, the pre-processing is realized in two stages, a stage of the correction of the line base by Morphological filtering and the top-hat transform for remove noises that are based on mathematical operators called derivation operators opening and closing morphology. Followed by the second step which is consisted of detecting the waves of the ECG signal and the cardiac murmurs of the PCG signal by morphology operators and a multi-scale structuring element.

2. Theory of mathematical morphology

2.1 The basic principle

The morphological transform is very widespread in the domain of signal processing and image processing because of its robustness and its simple and fast calculation [25, 26].

Mathematical morphology, based on set operations, provides an approach to the development of nonlinear methods of signal processing, in which the form of a signal's information is incorporated [27]. In these operations, the result of a data set transformed by another set depends on the shapes of both sets involved. A structuring element must be designed according to the characteristics of shape of the signal to be extracted.

There are two basic morphological operators: erosion ($\ominus$) and dilation ($\oplus$).

Opening and closing are derived operators defined in terms of erosion and dilation [28].

These operators are described in detail below with the corresponding mathematical expressions. Throughout this document denotes the discrete ECG signal of point size and the symmetrical structuring element of M points.

a. Erosion.

To obtain the eroded function of f(x), we attribute to f(x) its minimum value in the domain of the structuring element B and this, at each new displacement of B (**Figure 2**). The following formula illustrates the erosion of the function f(x) (original signal) by a structuring element *B* plane:

$$\varepsilon_B(f) = (f \ominus B)(n) = \min_{m=0,\ \dots M-1} \{ f(n) - B(m) \} \tag{1}$$

b. Dilation.

To obtain the dilated function of *f(x)*, we attribute to *f(x)* its maximum value in the field of the structuring element *B* and this, with each new displacement of *B* (**Figure 2**). The following formula illustrates the dilation of the function *f(x)* (original signal) by a structuring element *B* plane:

$$\delta_B(f) = (f \oplus B)(n) = \max_{m=0,\ \dots M-1} \{ f(n) + B(m) \} \tag{2}$$

Erosion shrinks peaks and the crest lines. The peaks narrower than the element structuring disappear. At the same time, it widens the valleys and the minima [29].

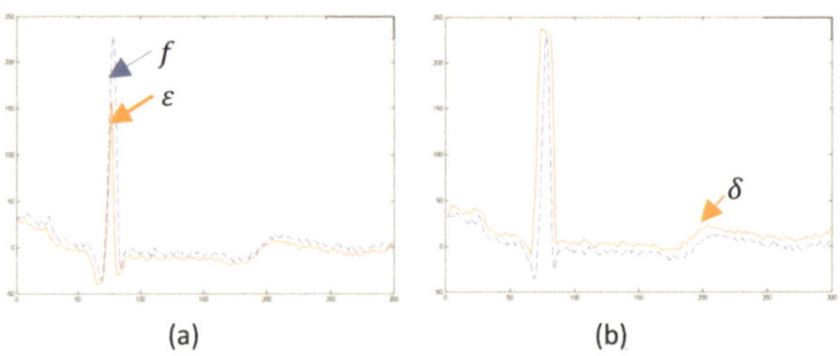

Figure 2.
a) Eroded ECG signal. b) Dilated ECG signal.

The dilation produces the opposite effects (fills in the valleys and thickens the peaks).

c. Opening.

As in mathematical morphology, the opening consists of the erosion followed by dilation. The opening of $f(x)$ by the structuring element B plane has the following consequences on the initial function (**Figure 3**):

The opening removes the peaks but preserves the valleys [30], according to the equation:

$$\gamma_B(f) = foB = f \ominus B \oplus B \tag{3}$$

d. Closing.

As in mathematical morphology, closing consists of dilation followed by erosion (**Figure 3**). The closing of $f(x)$ by the structuring element B plane, for its part, has the following consequences on the starting function [31]:

The closing fills the valleys [32] as follows:

$$\varphi_B(f) = f \bullet B = f \oplus B \ominus B \tag{4}$$

The "closing" and "opening" operators behave like filters; these are in the same time morphological Filters [33].

The opening and closing by adjunction create a simpler function than the initial function, by softening the latter in a nonlinear manner.

Opening (closing) eliminates positive (negative) peaks respectively that are narrower than the structuring element.

The opening (the closing) is located below (above) the initial function.

e. Structuring element.

After the selection of the morphology operator, the structuring element (SE) is the next component of the morphological analysis to be defined. Generally, only when the shape of the signal matches those of the structuring element that the signal can be preserved. Therefore, the shape, length (domain) and size (amplitude) of the structuring element should be chosen according to the signal to be analyzed. The shapes of the structuring element can vary regularly or irregularly, such as a triangle, line (flat), or a semicircle.

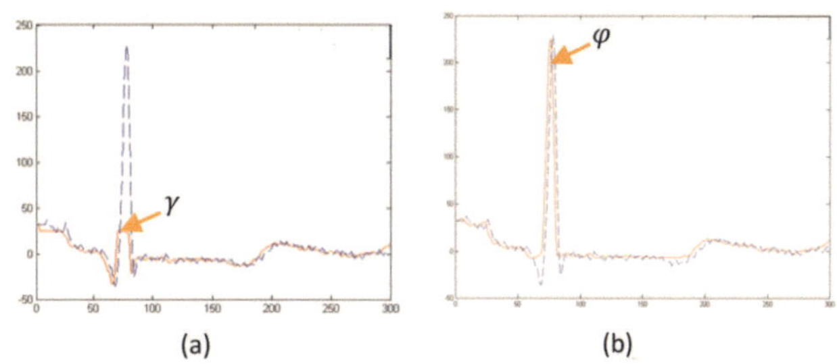

Figure 3.
a) Opening ECG signal. b) Closing ECG signal.

2.2 Filter construction

2.2.1 Morphological filter

In signal processing, the term "filter" is not very precise, it depends on the context in which it is used. It sometimes implies convolution, sometimes also any operation that produces a new function. On the contrary, mathematical morphology defines it very precisely [34–36]:

Any increasing and idempotent transformation on a trellis defines a morphological filter.

- Increase:

This hypothesis is the most fundamental. It ensures that the basic structure of the trellis, i.e. the order relation, is preserved during a morphological filtering.

This property causes the filter to generally lose information.

- Idempotence:

By definition, an idempotent transformation transforms the signal into an invariant.

This property often appears, but implicitly, in the descriptions. We say of an optical filter that it is red, or of an amp that its bandwidth is 50 kHz. Here, we will pose it as an axiom.

Idempotence is reached either after a single pass or as a limit by iteration. More generally, a sequence of operations, taken as a whole, can be idempotent.

Finally, note that when linear filters are idempotent, then they do not admit an inverse: they lose information, which brings them near to morphological filters.

2.2.2 Average filter

In practice, operators morphologic are based on different application scenarios in signal processing [37–42]. Sometimes it is difficult to obtain prior knowledge of the positive (positive peak) or negative (negative peak) pulse characteristics of the signal, especially when both positive and negative pulses are used. We can make by the combination of the four operators an average filter presented by the following formula:

$$AVG(f) = (f \bullet g + fog)/2 \tag{5}$$

Figure 4 illustrates the results obtained not used to flatten the positive and negative peaks.

2.2.3 Top hat transform

The concept of Top-Hat, due to F. Meyer, is a residue intended to eliminate the slow variations of the signal, or to amplify the contrasts. It therefore applies mainly to functions (**Figure 5**).

We call Top-Hat the residual between the identity and an invariant opening under vertical translation [43]:

$$\rho(f) = f - (foB) \quad (6)$$

We define in the same way a dual top-hat, residue between a closure and the identity:

$$\rho(f) = (f \bullet B) - f \quad (7)$$

2.2.4 Multi-scale morphology

f and *s*, represent respectively, a discrete signal and the structuring element (SE) for a morphological analysis. The morphology operator *R*, based on multi-scale analysis [44, 45], can be defined as a set $T_\lambda | \lambda > 0, \lambda \in N$, where $R_\lambda(f) = \lambda R(f/\lambda)$.

Multi-scale erosion and dilation are defined by:

$$(f \ominus s)_\lambda = \lambda[(f/\lambda) \ominus s] = f \ominus \lambda s \quad (8)$$

$$(f \oplus s)_\lambda = \lambda[(f/\lambda) \oplus g] = f \oplus \lambda s \quad (9)$$

and $\lambda g = s \oplus s \oplus \ldots \ldots . \oplus s(\lambda - 1\, times)$.

The original purpose of multi-scale morphology analysis is based on the morphology composition of the structuring element g is to improve the speed of morphology

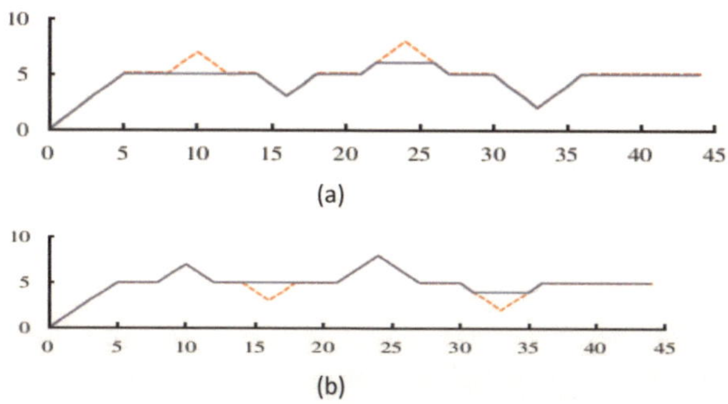

Figure 4.
a) Opening signal (lime draw f original*). b) Closing signal.*

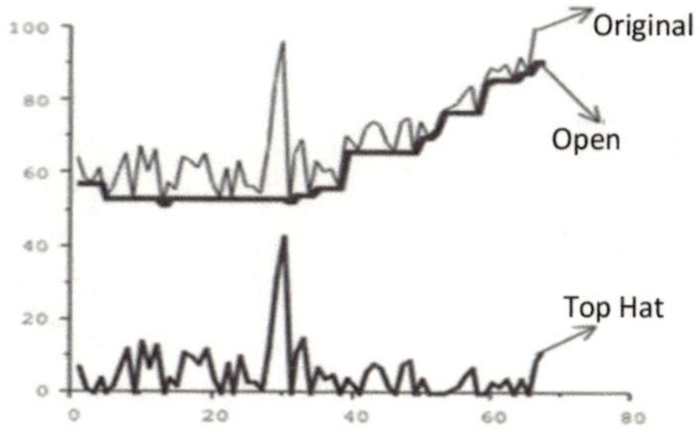

Figure 5.
Opening and top hat.

analysis by a large scale of structuring element and to expand the domains of application in signal processing.

The original purpose of multi-scale morphology analysis is based on the morphology composition of the structuring element g is to improve the speed of morphology analysis by a large scale of structuring element and to expand the domains of application in signal processing.

3. Application of morphological filtering to physiological signals

3.1 ECG signal filtering algorithm

The opening and closing operators proposed in this work for ECG signal processing, is shown in **Figure 6** below.

It consists of different phases. A first phase which consists in detecting variations in the baseline from the original noisy ECG signal. A second phase which consists in correcting these variations (correction of the baseline), and a third phase which consists in suppressing the remaining noises to finally generate the filtered ECG signal.

These different phases are realized through the development of a sequence of opening and closing operators.

This sequence is based on exploiting the different characteristics of baseline drift and noise contamination in ECG signals, different structuring elements and different morphological operators. For baseline correction, an opening operator followed by a closing operator is defined; as well as noise cancelation. They are described in detail in the following subsections.

3.1.1 Baseline correction algorithm

To correct for baseline variations, the variations of that line (f_b signal) detected from the original signal (f_o) are subtracted from that signal to generate the corresponding signal f_{cb} (i.e., an isoelectric line).

The signal f_b is obtained through a sequence of opening and closing operators with structuring elements B_o and B_f suitably chosen as the one described below.

$$f_b = f_o \bigcirc B_o \bullet B_f \quad (10)$$

$$= f_b \Theta B_o \oplus B_o \oplus B_f \Theta B_f$$

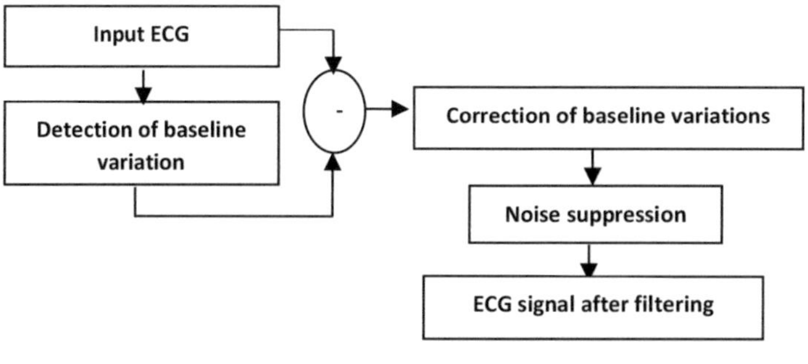

Figure 6.
Steps of the morphological filter algorithm.

$$f_{cb} = f - f_b \tag{11}$$

3.1.2 Noise suppression algorithm

The approach adopted for noise suppression appeal of Top-hat transformations, which are translated by the equations below.

$$\begin{aligned} f &= f_{cb} \bullet B - f_{cb} \circ B \\ &= (\mathrm{f_{cb}} \bullet \mathrm{B} - \mathrm{f_{cb}}) + (\mathrm{f_{cb}} - \mathrm{f_{cb}} \circ \mathrm{B}) \\ &= (\mathrm{f_{cb}} \oplus \mathrm{B_1} \Theta\, \mathrm{B_2} - \mathrm{f_{cb}}) + (\mathrm{f_{cb}} - \mathrm{f_{cb}} \Theta\, \mathrm{B_1} \oplus \mathrm{B_2}) \end{aligned} \tag{12}$$

$(f_{cb} \bullet B - f_{cb})$ and $(f_{cb} - f_{cb} \circ B)$ are of the type of morphological transformation by Top Hat. This transformation is a high pass filter.

$(f_{cb} \bullet B - f_{cb})$ and is called the black top hat transformation, which is used to extract negative pulses (or negative peaks); is called the white top hat transformation, which is used to extract positive pulses (or positive peaks). Thus the filter can be used to extract positive and negative pulses simultaneously [46].

Figure 7 represents the block diagram describing the structure of the top-hat transformation for noise suppression.

It consists of three steps: The first concerns the acquisition of ECG signals (f_{cb}: ECG signal after baseline correction).

This step is followed by another step that allows noise removal. This step uses the morphology operators defined in Eq. (12).

B1 and *B2* are structuring elements for opening and closing. These operators are employed simultaneously on the signal. The next step is the subtraction between the two closing and opening operators to generate a filtered ECG signal.

The proposed algorithm is implemented under MATLABR14 environment. It is tested on a set of ECG signals (noisy) from the MIT-BIH database [47].

3.2 PCG signal filtering algorithm

Figure 7 below illustrates the stages of noise suppression and heart murmurs.

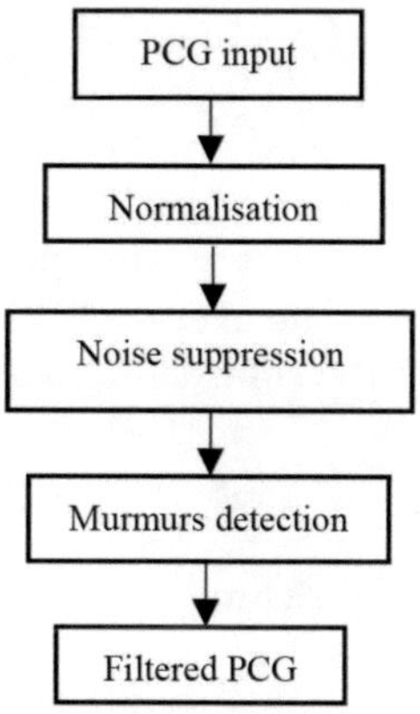

Figure 7.
Diagram of PCG filtering.

The first step is to normalize the PCG input signal. A second step is to remove noises, and a third step is to remove heart murmurs.

3.2.1 PCG signal normalization

The original signal has been normalized before performing any operation. The PCG signal is re-sampled at 8000 Hz with 16 bits of precision and converted to WAVE format and normalized by:

$$x_{Nor}(t) = \frac{x(t)}{max\,(|x(t)|)} \tag{13}$$

The aim of normalization is to reduce the amplitudes of the PCG signal.

3.2.2 Noise suppression algorithm

Noise suppression uses the morphological filter, which is presented by the following equations:

$$f_p = f \bullet B \bigcirc B \tag{14}$$

$$f_c = f - f_p \tag{15}$$

f_p represent the detection of the positive and negative peaks by the closing of the element.

B_1 followed by the opening of B_2 to finally generate the filtered signal f_c. So the signal f_c is the subtraction of the original signal and the signal f_p.

3.2.3 Heart murmur algorithm

The filter applied for the suppression of murmurs is the average filter; it is described in the equation below.

$$f_p = f \bullet B \bigcirc B \tag{16}$$

$$f_c = f - f_p \tag{17}$$

The detection of murmurs is based on two morphological operators, namely closing and opening, to suppress peaks. The average between the closing and opening operator gives the result f_p. After the subtraction between the f signal and f_p to generate a filtered signal f_c.

3.3 ECG signal wave detection algorithm

The detection of the RR interval can be accomplished only after a good detection of the R peak. This detection goes through three stages. A step which allows locating the positive peaks R by the opening operation and another step which allows locating the negative peaks R by the application of the closing operation. The final step to arrive at these peaks and valleys is the subtraction of the filtered ECG signal f with the two previous operations.

The following formula illustrates the extraction of R positive peaks:

$$Peaks\ (RR) = f - (foB) \tag{18}$$

And the following formula illustrates the extraction of valleys or negative peaks R:

$$Valleys(RR) = f - (f \bullet B) \tag{19}$$

Formula (18) and (19) are equivalent to:

$$Peaks(RR) + Valleys(RR) = f - (foB \bullet B) \tag{20}$$

Structuring element B is used to detect peaks and valleys. In this case it is considered as a geometric shape "horizontal segment of different lengths". The following formula shows the:

$$b(t) = \begin{cases} 1\ si\ |t| < k \\ 0\ si\ non \end{cases} \tag{21}$$

where K is a constant.

One of the problems of the morphological approach is to determine the optimal value of K. If it is too small, the transformation will be sensitive to high frequency noise, and the peaks are incorrectly determined. However, K which must be less than the peak width R. Research has shown excellent results by using values between [55–60] ms [48].

After detecting the RR rhythm, the next step is to detect the T wave. It uses the erosion operator to build maximum thresholding. Knowing that the amplitude of the T wave is enormously greater than the Q wave and the S wave in the normal or abnormal case of the ECG signal.

The following formula illustrates the detection of the T wave:

$$\begin{cases} (f \oplus \mathrm{B})(m) = \max\limits_{n=0,\ \dots,M-1} f(n) + B(m-n) \\ \text{for } N > M \text{ and } \mathrm{m} = \mathrm{M}-1,\ \dots\ \dots\ \dots,\mathrm{N}-1 \end{cases} \tag{22}$$

Where the sets f and B are underlined by $f(n) = \{0, 1, \dots, N-1\}$ and $B = \{0, 1, \dots, M-1\}$.

The next phase is the detection of the Q and S waves of the ECG signal. It uses a morphological operator called closing to detect the negative peaks. On the other hand, the morphology of Q and S waves in an ECG signal are of negative amplitudes. For this, we have chosen the most adapted closing operator to detect the negative peaks. Finally, the detection of the P wave is based on the opening operator which is combined with a structuring element of multi-scale, according to the equation:

$$f_p = f \bigcirc B_1 \bigcirc B_2 \tag{23}$$

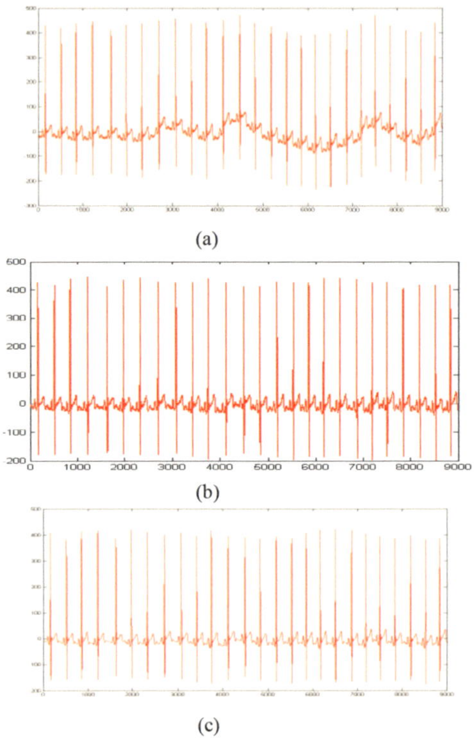

Figure 8.
a) Original ECG. b) Baseline correction. c) Filtered signal.

The signal is operated by two successive opening operators with a structuring element of an equal scale 2. This means that the number of opening operations and the number of the structuring element is two scales.

4. Results and interpretations

4.1 ECG signal filtering

The proposed morphological approach for baseline correction and noise suppression in the ECG signal was tested by the use of the MIT-BIH arrhythmia database.

Figure 8 illustrate respectively the noisy ECG signal, the ECG signal after baseline correction and the resulting filtered ECG signal.

After acquiring the ECG signal, the next step is baseline correction. It consists of the application of morphological operations: "opening and closing".

The signal is first opened by a structuring element $\boldsymbol{B_o}$, which means the application of two morphology operations "erosion + dilation", to remove the peaks and preserve the valleys. This "opening" operation generates a signal consisting of valleys which are suppressed, using the second operation which is the closing "dilation + erosion", so this operation uses another structuring element $\boldsymbol{B_f}$. We achieved to the signal that represents the estimate of the derivative of the baseline (or variations of the baseline).

The structuring element $(\boldsymbol{B_o}, \boldsymbol{B_f})$ is used for baseline correction. In this case $(\boldsymbol{B_o}, \boldsymbol{B_f})$ is chosen as a geometric shape corresponding to an horizontal segment of

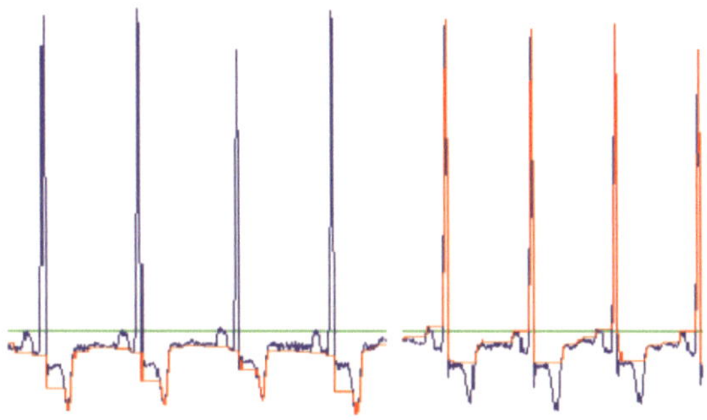

Figure 9.
Closing effect (to the left) and the opening operator (to the right).

different lengths. Different lengths of the structuring element B_o and B_f are employed considering that the construction of the structuring element for the correction of the baseline depends on the duration of the characteristic wave and the sampling frequency (F_s Hertz) of the ECG signal. If the length of a characteristic wave is T_L (***second***), the number of samples of this wave is $F_s * T_L$, which signify the structuring element B_o should have a length greater than $F_s * T_L$.

Figure 9 shows the closing operation which uses a structuring element to remove the valleys left by the opening operation. The length of the structuring element B_f must be longer than the length of the B_o.

The ECG signal, the most characteristic waves are the P wave, the T wave and the QRS complex, which are generally less than 0.2 second.

Therefore, L_o, the length of B_o is $0.2 * F_s$ and L_f, the length of B_f is typically chosen to be longer than the structuring element B_o, at approximately $1.5 * L_o$.

Since we employ $F_s = 360\ Hz$ as a sampling frequency, we get $L_o = 0.2 * F_s = 72$ and $L_c = 1.5 * L_o = 108$.

The final step to arrive at the baseline correction is the subtraction of the noisy ECG signal f_o with f_b (signal describing the baseline variations).

After baseline correction, the next step is noise removal. It consists of the application of morphology operators of the morphological transformation by top hat.

In fact, the input signal f_{cb} is processed simultaneously by the operations "close" and "open", followed by a subtraction, to end up with the filtered ECG signal f.

The morphological transformation by Hat-Top permits to extract the positive and negative impulses simultaneously by the application of the operations of opening and closing.

It should be noted that the shape of the structuring element in the noise suppression is different compared to the baseline correction. Indeed, it can take two different shapes and of equal lengths: a triangular shape B_1 for maintain peaks and valleys on a straight shape (segment of zero amplitude) B_2.

In our case, the size of the structuring element was fixed at 5 samples, with the value of the structuring element of $B_1 = (0, 1, 5, 1, 0)$ and $B_2 = (0, 0, 0, 0, 0)$. This value is set in an empirical way where the initial values of minimums and maximums are set to the optimal values in the noise removal step.

The algorithm is applied respectively to records 209 and 234 of the MIT-BIH Arrhythmia database. **Figures 10** and **11** illustrate, that the filtered ECG signal does not present any variation of the base line, also the different waves of the signal are clearly highlighted, and without any deformation.

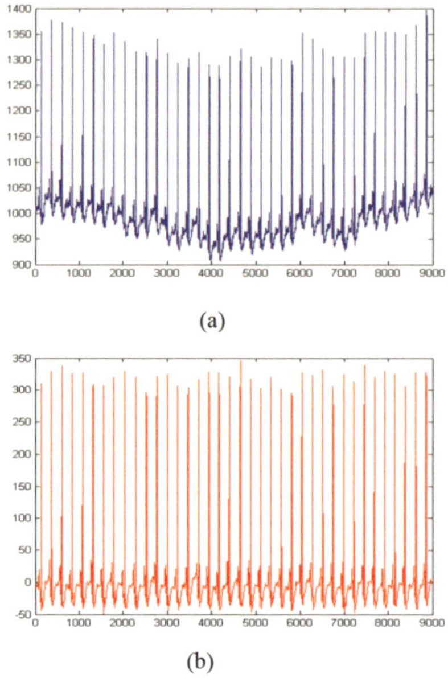

Figure 10.
a) Original ECG (record 234), b) filtered signal.

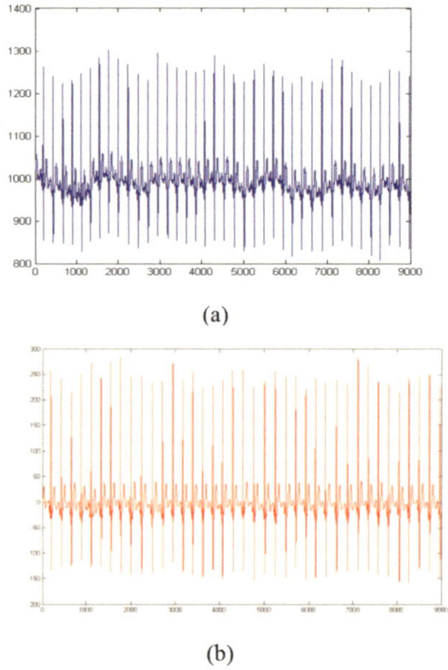

Figure 11.
a) Original ECG (record 209). b) Filtered signal.

4.2 PCG signal filtering

The proposed morphological approach for noise suppression and detection of heart murmurs from the PCG signal was tested from the Pascal Classifying Heart Sound Challenge [49].

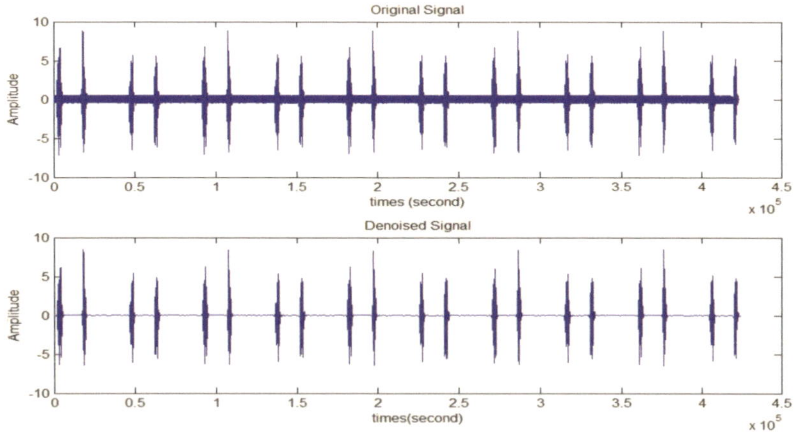

Figure 12.
Noise suppression of PCG signal.

Figure 12, shows a noisy signal that has been filtered by the morphological filter. This filter uses two successive operators including closing and opening.

These operators are combined with a single structuring element *B* to suppress noise. For this, the selection of the shape and size of *B* is very important so as not to distort the information of the signal.

In this context, the length *L* of *B* is *0.15*Fs* and the sampling frequency *Fs = 8000 Hz*, so we get *L = 1200*.

It depends on the duration of heart sounds S1 and S2 which are basic frequency (0.1–0.15) second, (70–0.14) ms, respectively.

After noise suppression, the next step is heart murmur suppression. It uses an average filter, which is combined with a structuring element *B*.

Knowing that heart murmurs are a frequency content above 100 Hz. Starting from this hypothesis, the length *L* of *B* = *0.15*f*, f = 100 Hz then we obtain that *L* = 15.

Figure 13 below shows heart murmur suppression.

4.3 ECG signal wave detections

The proposed morphological approach for detecting the beginnings and endings of QRS complexes, the T wave and the P wave of the ECG signal were tested from the MIT-BIH arrhythmia database.

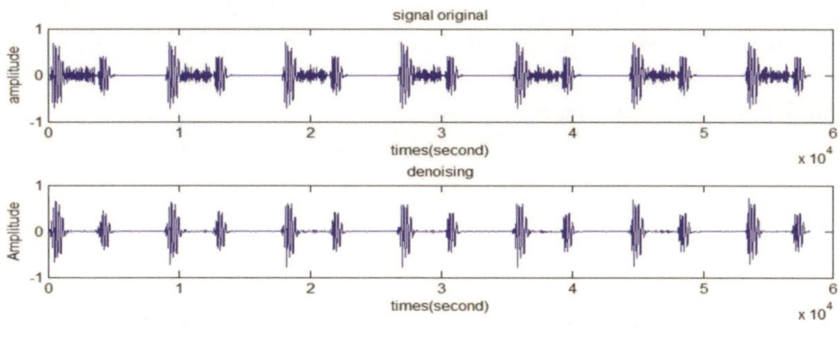

Figure 13.
Murmurs detection of PCG signal.

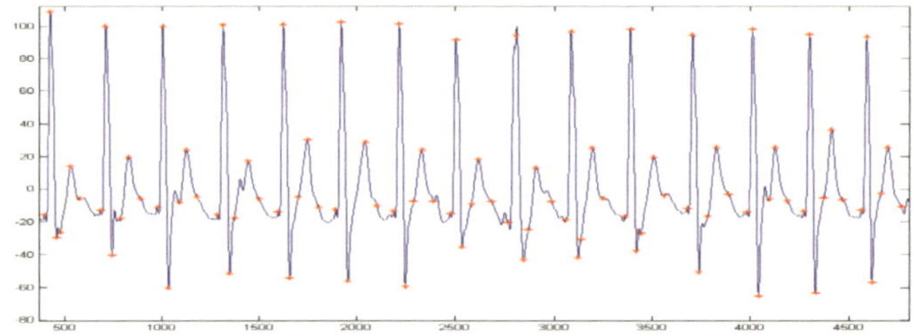

Figure 14.
Detection results (record 102).

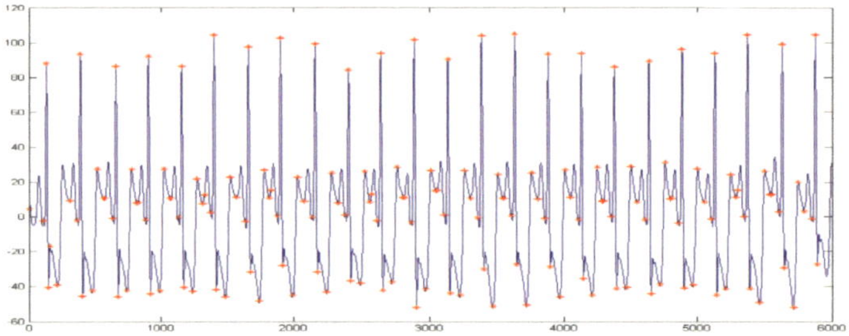

Figure 15.
Detection results (record 103).

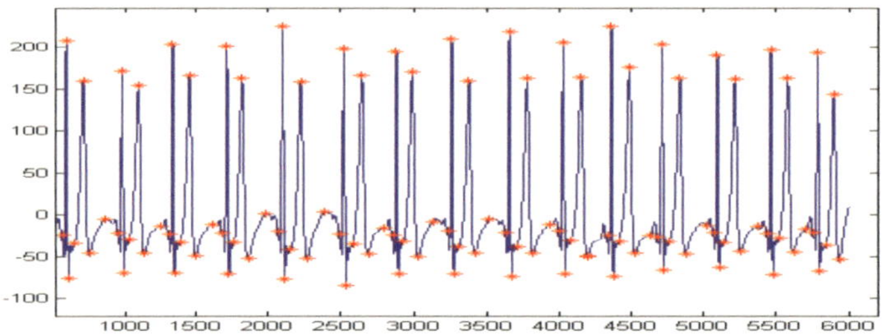

Figure 16.
Detection results (record 113).

For each (filtered) ECG input signal, the following procedures were performed:

(a) pre-processing the ECG signal; (b) detecting the RR heart rate by the morphological filter; (c) detection of the T wave by maxima of the erosion operator; (d) detection of the Q and S waves of the ECG signal by the closure operator; (e) the detection of the P wave is detected by the opening operator with a multi-scale structuring element.

Figures 14 to **16** illustrate the results obtained on three different recording representing different morphologies where the power of the morphological transformation algorithm is clearly shown.

5. Conclusion

The characteristic waves of an electrocardiogram (ECG) signal and the heart sounds of the phonocardiogram (PCG) signal provide important indicators for the diagnosis of heart disease; they reflect physiological processes of the heart and autonomic nervous system. The analysis and interpretation of these physiological signals make it possible to highlight new phenomena, which is sometimes possible to explain at the physiological level, and which leads to a better understanding of the overall functioning of the heart.

The automatic analysis of ECG and PCG signals provides the cardiologist with the information needed to diagnose cardiac pathologies. The implementation of reliable algorithms for the processing of ECG and PCG signals, making it possible to detect the useful information carried by the ECG and PCG signals remains a major concern for technicians.

A set of algorithms using morphology transforms has been developed. These algorithms concerning:

- On the one hand the pre-processing of ECG and PCG signals where an algorithm has been developed and implemented: one for the elimination of baseline ripples and the other for noise suppression.

- and on the other hand, the analysis of ECG and PCG signals where an algorithm has been developed for the detection of QRS complexes, the T wave, the P wave of the ECG signal and the murmurs of the PCG signal.

- The algorithms were evaluated by applying them to ECG and PCG signals from the universal database 'MIT-BIH' and Dataset from "Pascal Classifying Heart Sound Challenge, respectively.

Morphological filtering which uses two morphological operators opening and closing for the correction of the baseline.

In noise suppression, the Top Hat transformation was used. It combines the subtraction of the closing and opening morphology operators.

For the detection of ECG signal parameters, typically the QRS complex, the T wave, and the P wave, two techniques have been presented which are called multi-scale morphology and morphological operators.

At the PCG signal level, we used a morphological filter for noise suppression and heart murmur detection.

These techniques, which are based on mathematical morphology, are very effective in estimating rapid changes in the morphology of ECG and PCG signals.

Author details

Taouli Sidi Ahmed
Genie-biomedical Laboratory GBM, Faculty of Technology, Department of Genie-biomedical, University of Aboubekr Belkaid-Tlemcen, Tlemcen, Algeria

*Address all correspondence to: sidiahmed.taouli@univ-tlemcen.dz

References

[1] Einthoven W. Weiteres über das Elektrokardiogramm. Pflügers Archiv European Journal of Physiology. 1908; **122**:517-584. DOI: 10.1007/BF01677829

[2] Wilson FN, Johnston FD, Macleod AG, Barker PS. Electrocardiograms that represent the potential variations of a single electrod. American Heart Journal. 1934;**447**:471

[3] Wilson FN, acleod AG, Barker PS. The potential variations produced by the heart beat at the apices of einthoven's triangle. American Heart Journal. 1931; **207**:211

[4] Atbi A, Debbel SM. Segmentation of pathological signals phonocardiogram by using the Shannon energy envelogram. AJCM. 2013;**2**(1 and 2):1-14

[5] Serra J, Vincent L. An overview of morphological filtering. Circuits, Systems and Signal Processing. 1992;**11**: 47-108

[6] Lantuejoul C. Maisonneuve F. Geodesic methods in quantitative image analyses. Pattern Recognition. 1984;**17** (2):177-187

[7] Henry Chu CH, Delp EJ. Impulsive noise suppression and background normalization of electromagnetism signals using morphological operators. IEEE Transactions on Biomedical Engineering. 1989;**36**(2):262-272

[8] Thakor NV. Estimation of QRS complex power spectra for the sign of QRS Filte. IEEE Transactions on Biomedical Engineering. 1984;**11**:702-705

[9] Pan J, Tompkins WJ. A real time QRS detection algorithm. IEE trans. Biomedical Engineering. 1985;**32**(3): 230-236

[10] Lander P, Berbari EJ. Use of high-pass filtering to detect late potentials in the signal averaged ECG. Journal of Electrocardiology. 1989;**22**: 7-12

[11] Thakor NV, Zhu YS. Applications of adaptive filtering to ECG analysis: Noise cancellation and arrhythmia detection. IEEE Transactions on Biomedical Engineering. 1991;**38**:785-794

[12] Xue Q, Hu YH, Tompkins WJ, et al. Neural-network-based adaptive matched filtering for QRS detection. IEEE Transactions on Biomedical Engineering. 1992;**39**(4):317-329

[13] Hu Y, Palreddy S, Tompkins J. A patient-adaptable ECG beat classifier using a mixture of experts approach. IEEE Transactions on Biomedical Engineering. 1997;**44**(9):891-900

[14] Duro RJ, Santos J. Synaptic delay artificial neural networks and discrete time backpropagation applied to QRS complex detection. Proceedings of International Conference on Neural Networks ICNN97. 1997;**4**:2566-2570

[15] Li G. al. ECG beat recognition using fuzzy hybrid neural network. IEEE Transactions. 2001;**48**:1265-1271

[16] Laguna P, Thakor NV, Caminal P, Jane R, Yoon HR, Bayes A, et al. New algorithm for QT interval analysis in 24-hour Holter ECG: Performance and application. Medical & Biological Engineering & Computing. 1990;**28**(1): 67-73

[17] Laguna P, Jane R, Caminal P. Automatic detection of wave boundaries in multilead ECG signals: Validation with the CSE database. Computers and Biomedical Research. 1994;27(1):45:60

[18] Li C, Zheng C, Tai CF. Detection of ECG characteristic points using wavelet transforms. IEEE Transactions on Biomedical Engineering. 1995;**42**:21-29

[19] Daskalov IK, Christov II. Automatic detection of the electrocardiogram T-wave end. Medical & Biological Engineering & Computing. 1999;**37**(3):348-353

[20] Daskalov IK, Christov II. Electrocardiogram signal preprocessing for automatic detection of QRS boundaries. Medical Engineering & Physics. 1999;**21**(1):37-44

[21] Donoho DL, Johnstone IM. Ideal spatial adaptation via wavelet shrinkage. Biometrika. 1994;425:455. Vol. 81

[22] Ercelebi E. Electrocardiogram signals denoising using lifting-based discrete wavelet transform. Computers in Biology and Medicine. 2004;**34**:479-493

[23] Donoho DL, Johnstone IM. Adapting to unknown smoothness via wavelet shrinkage. Journal of the American Statistical Association. 1995;**90**:1200-1224

[24] Chang S, Yu B, Vetterli M. Adaptive wavelet thresholding for image denoising and compression. IEEE Transactions in Image Processing. 2000; **9**:1532-1546

[25] Chen CS, Wu JL, Hung YP. Theoretical aspects of vertically invariant gray- level morphological operators and their application on adaptive signal and image filtering. IEEE Transactions on Signal Processing. 1999; **47**(4):1049-1060

[26] Skolnick MM, Butt D. Cellular array algorithms for the analysis of EKG signals. In: Proceedings of the 1985 IEEE Workshop on Computer Architecture Pattern Analysis and Image Database Management, Atlantic, USA. 1985. pp. 438-443

[27] Serra J, Vincent L. An overview of morphological filtering. Circuits Systems and Signal Processing. 1992;**47**(108):11

[28] Serra J, Vincent L. Analysis and Mathematical Morphology. II: Theoretical Advances. London: Academic Press; 1998

[29] Soille P. Morphologische Bildverarbeitung. Berlin Heidelberg: Springer-Verlag; 1998

[30] Banon GJF. Characterization of translation invariant elementary operators for gray-level morphology. In Processing of SPIE, Neural, Morphological and Stochastic Methods in Image and Signal Processing, San Diego, USA. Vol. 2568. 1995. pp. 68-79

[31] Heijmans HJAM. In: Hawkes P, editor. Morphological Image Operators. Advances in Electronics and Electron Physics. Vol. 50. Boston: Ac. Press; 1994. p. 24

[32] Sedaaghi MH. ECG wave detection using morphological filters. Applied Signal Processing. 1998;**5**:182-194

[33] Breen E, Jones R, Talbot H. Mathematical morphology. A useful set of tools for image analysis. Statistics and Computing. 2000;**10**:105-120

[34] Crespo J, Serra J, Schafer R. Theoretical aspects of morphological filters by reconstruction. Signal Processing. 1995;**47**:201-225

[35] Maragos P, Shafer RW. Morphological systems for multidimensional signal processing. Proceedings of the IEEE. 1990;**78**(4): 690-710

[36] Keshet R. Mathematical morphology on complete semilattices and its applications to image processing. Fundamenta Informaticae. 2000;**33**:56. 41,1–2

[37] Serra J, Salembier P. Mathematical Morphology in Image Processing. Marcel Dekker, NY: Ch. 13, Ed. Dougherty (ed.). 1992;483-523. [D-42/92/MM]

[38] Serra J. Connections for sets and functions. Fundamenta Informaticae. 2000;**41**(1/2):147-186

[39] Soille P. Morphological Image Analysis. 2nd éd ed. Heidelberg: Springer-Verlag; 2003

[40] Serra J. Anamorphoses and function lattices (multivalued morphology). In: Dougherty E, editor. Mathematical Morphology in Image Processing. Marcel-Dekker; 1992. pp. 483-523

[41] Meyer FH, Heijmans J. From connected operators to leveling. In: Heijmans HJAM, Roerdink JBTM, editors. Mathematical Morphology and its Applications to Image and Signal Processing. de Computational Imaging and Vision. Vol. 12. Dordrecht: Kluwer Academic Publishers; 1998. pp. 191-198

[42] Matheron G. Treillis Compacts et Treillis Coprimaires. Rapport n°N-5/96/G. Centre de Géostatistique, École des Mines de Paris. 1996 ; Fontaine bleau. Google Scholar

[43] Gratin C. De la représentation Des Images au Traitement Morphologique d'images Tridimensionnelles [PhD Thesis]. Paris: Ecole des Mines de Paris; 1993

[44] Maragos P. Pattern spectrum and multiscale shape recognition. IEEE Transactions on Pattern Analysis and Machine Intelligence. 1989;**11**(7):701-716

[45] Wang J, Shu H, Chen X. Multiscale morphology analysis of dynamic power quality disturbances. Proceedings of the CSEE. 2004;**24**(4):63-67

[46] Taouli SA, Reguig FB. Noise and baseline wandering suppression of ECG signals by morphological filter. Journal of Medical Engineering & Technology. 2010;**34**(2):87-96

[47] Moody GB, Mark RG. The impact of the MIT-BIH Arrhythmia Database. IEEE Engineering in Medicine and Biology. 2001;**20**(3):45-50. PMID: 11446209

[48] Köhler BU, Hennig C, Orglmeister R. The principles of software QRS detection. IEEE Engineering in Medicine and Biology. 2002;**24**:57

[49] Available from: http://www.peterjbentley.com/heartchallenge/

Chapter 3

Applications of Quantum Mechanics, Laws of Classical Physics, and Differential Calculus to Evaluate Source Localization According to the Electroencephalogram

Kristin S. Williams

Abstract

Applications of quantum mechanics and physics-based calculus allow for advanced mathematical modeling of source localization estimations. Because EEG waveforms can be modeled as continuous or discrete quantum matter, algorithmic models that estimate current source density must also consider the statistical properties of the dipole fields that are etiologically relevant to the reflected waveforms. Further applications of quantum physics to the electroencephalogram (EEG) suggest that neurodynamic behavior that originates in thalamo-cortical regions compared to cortico-cortical regions yield divergent 3-dimensional dispersions of wave forms and quantum energy. Evaluations of the dispersion of quantum energy and dipole magnetic fields according to classical physics and electromagnetism indicate that the area of tissue by which the oscillatory mechanisms are thought to originate inherently influences the algorithmic modeling and estimations current source density. Principles and algorithms related to classical physics are included within this paper to evaluate limitations of algorithmic models of source localization and the inverse problem.

Keywords: EEG, electroencephalogram, physics, neurophysics, current source density

1. Introduction

The EEG is a neuroimaging device that reflects the electrophysiological activity of the cerebrum that is generated by the synchronistic firing of nerve cells [1, 2]. Because the EEG reflects dynamic neurocognitive processes according to millisecond variations, the statistical properties of neural activation and processes fluctuate according to time, depth, and orientation of the neural generators. Measurement of the electrical activity reflected by the EEG is best conceptualized as a nonlinear stochastic process that is inherently spatio-temporally dependent [1, 2].

Extracellular currents are derived from excitatory and inhibitory postsynaptic potentials allow for dipole moment per unit volume approximations [1, 3]. The dipole moment per unit volume approximations allow for the derivation of weighted estimations of current source density according to neural generators across and between local tissues and the orthogonal orientation of nerve cells within the neocortical layers [1].

While measurements of extracellular currents can be measured using divergent mathematical algorithms (i.e., phase shift, phase lock, coherence, and lagged coherence), the interaction between neurons that generate excitatory and inhibitory postsynaptic potentials must be evaluated according to time, frequency, and the location of the neural generators [4, 5]. Utilization of the Fast Fourier Transformation (FFT) allows for the derivation of EEG frequency bands from the raw signal according to time. FFT analyses elucidate phase angle and phase differences from the EEG frequency domains. When the phase angle is stable or constant, this indicates that coherence = 1.0 whereas coherence = 0 when there are phase differences due to moment to moment variations in the phase angle. Thus, coherence elucidates communication between distal and contiguous neuroanatomical regions and therefore, across and between functional networks via coupled neural oscillators [4, 5].

Mathematical modeling of current sources can be reflected as $P\ (r', t)$ when the estimation is derived according to dipole moment per unit volumetric approximations [1]. This algorithmic model asserts that r' is the estimated location of the neural source according to volume where t indicates time. Limitations of source localization methods are attributable to the inverse problem and assumptions related to the head volume conduction model [1–6]. The head volume conduction model is significantly flawed because there are multiple layers of biological material that the electrical current must surpass before it can be reflected on the scalp [1, 7]. Furthermore, because of the anisotropic conductivity of the brain, which is attributable to the inhomogeneous conductivity of the cerebrospinal fluid, dura and cerebral tissue, there are an infinite number of solutions to the inverse solution [1, 8–10].

2. Applications of Maxwell's law

Applications of Maxwell's equations to the EEG incorporate fundamental principles related to thermodynamics as derived by Faraday's law of electromagnetic induction and Gauss' law of electromagnetism [11–14]. Maxwell's equations establish that the electrical displacement of neural generators and the field produced by these neurophysiological generators inherently influence accurate estimations of current source density [14].

There are four algorithms that comprise Maxwell's equations [15–17]. Eq. (1) defines ∇ as a nabla operator [14]. The nabla must act upon the other variables denoted within the equation in order to derive estimations of current source density. E is defined as the electrical current. When E is considered as a cross product with the nabla, it is a mathematical constant that is derived as a function of the partial derivation, ∂, of the magnetic field, B, which varies according to temporal changes, t [14].

$$\nabla \times \boldsymbol{E} = -\frac{\partial}{\partial t}\boldsymbol{B}, \tag{1}$$

Considerations of Eq. (1) indicate that the nabla operator denotes a gradient of a scalar field when this operator is utilized to derive estimations of neural generators according to a Cartesian coordinate system [15]. Thus, this equation attempts to utilize statistical weighting to estimate Laplacian operators that are derived from electromagnetic fields at different points within the head volume conduction model. Because the activity reflected in an EEG recording is derived from the activity of orthogonally oriented neurons, estimations of current source density must account for the errors in estimation that are a result of the inability to determine the precise location of the neurobiological generators that produce dipole magnetic fields [15]. It is important to denote that $\nabla \times E$ represents a cross-product between these two factors and does not represent an order of multiplication [14].

Eq. (2) indicates that the cross product between the magnetic field strength, **H**, and the gradient of a scalar field, ∇, is equal to current source density, **J**, as it relates to a partial derivation, ∂, of time, *t*. The field of electric displacement is denoted as **D** [15].

$$\nabla \mathrm{x}\mathbf{H} = \mathbf{J} + \frac{\partial}{\partial t}\mathbf{D}, \tag{2}$$

Eq. (3) indicates that the gradient of a scalar field as a cross product between the electrical displacement, *D*, allows for the derivation of the unbounded charge density, *p* [15]. Eq. (3) is derived from Gauss' law of electromagnetism [15]. Gauss' law of electromagnetism indicates that the electrical flux that is reflected by a closed surface must be proportional to the total electrical charge within that surface [14, 16]

$$\nabla \cdot \boldsymbol{D} = p \tag{3}$$

Applications of Maxwell's law and Gauss' law of electromagnetism incorporate the divergence theorem [17]. The divergence theorem states that the properties of a continuous entity, such as electrical flux, within a closed circuit is equal to the spread of that continuous entity over the volume of the closed-circuit system. Thus, because the flow of a continuous entity must be calculated as a 3-dimensional dispersion, the calculation must consider the magnitude, directionality, and the time by which the divergence occurs. This theorem indicates that a geometric interpretation of the dispersion of a waveform that uses a 3-coordinate configuration system is equivalent to the derivation of current source density [17].

Eq. (4) indicates that the sum of the voltages within a closed-circuit loop must inherently sum to zero [15]. This assertion is consistent with Laplacian physics and Kirchhoff's Circuit Theory [18].

$$\nabla \cdot \boldsymbol{B} = 0 \tag{4}$$

3. Laplacian physics

Geometric models and calculus-based physics in EEG source localization include applications of Coulomb's inverse-square law [19]. Coulomb's law indicates that the magnitude of the electrical force between two particles is inversely related to the distance between the two charges. Thus, as distance increases, the magnitude of the two charges decrease. This law also indicates that electrical force increases as the charge of two particles increase. Coulomb's law can be applied to estimations of source localization if the difference in magnitude between divergent neural generators is considered similarly to the difference in charge of two particles. Specifically, as the distance between electrophysiological generators from the scalp increases, there is a decreased probability that this activity will be reflected on the surface. Coulomb's inverse square law is mathematically defined in Eq. (5) [19].

$$|FE| = k\frac{q1q2}{r^2} \tag{5}$$

Because the depth of a signal inherently influences the electrical field within a volume conductor, applications of Ohm's law to the EEG are also related to source localization [19]. Algorithmic modeling of Ohm's law can be reflected according to vector computations. Eq. (6) denotes that $E(r)$ is the electrical field represented at a specific location, p is resistance, and j is current source density [19].

$$E(r) = pj(r) \tag{6}$$

Gradient derivations are also employed to evaluate the Laplacian operators [19, 20]. Estimations of Cartesian coordinates to evaluate locations of electrical generators are determined by computations that derive the statistical term weights in vector space models. Eq. (7) indicates that the electrical field is computed as a vector function that fluctuates according to time. The derivation of the estimated coordinates account for the time and direction of the magnetic field which inherently affects the magnitude of power reflected by electrical generators. Eq. (7) defines $\boldsymbol{\partial}$ as a partial derivative of $V(r)$ according to its location and i, j, and k as individual Cartesian coordinates according to their orthogonal directionality. The orientation of the generator inherently affects the weighting or probabilistic influence of each coordinate in relation to the electrical signal. Grad indicates a gradient of $V(r)$ which is a measurement of the rate of change of electrical flux within a physical construct according to its radial direction [19, 20].

$$\text{Grad}\left(\mathrm{V}(\mathbf{r})\right) = \frac{\partial V(\mathrm{r})}{\partial x}\hat{\boldsymbol{i}} + \frac{\partial V(\mathrm{r})}{\partial y}\hat{\boldsymbol{j}} + \frac{\partial V(\mathrm{r})}{\partial z}\hat{k} \tag{7}$$

Computations of Laplacian operators require considerations of resistivity [1, 10, 21]. Because the resistivity of biologic materials within the EEG are anisotropic, estimations of Laplacian operators according to the head volume conduction model are inherently flawed. The head volume conduction model assumes isotropy or uniform conductivity. Weighted approximations of the resistivity within a biologic medium must account for the time, region, directionality and the type of tissue by which the electrical currents propagate. Because electrical currents indicate a non-uniform distribution, a cross-section within the brain may present divergent resistive properties dependent upon the Laplacian operator being cortical or subcortical in origin [21].

Further applications of Maxwell's equations include the Maxwell-Rayleigh algorithm [21]. This algorithm is utilized to calculate the resistive properties that occur within a spherical conductive model. Thus, the Maxwell-Rayleigh equation incorporates geometric configurations to estimate of gradations of resistivity that are attributable to a homogenous suspension that exists within a volume conductor. This application is directly related to the estimation of current source density as the brain is surrounded by cerebrospinal fluid. Eq. (8) defines η is resistance according to a specific medium, η_s is fluid resistivity, h is configured according to the geometrical shape of the volume conductor, and $\boldsymbol{\alpha}$ is the partial derivative of the volume by which the suspension occupies [21].

$$\frac{\eta}{\eta s} = \frac{\mathbf{1} + \boldsymbol{h}\alpha}{\mathbf{1} - \alpha} \tag{8}$$

Considerations of algorithms that attempt to model estimations of current source density according to the EEG must consider physiological constraints and mathematical limitations [1]. Derivations of the cumulative density function according to Eq. (9) does not consider the resistivity of the biological material by which the electrical signals must bypass. The resistivity of these biological materials alters the conductivity of the electrical signals that are reflected on the scalp. Eq. (9) defines **Φ** as the cumulative magnetic flux, for a given region, *r*, according to time, *t*. Determination of the cumulative magnetic flux is a function of the interaction between independent variables that vary according to time. This equation defines ∫ as the integral of *B*, the imaginary component, *GH* as the weighted term of volume conductance, $P\ (r', t)$ as the three-dimensional electrical field, and *dV* as the electrical flux according to density. V is defined as volume [1].

$$\phi \mathrm{S}(\mathbf{r},\mathrm{t}) = \int \mathrm{GH}(\mathbf{r},\mathbf{r'})\mathrm{P}(\mathbf{r'},\mathrm{t})\mathrm{dV}(\mathbf{r'}) \tag{9}$$

GH is a direct application of Coulomb's law of electrostatic force with regard to source localization. This equation indicates that *GH* is always larger for cortical generators compared to subcortical generators [1]. Thus, this is a direct application of Coulomb's law because as the distance between the electrophysiological generators and the scalp increases, the probability that the activity will be shown on the surface decreases. The reduced probability is attributable to Coulomb's law that indicates that the magnitude of electric force decreases as a factor of $1/r^2$ where *r* is defined as the distance between the two charges or generators that produce the dipole field [1, 19].

4. Quantum mechanics and Schrodinger equation applications

Applications of quantum mechanics indicate that linear models that are utilized to conceptualize EEG data are inherently flawed [22]. Linear models that attempt to model EEG signals according to volume conduction include the linear instantaneous time-invariant mixing algorithm [23]. The linear instantaneous time-invariant mixing model indicates that the generation of electrophysiological signals can be modeled as a linear function. This is attributable to the assertion that the cumulative electrical activity reflected on the scalp is a result of the mixing of underlying sources within the head volume conduction model. Congedo and Sherlin [23] indicate that the mixing coefficients or the individual sources do not vary according to time and are therefore fixed. Eq. (10) defines xi as the voltage, *ai* and *aiM* as the mixing coefficients, *s* as the source, and *t* as time [23].

$$xi(t) = ai1 \cdot s1(t) + ai2 \cdot s2(t) + \ldots + aiM \cdot sM(t) \tag{10}$$

Eq. (10) negates the inclusion of factors related to the resistivity of the biologic medium by which the electrical signals are derived [23]. Furthermore, this equation is inherently flawed in that the mixing coefficients are deemed as time invariant factors. Considerations of the inverse problem and Coulomb's law of electrical force indicate that the estimation of the electrical sources is dependent upon the depth, orientation, and number of neurons that generate the EEG rhythms that are reflected on the scalp [1, 7].

Applications of Heinsenberg's Uncertainty Principle and Schrodinger's equation further exemplify the error associated with conceptualizing the EEG as a linear function [22, 24]. These principles and algorithms indicate that EEG waveforms can be modeled as a summation of individual waves and quantum particles. Heinsenberg's Uncertainty Principle indicates that statistical modeling can be utilized in a priori estimations of the location and position of quantum objects as the precise location and momentum of particles cannot be simultaneously determined. Eq. (11) is a representation of the time independent derivative of the Schrodinger equation [22, 24].

$$i\hbar \frac{\partial \psi(\mathrm{x},\mathrm{t})}{\partial t} = -\frac{\hbar^2}{2m}\nabla^2 \psi(\mathrm{x},\mathrm{t}) + \mathrm{V}(\mathrm{x},\mathrm{t}) + \psi(\mathrm{x},\mathrm{t}) \tag{11}$$

Eq. (11) defines $i\hbar$ as energy, $\boldsymbol{\partial}$ as the partial derivative of the waveform according to time [24]. $\hbar$ is Plank's constant, $\boldsymbol{\Psi}$ indicates the wave function, and $\boldsymbol{\nabla}$ indicates the degree to which the wave function changes according to space relative to the conductor by which it is modeled. V is defined as the magnitude or force of the particle according to location and time where m represents the mass of the particle. Because the Schrodinger equation indicates that waveforms within the EEG can be conceptualized as quantum particles, this suggests that the energy or magnitude of the quanta that produce neuro-oscillatory behavior and EEG rhythms can be defined as a function of kinetic energy [24].

4.1 EEG application of Schrodinger equation

The Schrodinger equation exemplifies the inherent limitations of the head volume conduction model and, therefore, the inverse problem. Albeit Nunez and Srinivasan [21] have derived estimations of resistivity for divergent biological materials such as the skull, cerebrospinal fluid, dura, blood and the cortex, the Schrodinger equation indicates that the precise location of individual quantum particles and waveforms cannot be determined unless invasive procedures are utilized to isolate these particles [21, 22]. Postulates of the Schrodinger equation indicate that probability distributions are utilized to estimate the dispersion of each wave form [24]. This postulate can be applied to the EEG in relation to the derivation of dipole magnetic fields.

Because multiple 'neurorhythmicities' are generated at any given time, where each waveform will have its own probabilities and estimated dispersions of the dipole fields related to that wave, there is not a unique solution to the inverse problem. Derivation of the individual statistical weights for each waveform that is cortical or subcortical in origin is mathematically infeasible. These mathematical and physiological challenges that are specific to the head volume conduction model and inverse problem indicate the necessity to incorporate integrals and imaginary components to reduce statistical error in estimations of source localization.

5. Conclusion

The classification of EEG waveforms as continuous or discrete quantum matter and the output of the EEG as a linear or nonlinear function inherently affects algorithmic modeling for estimations of source localization [23, 24]. While Nunez and

Srinivasan [21] have estimated the degree to which specific biologic mediums and materials possess resistive properties, these parametric configurations do not provide a solution to the inverse problem. Applications of quantum mechanics indicate that neurodynamic behavior that originates in thalamo-cortical compared to cortico-cortical regions yield divergent 3-dimensional dispersions of wave forms and quantum energy [21].

The area of tissue by which the oscillatory mechanisms are thought to originate inherently determines the validity and applicability of Ohm's law to the EEG [1]. Specifically, the amount of tissue by which the neuro-oscillatory generators are thought to be dispersed distorts mathematical estimations of source localization. As the magnitude of space where neural generators are thought to originate increases, Ohm's law may only be applicable when estimates of current source density are calculated using matrices to account for the macroscopic and anisotropic heterogeneities that permeate calculations of resistivity in subcortical and cortical regions [21].

Applications of the Schrodinger equation and Heisenberg's Uncertainty Principle indicate that if EEG waveforms are considered as a summation of discrete particles and individual waveforms, the precise cytoarchitectural boundaries and power of the specific quantum particles that comprise these waveforms cannot be derived simultaneously. Estimations of current source density must obey laws of physics related to thermodynamics and electromagnetism. Thus, laws of classical physics and quantum mechanics such as Coulomb's inverse square law, Gauss's law of electromagnetism, and Maxwell's equations can be applied to derive estimations of the Cartesian coordinates that are utilized in 3-dimensional dipole electrical field per unit volumetric estimations of current source density [1, 19].

Author details

Kristin S. Williams
Columbia University, New York, USA

*Address all correspondence to: kw2994@cumc.columbia.edu

References

[1] Nunez MD, Nunez PL, Srinivasan R. Electroencephalography (EEG): Neurophysics, experimental methods, and signal processing. In: Ombao H, Linquist M, Thompson W, Aston J, editors. Handbook of Neuroimaging Data Analysis. London: Chapman & Hall/CRC; 2016. pp. 175-197

[2] Teleńczuk B, Baker SN, Kempter R, Curio G. Correlates of a single cortical action potential in the epidural EEG. NeuroImage. 2015;**109**:357-367. DOI: 10.1016/j.neuroimage.2014.12.057

[3] Olejniczak P. Neurophysiologic basis of EEG. Journal of Clinical Neurophysiology. 2006;**23**(3):186-189

[4] Thatcher RW. Coherence, phase differences, phase shift, and phase lock in EEG/ERP analyses. Developmental Neuropsychology. 2012;**37**(6):476-496

[5] Walter DO. Spectral analysis for electroencephalograms: Mathematical determination of neurophysiological relationships from records of limited duration. Experimental Neurology. 1963;**8**(2):155-181

[6] Riera JJ, Ogawa T, Goto T, Sumiyoshi A, Nonaka H, Evans A, et al. Pitfalls in the dipolar model for the neocortical EEG sources. Journal of Neurophysiology. 2012;**108**:956-975

[7] Łęski S, Wójcik DK, Tereszczuk J, Świejkowski DA, Kublik E, Wróbel A. Inverse current-source density method in 3D: Reconstruction fidelity, boundary effects, and influence of distant sources. Neuroinformatics. 2007;**5**(4):207-222

[8] Anastassiou CA, Perin R, Buzsaki G, Markram H, Koch C. Cell type- and activity-dependent extracellular correlates of intracellular spiking. Journal of Neurophysiology. 2015;**114**:608-623

[9] Lei X, Wu T, Valdes-Sosa PA. Incorporating priors for EEG source imaging and connectivity analysis. Frontiers in Neuroscience. 2015;**9**(284): 1-12. DOI: 10.3389/fnins.2015.00284

[10] Wagner T, Eden U, Rushmore J, Russo CJ, Dipietro L, Fregni F, et al. Impact of brain tissue filtering on neurostimulation fields: A modeling study. NeuroImage. Neuro-Enhancement. 2014;**85**(Part 3):1048-1057

[11] Burke WL. Applied Differential Geometry. Cambridge: Cambridge University Press; 1985

[12] Collell G, Fauquet J. Brain activity and cognition: A connection from thermodynamics and information theory. Frontiers in Psychology. 2015;**6**(818): 1-11. DOI: 10.3389/fpsyg.2015.00818

[13] Deschamps GA. Electromagnetics and differential forms. Proceedings of the IEEE. 1981;**69**(6):676-696

[14] Doschoris M, Kariotou F. Mathematical foundation of electroencephalography. In: Sittiprapaporn P, editor. Electroencephalography. London: IntechOpen; 2017. DOI: 10.5772/68021

[15] Gratiy S, Halnes G, Denman D, Hawrylycz M, Koch C, Einevoll G, et al. From Maxwell's equations to the theory of current-source density analysis. European Journal of Neuroscience. 2017;**45**:1013-1023

[16] Nave R. Maxwell's Equations. 2016. Available from: http://hyperphysics.

phyastr.gsu.edu/hbase/electric/maxeq.html

[17] Warnick K, Selfridge R, Arnold D. Teaching electromagnetic field theory using differential forms. IEEE Transactions on Education. 1997;**40**(1):53-68

[18] Feldmann P, Rohrer R. Proof of the number of independent Kirchhoff equations in an electrical circuit. IEEE Transactions on Circuits and Systems. 1991;**38**(7):681-684. DOI: 10.1109/31.13573

[19] Carvalhaes C, Barros JAD. The surface Laplacian technique in EEG: Theory and methods. International Journal of Psychophysiology. 2015;**97**(3):174-188. DOI: 10.1016/j.ijpsycho.2015.04.023

[20] Schleifer N. Differential forms as a basis for vector analysis—With applications to electrodynamics. American Journal of Physics. 1983;**51**(12):1139-1145

[21] Nunez P, Srinivasan R. Electric fields and currents in biological tissue. In: Electric Fields of the Brain: The Neurophysics of EEG. 2nd ed. New York: Oxford University Press; 2006. pp. 147-202

[22] Gandhi V, Prasad G, Coyle D, Behera L, McGinnity TM. EEG-based mobile robot control through an adaptive brain-robot interface. IEEE Transactions on Systems, Man, and Cybernetics: Systems. 2014;**44**(9):1278-1285

[23] Congedo M, Sherlin L. EEG source analysis: Methods and clinical implications. In: Neurofeedback and Neuromodulation Techniques and Applications. San Diego: Academic Press; 2011. pp. 25-44

[24] Thornton ST, Rex A. Modern Physics for Scientist and Engineers. Boston: Brooks/Cole; 2013

Chapter 4

Protecting Bioelectric Signals from Electromagnetic Interference in a Wireless World

David Marcarian

Abstract

The exponential growth of wired and wireless technologies which generate Electromagnetic Interference (EMI) has made obtaining microvolt-level bioelectric signals challenging. While digital filtering algorithms provide a wealth of information and allow Artificial Intelligence (AI) to interpret the data, the process may denigrate the integrity of the original signal. Busy clinicians and researchers have relied on computer-analyzed ECG, losing their ability to discriminate between data of high quality and data contaminated with EMI (noise). Resolving an EMI issue with a microphone is one way to learn the methodology. A step-by-step process of troubleshooting EMI in an audio application provides a framework for understanding the fundamental variables that generate EMI and a better understanding of analog electronics. The troubleshooting methodology applies to resolving EMI issues with all biologic signals including Surface Electromyography (SEMG), EEG, ECG, and Needle EMG. As we enter the age of extended range WIFI and cellular technologies, understanding analog electronics is crucial in ensuring we obtain clean data for more clinically meaningful results.

Keywords: electromagnetic interference, EMI, EMF, surface EMG, SEMG, electrical interference, shielding, EMF reduction, digital signal processing, filtering EMI, microphone, USB-powered microphone

1. Introduction

The development and widespread use of electrically powered technology has grown exponentially since the 1960s. Modern homes and offices routinely have flat-screen TVs, microwave ovens, WIFI, and air conditioning systems. Technology requires power in either Alternating Current (AC) or Direct Current (DC) form. Cellular, WIFI, satellite, and other Radio Frequency (RF) devices provide communication between technologies. The widespread use of wired and wireless technologies has led to increased Electromagnetic Interference (EMI) due to Electromagnetic Fields (EMF) in its many forms. Electromagnetic Fields (EMF) are generated by both the source of power, and the technology device that is powered. Electromagnetic

Interference (EMI), or "electrical noise" is the unwanted disturbance in a circuit caused by EMF [1].

EMI creates problems for the electrophysiologist attempting to extract bioelectric signals from the body, especially when those signals are in the microvolt (μV) range such as Surface Electromyography (SEMG), ECG and EEG [2]. Wireless devices have been quickly replacing wired devices in every area of technology. Smart meters are replacing water, gas and power meters in both residential and commercial applications. WIFI routers and microwave based WIFI blanket many towns and cities. Cellular towers, cellular phones and Bluetooth devices all contribute to EMI. In addition to wireless signals, the impact of the electric vehicle has led to an increase in the transmission of high levels of AC power with powerlines the area we live and work. Wireless devices along with EMF generated by power sources contribute to EMI or EMF, potentially damaging the integrity of bioelectric signals as measured at the human body.

In the past decade, there has been a disturbing trend toward clinicians relying upon computer-analyzed ECG/ECG bioelectric data and making clinical decisions based on erroneous results [3]. Unfortunately, many clinicians no longer understand ECG graphs or understand the subtle meaning of the graphed analog signal. This lack of knowledge means there is a higher probability that they will not be aware of the impact of EMI on electrophysiologic evaluations, and the importance of obtaining a clean signal before being processed by the computer.

There are many methods of filtering out EMI, from hardware-based filtering to software algorithms. The best method of preserving the integrity of a bioelectric signal is to reduce the impact of EMI at the source of the biological signal.

Surface Electromyography (SEMG) is a measurement of muscle activity. A pubmed.gov search of the term yields over 13,500 peer-reviewed studies, including the evaluation for presence or absence of back pain and soft tissue injury [4] and workplace ergonomics evaluations. Since this technology measures muscle activity in the microvolt range, it is extremely susceptible to EMI and is a good tool to use when evaluating a location for EMF/EMI. The device utilizes high gain differential amplifiers, and sensors comprised of a metallic electrode with conductive medium which is placed on the skin above the muscles of greatest interest. When performed with the proper equipment and controlling for EMI, the device can extract a microvolt level signal produced by motor units beneath the skin [5].

EMI can make SEMG extremely difficult to measure, making it a perfect tool for evaluating methods of eliminating EMI. The microphone is another device that allows you to"hear" the presence of EMI (constant "hum" in the speakers), and quickly determine when EMI has been removed. Troubleshooting EMI with a commercially available microphone requires the same troubleshooting steps that apply to eliminating EMI's impact on bioelectric signals.

2. Problem-solving techniques: methods for removing EMI in practical use-case scenarios

With the significant advancements in sensor technology over the past 10 years, EMI is less of an issue as in the past. That being said, there are additional variables beyond the measurement instrument itself which determines the quality of bioelectric signal obtained. One of these variables is the increasing level of EMI in our environment.

2.1 Obtaining quality signals: Practical examples

Described below are practical examples demonstrating methods of reducing or eliminating EMI in actual practice.

2.1.1 Practical example 1: The CT angiogram and ECG

The author was required to have a CT Angiogram, and arrived for the exam with my own pack of ECG electrodes. At the time, the CT was timed based upon the ECG, and without a clean ECG signal, the test could not be performed.

After looking at the electrodes they were using, I asked the nurse if they had difficulty obtaining a stable ECG signal. She acknowledged that they were having significant challenges with the ECG, and did not know why. They had the ECG serviced, but the difficulties continued. What was wrong?

The hospital-supplied electrodes had a very high viscosity "gummy bear" type conductive medium. The author-supplied electrodes had a low viscosity gel form of conductive medium. Having the most high-tech ECG would not matter, as the weakness in this system was in the $5.00 pack of electrodes.

To obtain a clean signal, the skin-electrode interface has to have a low enough impedance that the ECG amplifiers would be capable of acquiring the ECG signal without being "saturated" with EMI from all the other electronics in the room. I explained that the hospital supplied electrodes may work if given enough time for the conductive medium to heat up enough to permeate the skin. The gel-type medium on the author supplied electrodes instantly permeated the skin due to its low viscosity.

2.1.2 Tools for evaluating and reducing EMI

These first two devices are crucial in detecting EMI/EMF issues at the physical location of data collection. The inverse square law applies to EMI. In other words, by moving a few feet away from the source of the EMI may resolve the problem. Therefore, you must test for EMI at the location where you will be performing the data collection. You will see the manufacturer and model number of the devices used in troubleshooting.

1. A simple electrical outlet ground tester confirms the AC outlets are properly grounded.

2. An EMF meter measures RF, EMI, Powerline EMF, and cellular EMI.

3. A Faraday Cage or EMI shielding. There are commercially available shielding paints and cloth.

4. Smart-meter shield, if a smart meter is close to your data collection site.

2.1.3 Resolving EMI issues with a commercially available USB-powered microphone

A demonstrative method of eliminating EMI was in resolving an EMI issue with one of the most popular, commercially available microphones (Blue Microphones model: Yeti). The popularity of this microphone is based upon its simplicity and excellent sound quality (once EMI is removed). It is USB-powered and does not rely upon a separate amplification system.

The approach to resolving EMI issues with a microphone is identical to resolving EMI issues with SEMG or any low-level bioelectric signal. The microphone is a perfect example, as the process for eliminating EMI is the same for the microphone for bioelectric signals. There is no need to learn to operate an oscilloscope as the human ear can hear the change in sound quality when the EMI issue is resolved.

Upon plugging the device into my computer, and attempting to record, I immediately noticed a problem with a low-frequency" hum". In an online search, I found every expert on the microphone recommending the use of audio editing software with a noise reduction algorithm.

The resultant processed audio demonstrates the exact problem with digital signal filtering: The digital noise reduction definitively removed the hum, but concomitant with this approach was the removal of the subtle, rich, and warm qualities of the human voice heard in the original recording. The use of sound as an analogy demonstrates the impact digital signal processing may have on biologic signals, as sound has much of the same spectral and amplitude characteristics.

In a google search, the experts on this microphone almost unanimously recommended using audio editing software filters and equalizers to recover the unique vocal attributes removed during the noise reduction processing. In following this approach, the resultant output although improved lacked all the qualities of the original recording, degrading the sound quality along with removing the hum. Is there a better way than to use software to filter out the EMI?

Ideally, if we could remove the source of EMI, there would be no need for post-recording filtering. The problem-solving process presented below applies to any bioelectric signal contaminated by EMI (e.g. SEMG, EMG, ECG etc.) As with all problem-solving, it is essential to change one variable at a time (**Figures 1–5**).

These are the steps I followed in resolving the EMI issue:

1. Use an electrical ground tester (Klein Tools Model RT 310) to confirm that all electrical outlets are tied to earth ground. Although this issue is more likely to occur in an older residential home, it is still possible the location was not properly wired. An ungrounded AC circuit is a source of EMI and needs to be

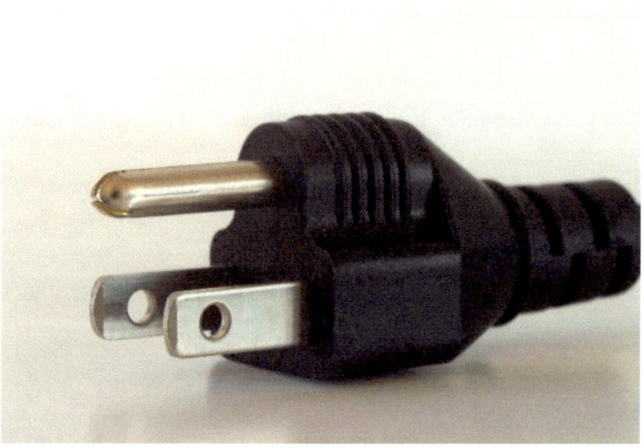

Figure 1.
Grounded 3 prong AC adapter.

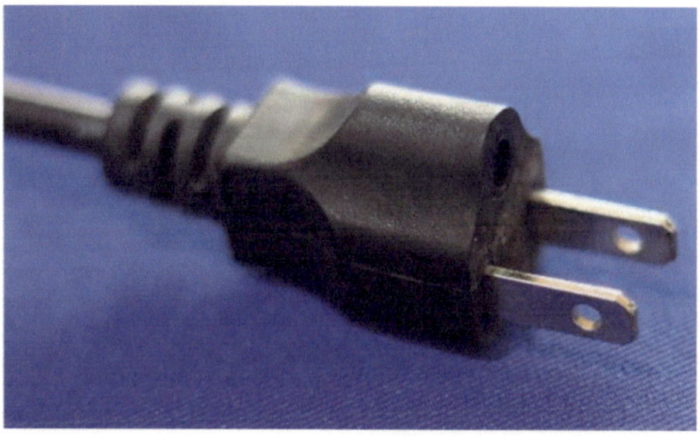

Figure 2.
Ungrounded AC adapter.

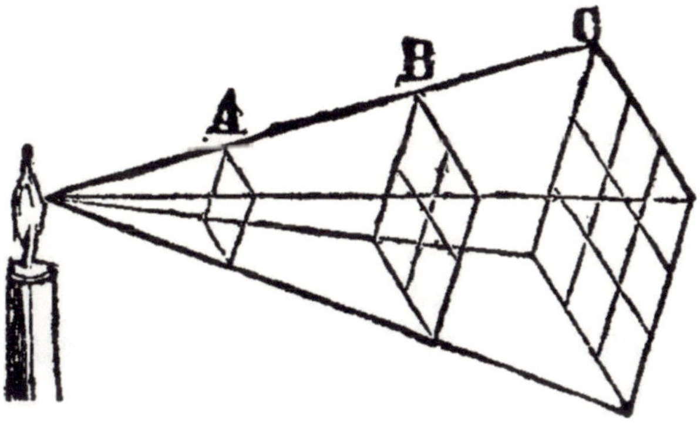

Figure 3.
The Inverse Square law.

resolved immediately. The ground appeared good in all outlets throughout my office setting.

2. The laptop had an ungrounded AC Adapter (a two-prong plug). An ungrounded AC adapter can be a significant source of EMI, as there is no path to ground. As many computers are utilizing the USB-C connector for power, finding a replacement grounded AC adapter was easy. Another approach while waiting for the AC adapter to arrive was to run the computer on battery power. It is crucial to have t he AC adapter unplugged from the AC outlet and the computer. The only problem is when operating on battery power, the internal power supply may generate enough EMI to cause interference. It is always best to have the system grounded. Unfortunately, upgrading to a grounded AC adapter did not resolve the problem. NOTE: Many believe that there is an adapter that allows conversion from ungrounded AC plug to a grounded AC plug. This is false. There is an adapter which allows conversion from grounded to ungrounded (3 prong to 2 prong plug) but it is impossible to add a ground connection.

3. The Faraday cage is essentially a metal box surrounding the subject with the metal connected to the earth ground connection on the wall outlet. The Faraday cage essentially shields the subject from EMI, drawing it to earth ground. In

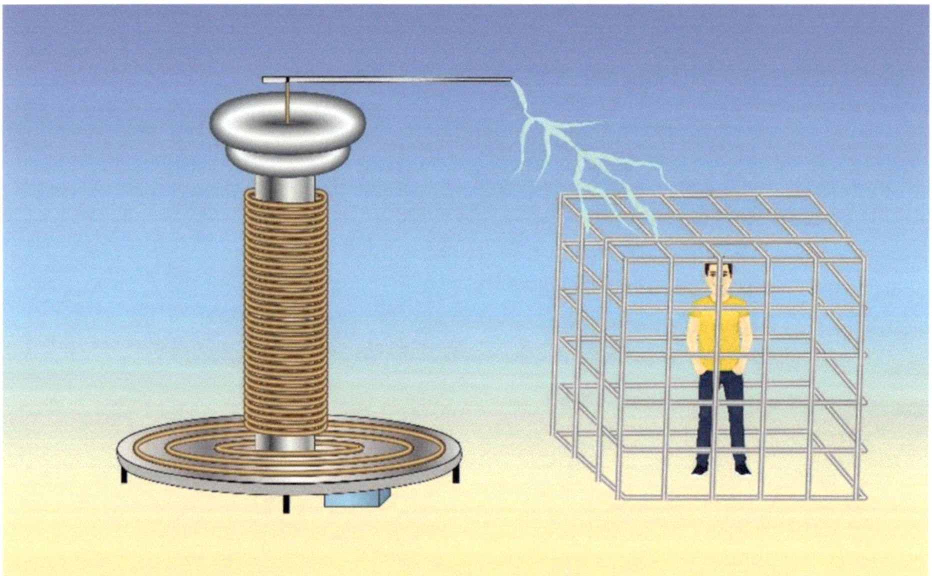

Figure 4.
Faraday cage concept.

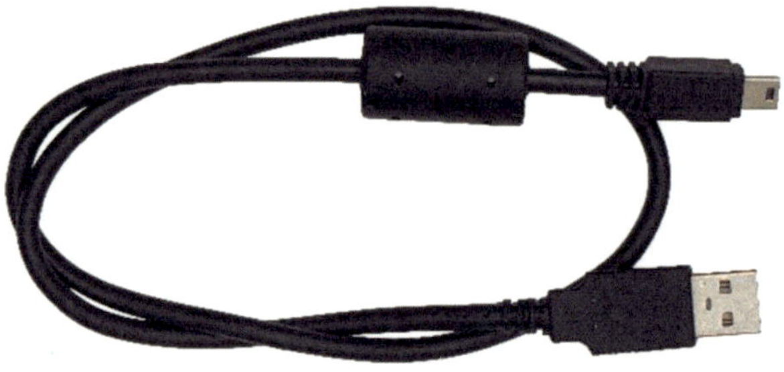

Figure 5.
Ferrite Core mini USB cable.

a location with severe EMI issues, the lab room was painted with a commercially available shielding paint designed with a grounding plate (e.g. Gigahertz Solutions Manufacturer number 863–091 with grounding plate 863–138). It is recommended that a professional perform the installation of such paint. Also, there are manufacturers who provide cloth that can be used to build a Faraday Cage (JJ Care part FF44x20), but the process of building a proper Faraday cage is more complex than it appears [6], and without proper understanding of the principles it is the position of the author that these should be limited to use in clinic or lab settings. The Faraday cage I built for the microphone was unsuccessful.

4. Testing the microphone/computer system at a different location was done to eliminate any source of EMI not obvious. Changing locations has exposed issues for other offices, but did not eliminate the EMI issue with the microphone. In one scenario the dry cleaner next door was using industrial size washers

and dryers generating so much EMI that the only solution was to move the entire SEMG system to the opposite end of the office. The good news is that the inverse square law applies to EMI (the impact of EMI drops off rapidly the further you move away from the source of interference).

5. Lights may be a significant source of EMF. Fluorescent lights have always been a source of EMI. Newer LED lighting systems generate significant EMI as well. It is most likely the power supplies which generate the EMI but turning off LEDs can reduce EMI significantly. In my testing with the hum, I also connected a SEMG system to evaluate the EMI of LED lights [7]. Turning off the lights had no impact on the low frequency hum, but did cause significant EMI in the SEMG signal.

6. The next step involved unplugging all electronics in the office, whether near the microphone or not. The most likely culprit? The flat screen TV: If a Plasma TV, the power supplies generate quite a bit of EMI. You will note that plasma TV manufacturers typically equip all important cables including both power cords and those for connection to the source of entertainment (e.g. HDMI cables for DVD players) with ferrite wrapped cores to reduce the impact of EMI [8].

7. Many TV manufacturers have been shipping large screen TVs with ungrounded 2 prong AC power plugs. This makes them the most likely source of EMI when performing any low-level signal measurement. Since monitors and TVs have always been a source of EMI, but I simply made sure to move the microphone at least 8 feet from the large screen TV I was using as a monitor. Moving a few feet away from the screen drops the EMI dramatically as the inverse square law applies.

8. Cellular phones generate significant EMI. It is important when gathering any low-level biologic signal to keep the phone at least 6–8 feet away from the sensors. Many believe if the ringer is off, that the phone will not generate EMI. When a call comes in, whether the ringer is on or off, the wattage increases significantly and can be seen directly on the graph of an SEMG measurement. I also moved my cellular phone at least 6 feet from the microphone but this had no affect.

9. Any device with a motor may be a source of EMI whether it is turned on or not. Massage chairs or motorized tables as found in a chiropractic or physical therapy office need to be unplugged as part of the process of eliminating them as a source of EMI. With the lights off, the laptop powered by a grounded AC adapter and after unplugging all electronics including the massage chair and TV, the microphone issue was not resolved.

10. The next variable involved the Smart Meter proliferating throughout the US. The device sends data to the utility company but appears to generate significant EMI. I measured the level of EMI using an EMF meter (GQ Electronics, Inc. Model EMF-390), and found the smart meter was generating such significant EMI that I felt the need to apply a shield. Initially I was skeptical of these forms of Faraday cages, as the claims being made by some seemed ludicrous. I was wrong. The measured level of EMI dropped by 14 times with the shield in-

stalled and grounded (Smart Meter Guard, Model SMG1). The smart meter still functioned properly, but the microphone EMI issue was not resolved.

11. I decided to take an inventory of the system disconnected to evaluate possible sources of EMI that were inherent in the design. What I immediately noticed was that the USB A cable to Mini USB cable (which powered and transmitted data from the microphone to the PC) was a standard cable without a ferrite core. I purchased a male USB-2.0 A to male Mini USB cable (Monoprice model 105,447), manufactured with a ferrite core wrapped around the Mini-USB end of the cable. The problem was resolved, and this wonderful microphone was now usable without any digital filtering. Attenuating EMI at the source will always lead to a cleaner, more clinically valuable signal and reduce the need for as much signal processing. The process above applies to any EMI issue with any device.

2.1.4 Miscellaneous means of reducing EMI

Improving the interface between the human and measurement sensor is always critical. Without proper conductivity, bioelectric signals are difficult to measure.

3. Conclusions

The current trend in biomedical engineering is to focus on development of algorithms that provide the healthcare provider, researcher and layperson with valuable biological data to aid in maintaining better health and automating the evaluation of bioelectric signals. The focus of this chapter provides a reminder to be aware of the environmental effects on any biologic signal and not to completely rely upon computers for automated analysis. Although the computer will definitively do a much better job in the future, there may be a variable not taken into consideration.

Additionally, it is important to always attempt to properly attach sensors to the body. By doing so, we increase the probability of obtaining a clean signal at the sensor/human interface such that the original signal is faithfully reproduced in digital format. With the proliferation of wireless technologies throughout the globe, the importance of preventing Electromagnetic Interference (EMI) from contaminating the biologic signal is of utmost importance.

The process of eliminating EMI is presented in the simple case study of a microphone, but the algorithm applied to resolving EMI issues with a microphone apply to all human bioelectric signals. It is the hope that this chapter provide some a different perspective that may aid the researcher and clinician in developing a methodology which leads to the cleanest, noise-free signal possible when gathering bioelectric signals.

Author details

David Marcarian
Precision Biometrics, Inc., Lynnwood, Washington, USA

*Address all correspondence to: david@myovision.com

References

[1] Ozdemir F, Kargi A. Electromagnetic Waves and Modern Health. London, UK: IntechOpen; 2011. DOI: 10.5772/16343

[2] Kibret B, Teshome AK, Lai DTH. Human body as antenna and its effect on human body communications. Progress in Electromagnetics Research. 2014;**148**:193-207. DOI: 10.2528/PIER14061207

[3] Schlapfer J, Wellens HJ. Computer-interpreted electrocardiograms: Benefits and limitations. Journal of the American College of Cardiology. 2017;**70**(9):1183-1192. DOI: 10.1016/j.jacc.2017.07.723

[4] Geisser ME, Ranavaya M, Haig AJ, Roth RS, Zucker R, Ambroz C, et al. A meta-analytic review of surface EMG among persons with low back pain and normal, healthy controls. The Journal of Pain. 2015;**6**(11):711-726. DOI: 10.1016/j.jpain.2005.06.008

[5] Basmajian JV. Muscles Alive: Their Functions Revealed by Electromyography. Baltimore, MD, USA: Lippincott Williams & Wilkins; 1979. ISBN: 0683004131

[6] Panagopoulos DJ, Chrousos GP. Shielding methods and products against man-made Electromagnetic Fields: Protection versus risk. Science of the Total Environment. 2019;**667**:255-262. DOI: 10.1016/j.scitotenv.2019.02.344

[7] Milham S, Stezer D. The electronics in fluorescent bulbs and light emitting diodes (LED), rather than ultraviolet radiation, cause increased malignant melanoma incidence in indoor office workers and tanning bed users. Medical Hypotheses. 2018;**116**:33-39. DOI: 10.1016/j.mehy.2018.04.013

[8] Suarez A et al. Performance study of Split ferrite cores designed for EMI suppression on cables. Electronics. 2020;**9**:1992. DOI: 10.3390/electronics9121992

Section 2

Biosignal Processing Algorithms and Applications

Chapter 5

Non-Invasive Approach for Glucose Detection in Urine Quality Using Its Image Analysis

Anton Yudhana, Liya Yusrina Sabila, Arsyad Cahya Subrata, Hendriana Helda Pratama and Muhammad Syahrul Akbar

Abstract

Human health can be detected through urine content, where metabolic waste in the body is excreted through urination. Glucose in the urine is caused by high levels of glucose in the blood, which can cause poor kidney function. This study aims to detect glucose in urine using non-invasive image analysis. The three measurement parameters in this research consist of Hue (H) is the color portion of the model that is expressed as a number from 0°C to 360, saturation (*S*) is the amount of gray in a particular color from 0% to 100%, and value/brightness (*V*) is the intensity of the color from 0% to 100%. Reagent strips for urinalysis with 10 variables are applied in this research, including glucose, bilirubin, ketone, specific gravity, blood, pH, protein, urobilinogen, nitrite, and leukocytes. All reading data from the system is sent to the monitor layer, which uses the python platform with the additional library Open-cv. The results obtained that the urine color is getting dimmer with the addition of 1 g of glucose in each test. This study was able to detect glucose in urine using image analysis.

Keywords: glucose detection, non-invasive, urine quality, image processing, Arduino microcontroller

1. Introduction

Health is one of the important things that need to be maintained and considered. However, the pattern of human consumption of various types of food and beverages is often a major problem for individual health—especially the frequent habits of individuals when consuming food with glucose levels on an irregular basis. The composition of substances in urine varies depending on the type of food and water drunk [1]. One way to find out if the body is healthy can be done by detecting urine. Normal human urine consists of water, urea, uric acid, ammonia, creatinine, lactic acid, phosphoric acid, sulfuric acid, chloride, and salt, under certain conditions, excess substances such as vitamin C, drugs [2, 3].

Glucose in the urine (called glucosuria) is a disease. If diabetes is accompanied by hyperglycemia (increased blood sugar levels), it can be diabetes mellitus (DM), pancreatic disease, central nervous system disease, severe metabolic disorders, or due to corticosteroid drugs, thiazides, oral contraceptives. Diabetes without hyperglycemia is found in situations of abnormal renal tubular function, pregnancy, sugar other than glucose in the urine, or eating lots of fruit.

The renal glucose threshold is in the range of 60–180 mg/dl, and the urine will immediately show a higher number than the glucose value. Therefore, if the positive value is reduced by one (+1), it is estimated that it will enter the range of 160–180 mg/dl, two (+2) range of decrease in blood glucose estimated 180–250 mg/dl, three positive decreases (+3) estimated range of blood glucose 250–300 mg/dl, four positive range of decrease (+4) estimated range of blood glucose >300 mg/dl.

Urine can be used to diagnose several diseases such as diabetes, liver disease, kidney disease, and others. One of the causes of these diseases is high glucose levels [4–7]. Therefore, the need for early detection of glucose levels in the urine. There are many ways to detect glucose levels in the body in the medical field, including invasively, namely taking blood samples which are analyzed through clinical laboratory procedures. However, this method requires medical action by injuring the limbs using a syringe [8]. Then the second method is non-invasive, which is the opposite of the first method, namely, without any medical action to injure the human body. The non-invasive is an option that has not been widely supported by detector/technology that are devoted to detecting/analyzing glucose content, even if it is available on the market but requires a large purchase cost (high cost) [9–11].

Various studies have developed non-invasive methods for glucose detection with various target sites. Some of these studies include reverse iontophoresis and bioimpedance spectroscopy [12, 13] with target site is wrist skin, ultrasound, electromagnetic and heat capacity [14] with target site is ear lobe skin, near-infrared spectroscopy, and photoacoustic spectroscopy [15, 16] with target site is fingertip skin, Raman spectroscopy [17] with target site is fingertip skin, optical coherence tomography [18] with target site is skin, fluorescence technology [19] with target site is intravascular, and thermal emission spectroscopy [20] with target site is tympanic membrane.

The non-invasive method is recommended because it is carried out without medical action that injures the body. However, to overcome the problem of cost due to the large size of the equipment used, a device for detecting glucose in urine that is easy to move has been developed. This detector, which is designed in the form of a mobile detector, is specifically designed to analyze glucose content non-invasively through urine. This detector is in the form of a storage box that is easy to use without the need to be attached to a member of the body by utilizing a temperature sensor to detect glucose content through urine. The urine waste detector system uses infrared spectroscopy in real-time. From the claims of this study, it shows the difference from using a detector system, namely analyzing the signal-to-noise ratio from the input of the IR thermal sensor resulting from the reflection of light in the urine fluid. Therefore, the proposed research does not require light to detect the glucose content in urine.

A robust analysis is needed to obtain accurate results of glucose detection in urine. One of the analytical techniques that are often used is image analysis through image processing techniques. Urine strip test results can be detected using image processing techniques [21]. The results showed that the image quality of the system is quite low because the system uses a webcam that is experiencing interference. In addition, image processing techniques are used for glucose detection for accurate results [22]. Several studies have shown that image processing techniques can be recommended for various needs, such as monitoring the growth of corn sprouts, comparison of image segmentation, batik identification, and others [23–25]. The detector made in this study will be a solution to the shortage of existing detectors with image analysis.

2. Material and methods

2.1 Non-invasive glucose monitoring

The detector will be known as a non-invasive glucose detector as an early diagnosis of glucose content as an alternative to conventional invasive glucose detectors. Technologies used for non-invasive glucose monitoring include optical, transdermal, and thermal techniques [26]. Non-invasive methods are highly sought after to replace traditional fingerprinting methods because they can facilitate continuous glucose monitoring. The research group has been working on developing practical and non-invasive glucose for decades. The challenges associated with non-invasive glucose monitoring are the many factors that contribute to inaccurate measurements [27].

2.2 Microcontroller

Arduino Nano is a complete small microcontroller board that supports the use of PCB boards. Arduino Nano is based on the Atmel AVR microcontrollers. This microcontroller is open source with Arduino Language programming language, which resembles C++. The Arduino Nano doesn't include a barrel jack, but it connects to a computer using the MiniB USB connector. Arduino Nano is equipped with 8 analog pins and 22 digital pins (6 of which is PWM pin) with 16 MHz of clock speed. **Figure 1** shows the shape of the Arduino Nano.

2.3 Adapter microSD card module

This microSD card adapter module is a microSD card reader module. Through the file system and SPI driver interface, the MCU completes the file system read and write operations of the microSD card. Arduino users can directly use the Arduino IDE,

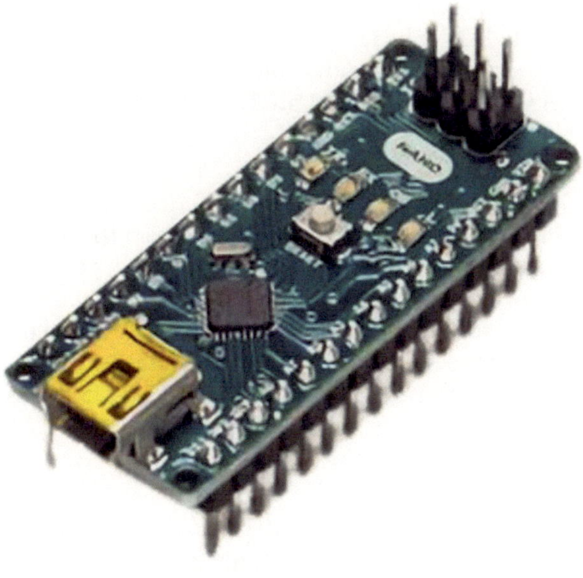

Figure 1.
Arduino Nano.

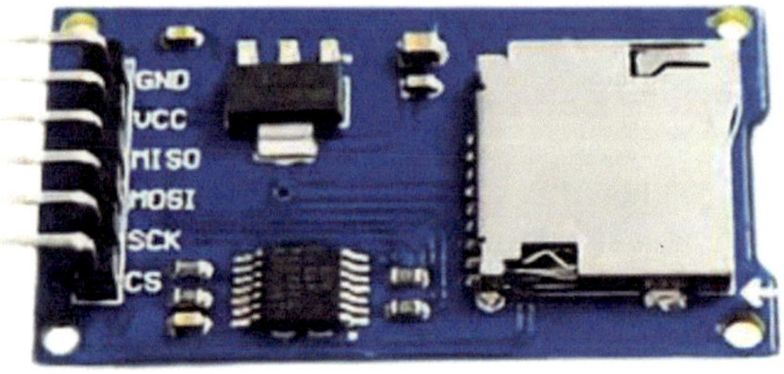

Figure 2.
MicroSD card module.

which is equipped with an SD card. The figure of the microSD card module is shown in **Figure 2**.

This communication model is indeed more wasteful in terms of the use of data lines, but it is safer when synchronizing data between data sent from the signal processing module and data received by the data storage module. This is because this model uses synchronous communication with a single clock source originating from the Arduino Nano module. In this study, the data is stored in the form of text files on a microSD card with a capacity of 4 GB. The pins between the Arduino and the microSD card module are VCC to 5 V, GND to ground, Mosi to pin 11, Miso to pin 12, SCK to pin 13, CS to pin four from Arduino.

2.4 I2C (inter integrated circuit) module and LCD 16×2

I2C liquid crystal display (LCD) is an LCD module that is controlled serially synchronously with the I2C/IIC (inter-integrated circuit) or TWI (two wire interface) protocol. The figure of I2C is shown in **Figure 3**. The LCD module is controlled in parallel for both the data and control lines. However, parallel lines will take up a lot of pins on the controller side, so an I2C is needed to save on PIN usage on Arduino. The Arduino is supported I2C. The I2C pin is on pin A4 for serial data and pins A5 for serial clock. The pins between the Arduino and the I2C module are GND to ground, VCC to 5 V, SCL to A5 pin, and SDA to A4 pin from Arduino.

2.5 LCD 16×2

LCD, as shown in **Figure 4**, is an electronic component that can display data in the form of characters, letters, or graphics. The LCD replaces the role of the seven-segment display by providing many advantages, such as a good display form, high energy efficiency, and a small form factor. The features presented in the 16×2 LCD consist of 16 characters and 2 lines, have 192 stored characters, there is a programmable character generator, can be addressed in 4-bit and 8-bit modes, and is equipped with a backlight.

2.6 IR thermal camera sensor

Thermal imaging is a tool that uses heat energy to detect the surface of an object. Currently, thermal imaging technology has been used in various fields, including engineering, health, military, environment, to health.

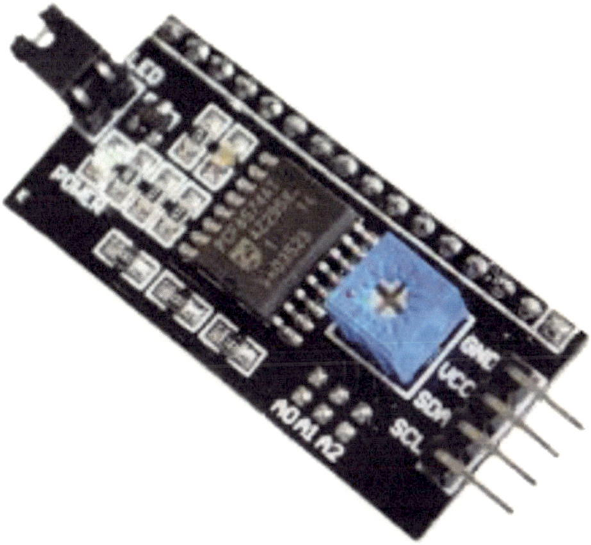

Figure 3.
I2C LCD module.

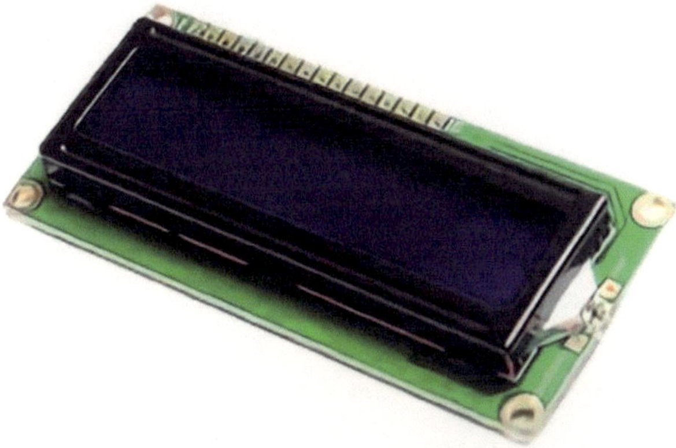

Figure 4.
LCD 16×2.

IR Thermal Camera is a non-contact sensor device that can detect heat or infrared energy and convert it and convert it into electrical energy or electronic signal, which can then produce a thermal image. In addition to generating thermal images, these electronic signals can also be used to perform temperature calculations or measurements.

Visualization of AMG8833 sensor is shown in **Figure 5**. The AMG8833 is a thermal imaging camera sensor with an 8×8 pixel thermal sensor family manufactured by Panasonic. The AMG8833 only supports I2C and has a configurable interrupt pin, which can be activated when each pixel is above or below the required threshold.

The detector on the AMG8833, as shown in **Figure 6**, consists of a thermopile sensor using MEMS (micro electro mechanical system) technology which is arranged in an 8×8 pixel array. A thermopile is a temperature sensor composed of a layer of the silicon film, which contains many thermocouples so that the infrared energy

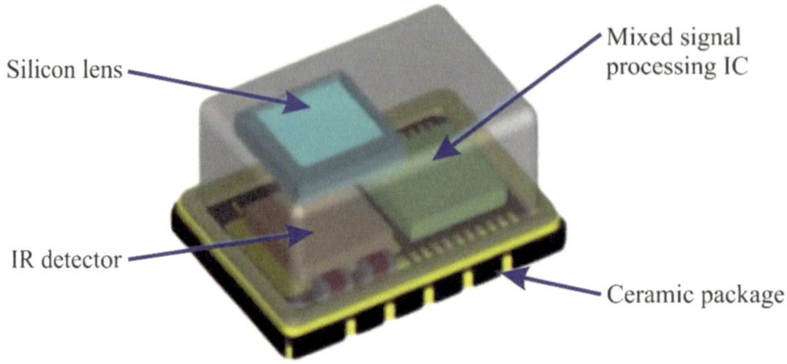

Figure 5.
Visualization of AMG8833 sensor.

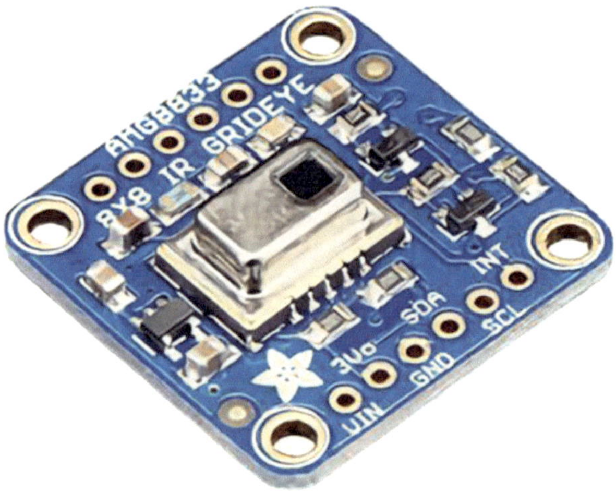

Figure 6.
Sensor IR thermal camera AMG8833.

emitted from the object will be absorbed and converted into electrical energy. After turning into electrical energy, signal processing is carried out. In the signal processing process, first, amplify the electrical energy or electrical signal obtained, then use an analog-to-digital converter (ADC) to convert it into a digital signal. Then the digital signal enters the control system for calculation, comparison, and correction so that the output temperature is Celsius.

2.7 UBEC regulator module

UBEC, as shown in **Figure 7**, is a circuit to change the voltage, high to low or vice versa, requires the right circuit, so that power can be delivered with the highest possible efficiency level. However, there is also switching battery elimination circuit (SBEC) where the overall use is the same as UBEC, and only SBEC has quality below UBEC. The 7805 regulator IC is very commonly used to lower the voltage. This regulator has the ability to handle currents up to 3 A, with a V_{in} of 5.5–26 V, for 5–6 V output.

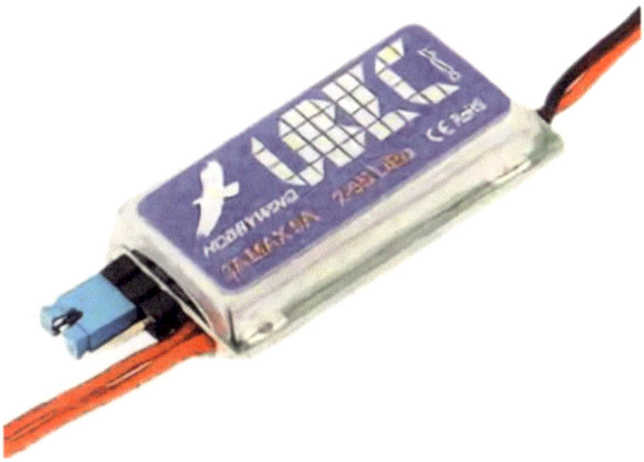

Figure 7.
UBEC regulator module 3 A 5–6 V.

2.8 Block diagram and flowchart portable urine quality detector

Figure 8 shows that the tool is fully integrated with all the components used. The thermal sensor has an 8×8 infrared sensor array that measures the temperature of urine in a non-contact container by detecting infrared energy or thermal energy emitted from the urine sample. The reading results produce an electrical signal and amplify it and then convert it into a digital signal using ADC.

A digital signal is sent to the control system for calculation, comparison, and correction so that the output temperature is expressed in degrees Celsius (°C). When connected to the Arduino Nano microcontroller, it displays an array of individual infrared temperature readings of 64 pixels per pixel display the Arduino readings. There is an interpolation scheme that connects to Matlab via serial communication and improves pixel scaling from 8×8 to 100×100.

Flowchart portable urine quality detector can be seen in **Figure 9**. The first stage is to take a urine sample and put it in a reservoir. Urine was taken in three variations, namely urine taken in the morning, urine taken at any time, and postprandial urine with urine composition consisting of mineral water and some drinks containing glucose. Inside the portable detector, the IR Thermal sensor will detect the urine temperature. Furthermore, the system will analyze the temperature data captured by the IR Thermal sensor. The diagnosis results will be displayed through the Matlab software and also the LCD.

2.9 Schematic diagram of portable urine quality detector

Figure 10 shows a schematic of the portable urine quality detector circuit using the Proteus application software. In the schematic of the circuit, the voltage source

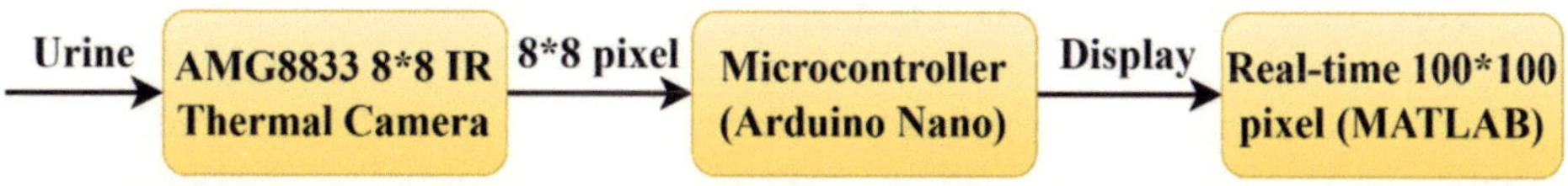

Figure 8.
Block diagram of portable urine quality detector.

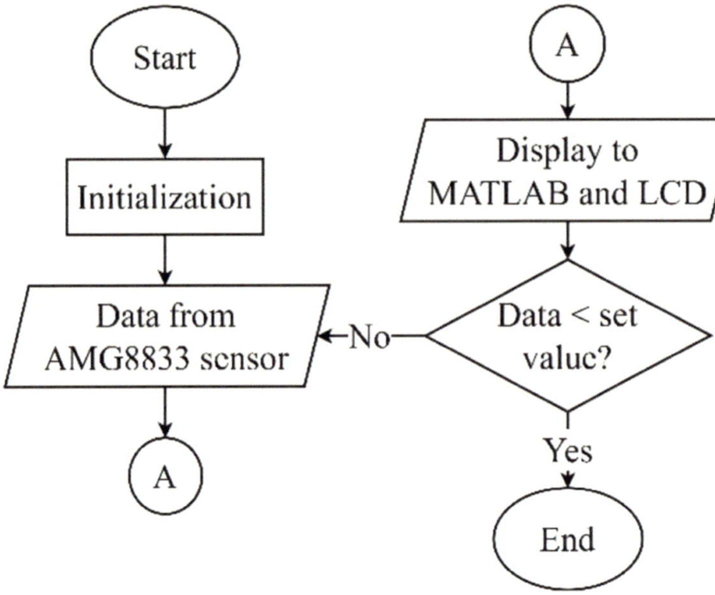

Figure 9.
Flowchart portable urine quality detector.

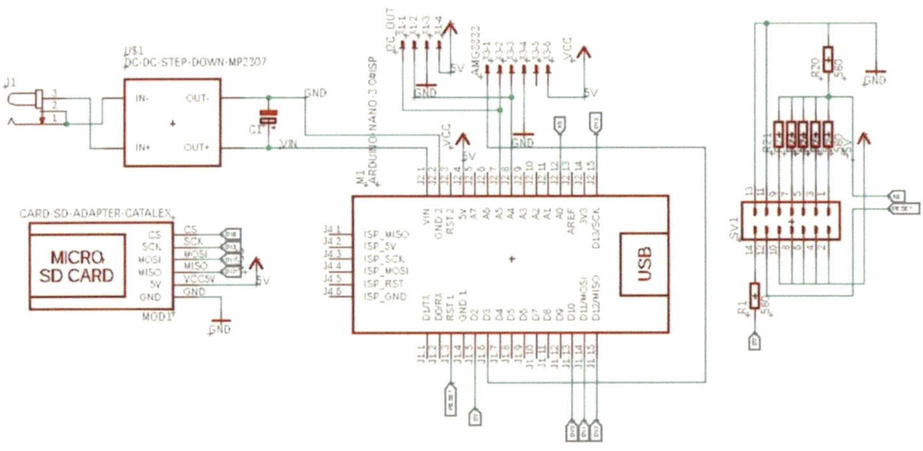

Figure 10.
Circuit schematic of portable urine quality detector.

in the circuit is lowered using a DC-to-DC step-down, then the AMG8833 sensor is connected to the Arduino Nano microcontroller after that from the Arduino Nano, it is connected to the microSD card.

2.10 Urine quality detector portable design

This device as shown in **Figure 11** has a fairly small form which has the advantage of being easy to move so that it can be used anywhere. The closed box enables this invention to work without being affected by the external light intervention. The sensor used is a camera sensor as a component to take pictures from the reaction strip.

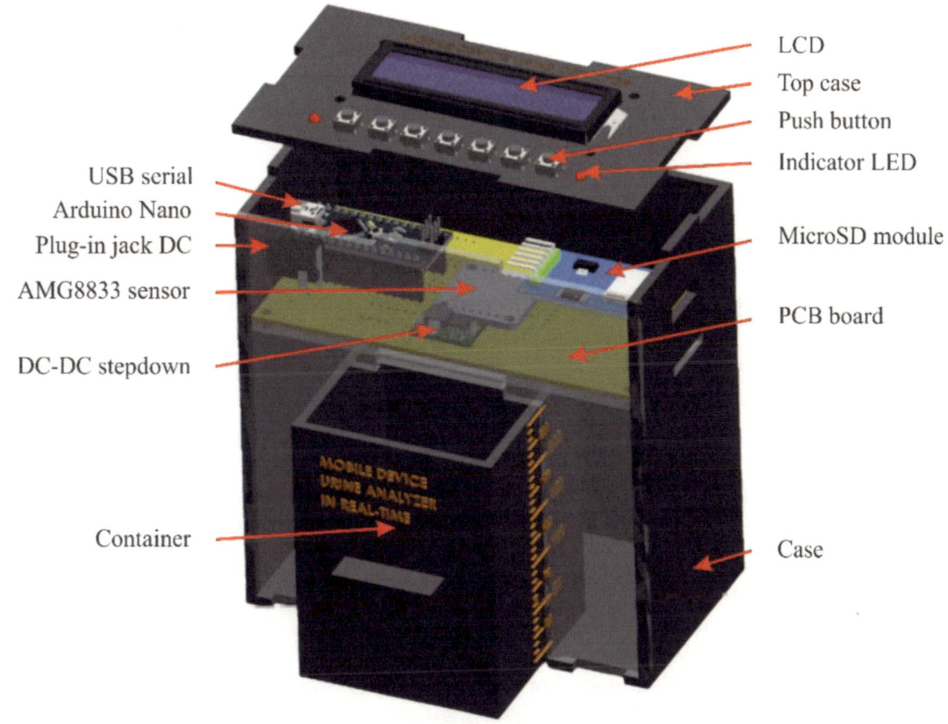

Figure 11.
Design of urine quality detector portable.

This urine glucose detector hardware is integrated with software that functions to analyze the data that has been obtained.

The device consists of a camera sensor, an LED module, a filament box, and a reaction strip slider. The ELP USB industrial camera type camera sensor is used as a sensor to take image data obtained from the reaction strip. The reaction strip consists of 10 variables, namely glucose, bilirubin, ketones, specific gravity, blood, pH, protein, urobilinogen, nitrite, and leukocytes. The reaction strip slider is made in such a way that its size matches the medical standard reaction strip. The camera sensor is equipped with a convex lens so that it can cover a wide area and can capture data from 10 variables simultaneously. The LED used in the LED module is a Super Bright LED type with a diameter of 3 mm. The LED module acts as a reaction strip light and adds light that enters the camera sensor. The LED module is also used to minimize the intervention of light entering the glucose detector in the urine. The LED module gets a voltage supply through an AC to DC power source with a working voltage of 12 V. The input of the power source is an alternating voltage type with a voltage value of 220 V. The output of the power source is a direct voltage of 12 V, 2 A. The camera sensor does not is always on to retrieve data, but the camera sensor starts capturing data on a command from the software. The test strip is dipped in a tube containing urine, and then the test strip enters the glucose detector through the test strip slide. When the reaction strip is in the correct position, the software will instruct the camera sensor to start taking pictures. The software takes an image through the camera sensor for 30 s from the moment the test strip is inserted into the glucose detector. The data that has been taken is stored on the computer. The software has been equipped with an algorithm to analyze the data that has been taken.

The software converts image data into value data from the 10 variables mentioned above. The output of this system is an early diagnosis of diabetes. The software will provide analysis results in the form of two choices, namely diabetes, and non-diabetes. The data that has been obtained in the software is also uploaded to the server, which will be used as a machine learning data set. The system on the server continues to study the data that has been collected, which is then used as a parameter in making decisions for the early diagnosis of diabetes. The box is made of a 3-dimensional mold with the type of PLA+ material. The box is made in such a way that it can accommodate the components used. Furthermore, the box also functions to reduce the intervention of light from outside so that the glucose detector in urine can be used anywhere and anytime.

3. Result and discussion

The test is carried out using three types of urine, namely morning urine, which is the first urine excreted in the morning when you wake up. This urine is more concentrated than urine that comes out during the day, so it's great for checking sediment, specific gravity, protein, etc., and also great for pregnancy tests based on the presence of HCG (human chorionic gonadotrophins) in urine. Urine at any time where this urine can be used for various instantaneous tests, i.e., urine excreted at an unspecified time. Urine at this time is usually good enough for examination. Then the postprandial urine, where this urine sample can be used to check for glucosuria. Postprandial urine is the first urine excreted 1½–3 h after eating.

Test results data on urine temperature from several samples of the morning urine, urine at any time, postprandial urine. The urine sample is accommodated 20–30 ml in a urine collection container that is directly removed from the urethra and in real-time can be seen in **Figure 12**. In testing sample 1, urine collection was taken in the morning at 06.14, random urine at 13.20, postprandial urine at 20.13. The result for consumption of water and drinks containing glucose 1 × 24 h, namely 600 ml bottled water, 15 g warm tea, 10 g iced tea, 22 g Velluto Tango Drink, can be seen in **Figure 13**. It is known that the temperature of the morning urine is 28°C, the urine at any time is 27°C, and the postprandial urine is 30°C.

The next data is the test of sample 2 with the same dose directly removed from the urethra and in real-time in **Figure 14**. In the second sample test, urine collection was taken in the morning at 05.34, random urine at 16.20, postprandial urine at 22.07

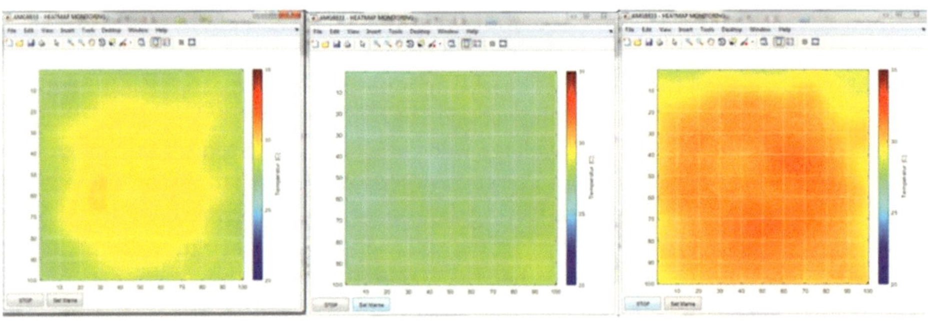

Morning urine | Urine at any time | Postprandial urine

Figure 12.
Temperature display on sample 1.

WIT. The result for consumption of water and drinks containing glucose 1 × 24 h, namely one glass of 330 ml bottled water, good day cappuccino 25 g, iced tea 15 g, orange ice 10 g, soya bean V-soy 19.8 g, that can be seen in **Figure 15**. It is known that

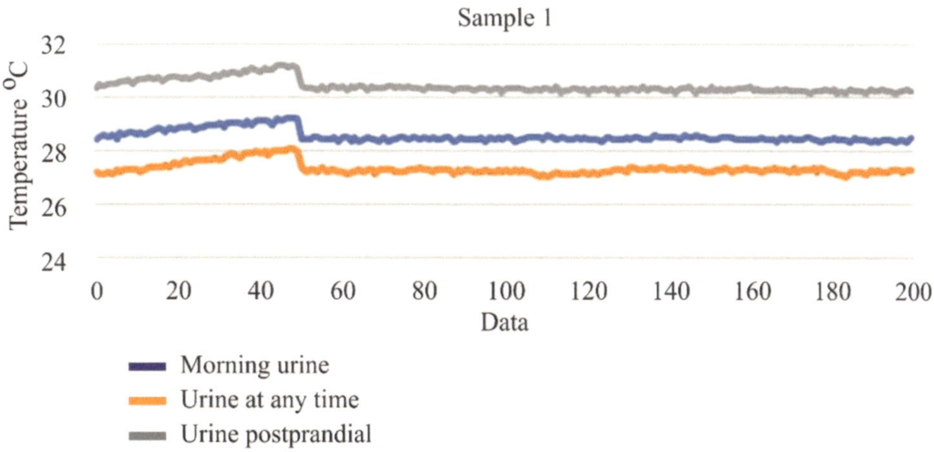

Figure 13.
Graph of sample test results 1.

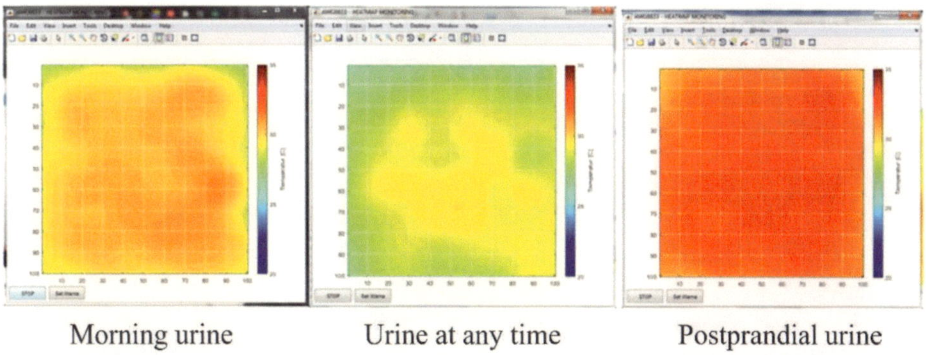

Figure 14.
Temperature display on sample 2.

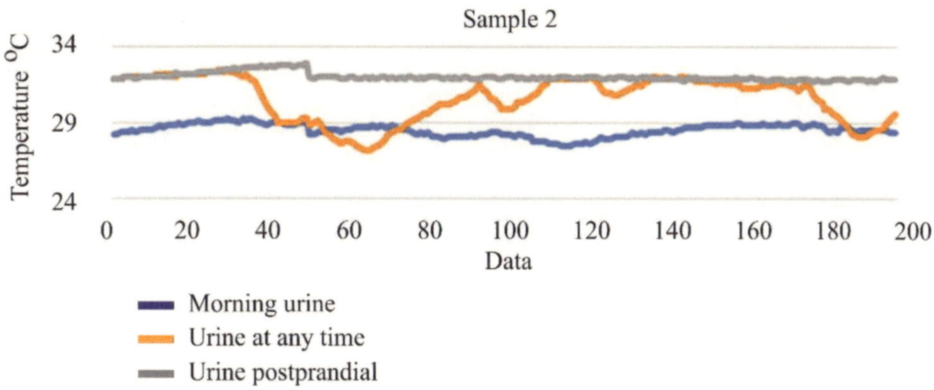

Figure 15.
Graph of sample test results 2.

the temperature of morning urine is 28°C, intermittent urine is 31°C, postprandial urine is 32°C.

The next data is testing sample 3 with the same dose directly removed from the urethra and in real-time in **Figure 16**. In the third sample test, urine collection was taken in the morning at 06.47, random urine at 21.46, postprandial urine at 16.44. The result for consumption of water and drinks containing glucose 1 × 24 h, namely 250 ml of water, 15 ml of reject wind, 23 g of Kopiko Coffee, can be seen in **Figure 17**.

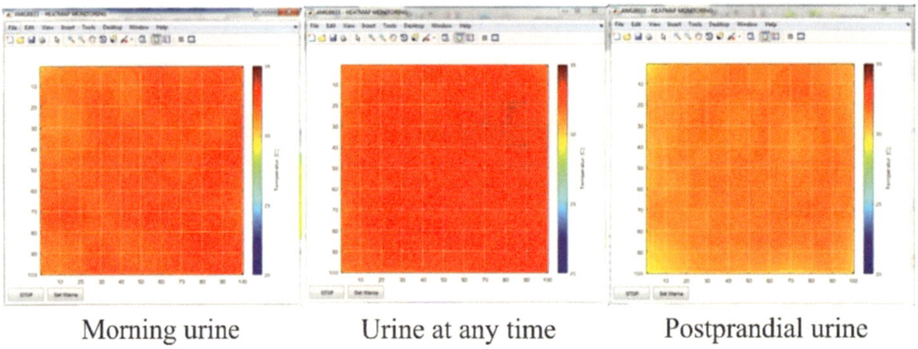

Figure 16.
Temperature display on sample 3.

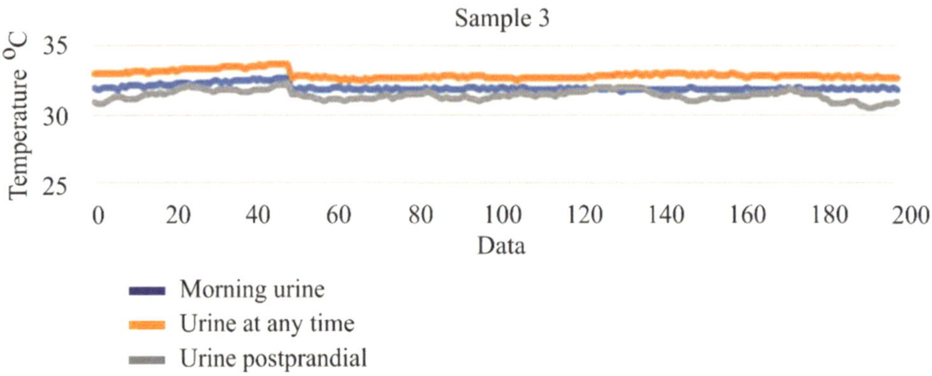

Figure 17.
Graph of sample test results 3.

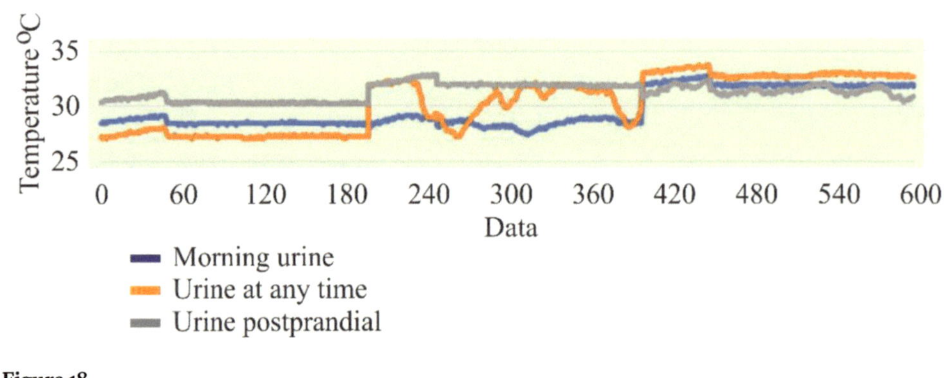

Figure 18.
Graph of measuring average.

It is known that the temperature of morning urine is 32°C, intermittent urine is 33°C, postprandial urine is 32°C.

The data from the test results of the Urine Quality Detector tool have an average conductivity value which can be seen in **Figure 18**. **Figure 18** is a graph of the average temperature conductivity value in urine from three different samples with consumption of various types of drinks that contain glucose. The graph shows that postprandial urine temperature has the highest average temperature value, which is between 30°C and 32°C compared to morning urine and occasional urine.

Captured samples were processed in the HSV color space. **Figure 19** shows the HVS values generated in several types of samples, including without artificial glucose, with artificial glucose of 1, 2, and 3 g. At the same time, the distribution of HVS values is shown in **Figure 20**.

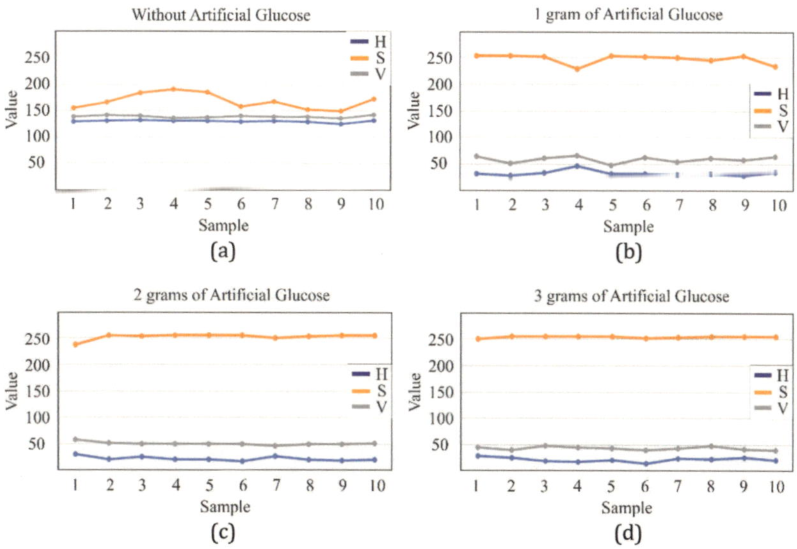

Figure 19.
HSV value of samples, (a) without, (b) 1 g, (c) 2 g, and (d) 3 g of artificial glucose.

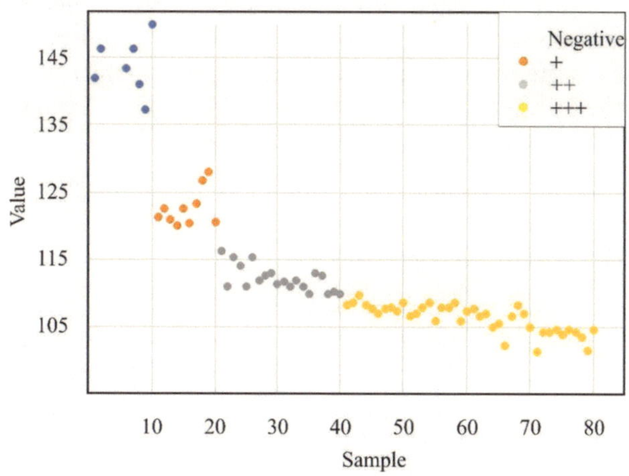

Figure 20.
Distribution of HSV values.

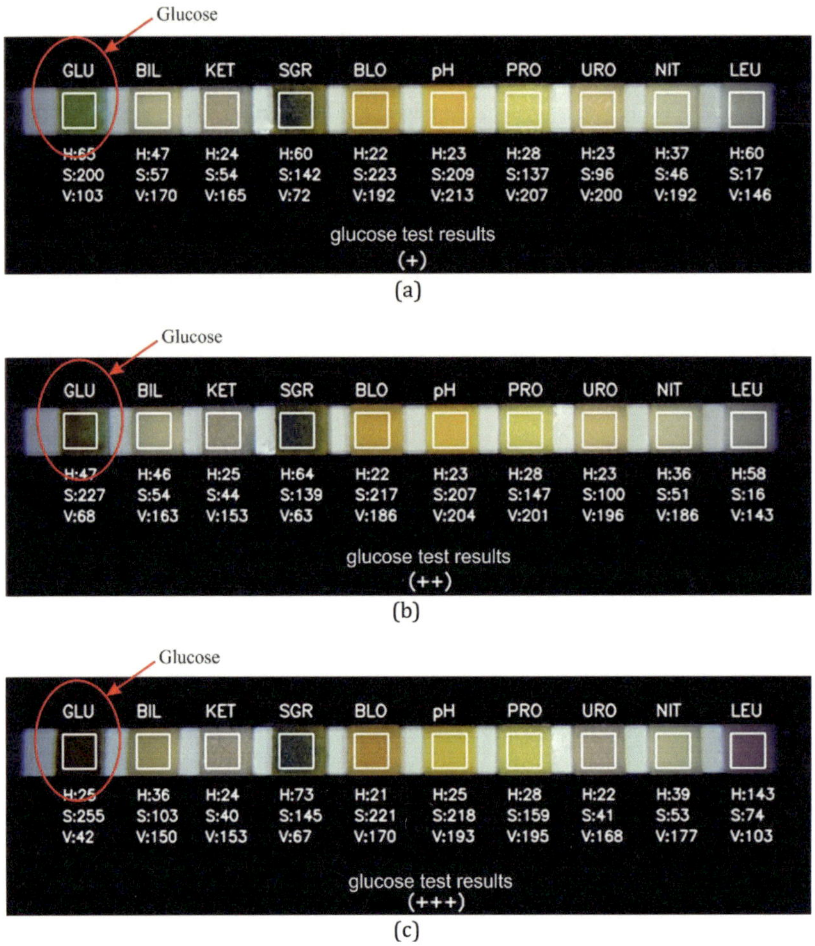

Figure 21.
Glucose test result with three different levels (a) level 1 or +, (b) level 2 or ++, and (c) level 3 or +++.

Finally, a urine test strip treated with a urine sample can be detected. Glucose levels can be detected through the color on the glucose indicator box (GLU). It can be seen the difference in the color of the GLU indicator affects the HSV combination. **Figure 21** shows the different levels of glucose levels, (a) level 1 is indicated by "+", (b) level 2 is indicated by "++", and (c) level 3 is indicated by "+++".

4. Conclusion

The IR Thermal Camera sensor AMG8833 was applied in this study to detect urine temperature from the experiment. Three experimental conditions were carried out, namely morning urine, intermittent urine, and postprandial urine, with a combination of drink consumption on the respondents. Postprandial urine showed the highest temperature in samples 1 and 2, around more than equal to 30°C, while urine at any time showed the highest temperature in sample 3 with a value of 30°C. This proves that the glucose detector in the urine can function properly.

Author details

Anton Yudhana*, Liya Yusrina Sabila, Arsyad Cahya Subrata,
Hendriana Helda Pratama and Muhammad Syahrul Akbar
Department of Electrical Engineering, Ahmad Dahlan University, Yogyakarta,
Indonesia

*Address all correspondence to: eyudhana@ee.uad.ac.id

References

[1] Li N, Ho KWK, Ying GG, Deng WJ. Veterinary antibiotics in food, drinking water, and the urine of preschool children in Hong Kong. Environment International. 2017;**108**(April):246-252. DOI: 10.1016/j.envint.2017.08.014

[2] Zulyadi R. Obstacle factors on evidence system of urine test result on drugs cases in national narcotics board of North Sumatera Province, Indonesia. Budapest International Research and Critics Institute. 2020;**3**(2):1316-1324. DOI: 10.33258/birci.v3i2.976

[3] Mir C et al. Analysis of urine composition from split 24-h samples: Use of 12-h overnight samples to evaluate risk factors for calcium stones in healthy and stone-forming children. Journal of Pediatric Urology. 2020;**16**(3):371.e1-371.e7. DOI: 10.1016/j.jpurol.2020.02.011

[4] Rowe I et al. Defective glucose metabolism in polycystic kidney disease identifies a new therapeutic strategy. Nature Medicine. 2013;**19**(4):488-493. DOI: 10.1038/nm.3092

[5] Hu T et al. Portable and intelligent urine glucose analyzer based on a cdte qds@gox aerogel circular array sensor. ACS Omega. 2021;**6**(48):32655-32662. DOI: 10.1021/acsomega.1c03449

[6] Fünfstück R, Nicolle LE, Hanefeld M, Naber KG. Urinary tract infection in patients with diabetes mellitus. Clinical Nephrology. 2012;**77**(1):40-48. DOI: 10.5414/CN107216

[7] Bechmann LP, Hannivoort RA, Gerken G, Hotamisligil GS, Trauner M, Canbay A. The interaction of hepatic lipid and glucose metabolism in liver diseases. Journal of Hepatology. 2012;**56**(4):952-964. DOI: 10.1016/j.jhep.2011.08.025

[8] Gonzales WV, Mobashsher AT, Abbosh A. "The progress of glucose monitoring—A review of invasive to minimally and non-invasive techniques, devices and sensors", Sensors (Switzerland). 2019;**19**(4)

[9] Shokrekhodaei M, Quinones S. Review of non-invasive glucose sensing techniques: Optical, electrical and breath acetone. Sensors (Switzerland). 2020;**20**(5). DOI: 10.3390/s20051251

[10] Tang L, Chang SJ, Chen CJ, Liu JT. Non-invasive blood glucose monitoring technology: A review. Sensors (Switzerland). 2020;**20**(23):1-32. DOI: 10.3390/s20236925

[11] Yudhana A et al. Multi sensor application-based for measuring the quality of human urine on first-void urine. Sensing and Bio-Sensing Research. 2021;**34**:100461. DOI: 10.1016/j.sbsr.2021.100461

[12] Leboulanger B, Guy RH, Delgado-Charro MB. Reverse iontophoresis for non-invasive transdermal monitoring. Physiological Measurement. 2004;**25**(3):R35

[13] Hillier TA, Abbott RD, Barrett EJ. Hyponatremia: Evaluating the correction factor for hyperglycemia. The American Journal of Medicine. 1999;**106**(4):399-403

[14] Lee S, Nayak V, Dodds J, Pishko M, Smith NB. Glucose measurements with sensors and ultrasound. Ultrasound in Medicine & Biology. 2005;**31**(7):971-977

[15] Allen TJ, Cox BT, Beard PC. "Generating photoacoustic signals using high-peak power pulsed laser diodes," In: Photons Plus Ultrasound: Imaging

and Sensing 2005: The Sixth Conference on Biomedical Thermoacoustics, Optoacoustics, and Acousto-Optics. 2005;**5697**:233-242

[16] Alavi SM, Gourzi M, Rouane A, Nadi M. "An original method for non-invasive glucose measurement: Preliminary results," In: 2001 Conference Proceedings of the 23rd Annual International Conference of the IEEE Engineering in Medicine and Biology Society. Istanbul, Turkey. 2001;**4**:3318-3320

[17] Ellis DI, Goodacre R. Metabolic fingerprinting in disease diagnosis: Biomedical applications of infrared and Raman spectroscopy. Analyst. 2006;**131**(8):875-885

[18] Larin KV, Eledrisi MS, Motamedi M, Esenaliev RO. Noninvasive blood glucose monitoring with optical coherence tomography: A pilot study in human subjects. Diabetes Care. 2002;**25**(12):2263-2267

[19] Fusman R et al. Image analysis for the detection of increased erythrocyte, leukocyte and platelet adhesiveness/aggregation in the peripheral blood of patients with diabetes mellitus. Acta Diabetologica. 2001;**38**(3):129-134

[20] Khalil OS. Noninvasive photonic-crystal material for sensing glucose in tears. Clinical Chemistry. 2004;**50**(12):2236-2237 Oxford University Press.

[21] Ongkum C, Keawmitr K, Boonchieng E. "Analysis system for urine strip test using image processing technique," In: BMEiCON 2016 - 9th Biomedical Engineering International Conference. Laung Prabang, Laos. pp. 3-7. DOI: 10.1109/BMEiCON.2016.7859610

[22] Xia ML, Wang L, Yang ZX, Chen HZ. A novel digital color analysis method for rapid glucose detection. Analytical Methods. 2015;**7**(16):6654-6663. DOI: 10.1039/c5ay01233c

[23] Yudhana A, Umar R, Ayudewi FM. The monitoring of corn sprouts growth using the region growing methods. Journal of Physics Conference Series. 2019;**1373**(1). DOI: 10.1088/1742-6596/1373/1/012054.

[24] Yudhana A, Sunardi S, Saifullah S. Segmentation comparing eggs watermarking image and original image. Bulletin of Electrical Engineering and Informatics. 2017;**6**(1):47-53. DOI: 10.11591/eei.v6i1.595

[25] Surya RA, Fadlil A, Yudhana A. Identification of Pekalongan Batik images using Backpropagation method. Journal of Physics Conference Series. 2019;**1373**(1). DOI: 10.1088/1742-6596/1373/1/012049

[26] Lin T. Non-invasive glucose monitoring: A review of challenges and recent advances. Current Trends in Biomedical Engineering & Biosciences. 2017;**6**(5):1-8. DOI: 10.19080/ctbeb.2017.06.555696

[27] Soni A, Jha SK. A paper strip based non-invasive glucose biosensor for salivary analysis. Biosensors & Bioelectronics. 2015;**67**:763-768. DOI: 10.1016/j.bios.2014.09.042

Chapter 6

Deep Learning Algorithms for Efficient Analysis of ECG Signals to Detect Heart Disorders

Sumagna Dey, Rohan Pal and Saptarshi Biswas

Abstract

Electrocardiography (ECG) has been a reliable method for monitoring the proper functioning of the cardiovascular system for decades. Recently, there has been a lot of research focusing on accurately analyzing the heart condition through ECG. In recent days, numerous attempts are being made to analyze these signals using deep learning algorithms, including the implementation of artificial neural networks like convolutional neural networks, recurrent neural networks, and the like. In this context, this chapter intends to present some important techniques for classifying heartbeats based on deep neural networks with 1D CNN. Five ECG signals (N, S, V, F, and Q) standardization are based on the AAMI EC57 standard. The primary focus of this chapter is to discuss the techniques to classify ECG signals in those classes with promising accuracy and draw a clear picture of the current state-of-the-art in this sphere of study.

Keywords: signal processing, electrocardiography, deep learning, 1D convolutional neural network, recurrent neural network

1. Introduction

Cardiac problems are one of the most important problems across the globe. According to autopsy studies, heart disease has increased since the 1960s due to a rise in the frequency of coronary atherosclerosis with resultant coronary heart disease. The number of CVD deaths in India each year is anticipated to increase from 2.26 to 4.77 million between the years 1990 and 2020. The coronary heart disease frequency rates in India have fluctuated from 1.6 to 7.4% in rural populations whereas from 1 to 13.2% in urban populations during the last several decades [1]. Heart disease claims the lives of about 17 lakh individuals in India each year, and the number is estimated to rise to 2.3 crores by 2030. This rise is linked to an increase in smoking and dietary changes, resulting in higher blood cholesterol levels. The symptoms like angina, chest pain, difficulty breathing, edema, fatigue, and lightheadedness may indicate a heart problem or heart attack. Heart attack can lead to cardiac arrest, which occurs when the heart's rhythm is disrupted, or the heart stops beating, and the body can no longer function [2].

Any disorder that affects the cardiovascular system is alluded to as heart disease [3]. Heart disease comes in various forms, each of which affects the heart and blood arteries in distinct ways. The most typical kinds of heart disease are coronary artery disease, arrhythmia, heart valve disease, and heart failure [4]. Coronary artery disease is the most noticeable type of heart disease. It happens when plaque accumulates in the arteries that deliver blood to the heart. It can cause a reduction in blood flow to your heart muscle, preventing it from receiving the oxygen it requires. Atherosclerosis, often known as artery hardening, is the most common cause of the illness. Arrhythmia refers to an improper beating of the heart [5]. It happens when the electrical impulses that regulate the heartbeat do not even function properly. As a result, the heart may beat excessively fast, too slowly, or in an irregular pattern. Heart valve disease occurs when a heart valve is damaged [6]. Infectious diseases such as rheumatic fever, congenital heart disease, excessive blood pressure, coronary artery disease are all causes of heart valve disorders. Heart failure does not imply that the heart has ceased to beat. A condition in which the heart is not pumping blood as efficiently as it should be to satisfy the body's demands. There are some more heart diseases like pericardial disease, myocardial infarction [7], cardiomyopathy, mitral valve regurgitation, congenital heart disease, etc.

Over the last several decades, the rapid advancement of cardiology has profoundly changed the natural course of cardiac patients. Cardiac care has evolved, with technology playing an increasingly significant role. With the appropriate technology and artificial intelligence (AI) and machine learning, cardiac care providers have been motivated to improve treatment methods [8]. Then there's remote care that enables electrocardiogram (ECG) diagnosis [9], which uses cloud technology and Bluetooth-enabled cardiac devices to test the parameters and send them back to healthcare practitioners without attending the clinic. Some emerging technologies used every day in cardiology are transcatheter mitral and tricuspid valve interventions, artificial intelligence, wearable devices, big data, structured reporting, robots in the cath lab, virtual and augmented reality, FFR technologies, holographic procedural navigation in the Cath Lab, etc. [10].

There are many cardiac implantable electronic devices like pacemakers, implanted cardioverter defibrillators (ICDs), biventricular pacemakers, and cardiac loop recorders, which are used to control or monitor irregular heartbeats in persons with specific heart rhythm problems and heart failure. An implanted cardioverter-defibrillator is a device that can do cardioversion, defibrillation, and cardiac pacing. ICD is capable of rectifying the majority of life-threatening cardiac arrhythmias. A pacemaker is a device that is implanted beneath the skin and communicates with the heart through electrical leads. Pacemakers are used to treat bradycardia, a condition where the heart beats too slowly (less than 60 times per minute). The pacemaker sends electrical pulses to the heart to maintain it beating normally. A biventricular pacemaker is a compact, battery-operated device and light. This gadget aids with the proper pumping of your heart. It also protects from harmful cardiac arrhythmias. An implantable loop recorder is a heart-monitoring device implanted beneath the chest skin. It has a variety of applications. Searching for reasons of fainting, palpitations, very rapid or slow heartbeats, and hidden rhythms that might cause strokes are among the most prevalent. Computer-aided diagnosis (CAD) [11] refers to software that helps clinicians understand medical images. The radiologist or other medical expert must assess and evaluate a large amount of data in a short amount of time using imaging modalities such as X-ray, MRI, and ultrasound diagnostics. The Kurt Rossmann Laboratories for Radiologic Image Research in the Department of

Radiology at the University of Chicago began large-scale systematic research and development of several CAD methods in the early 1980s. The idea of computer-aided design was established in 1966 and has been completely implemented since 1980.

Nowadays, computer-aided diagnosis has become a contentious research topic in medical imaging and diagnostic radiology research. CAD technology aids in the improvement of the performance of radiologists in increasing productivity by cost-effectively enhancing sensitivity rate. CAD can improve image diagnostic accuracy by detecting illnesses that are too premature to be detected by naked eyes. It enables early detection, which can lead to better treatment results. Computer-aided detection is a relatively new advancement in the area of breast imaging that aims to increase the throughput of radiologists to identify diseases like breast cancer [12] even at an early stage. In recent times, computer-aided diagnosis is used to diagnose acute lymphoblastic leukemia, which suggested a solution to the flaws in manual diagnosis techniques. Even ECG-based computer-aided diagnosis [13] is also used for cardiovascular diseases which have the potential to improve diagnosis accuracy while also lowering costs.

Medical images nowadays play a crucial role in the identification and diagnosis of awide range of disorders. To aid in the interpretation of medical images, a variety of computer-aided detection and diagnosis technologies have recently been developed in order to achieve a more reliable and accurate diagnosis. CT, MR imaging, digital radiography, biomagnetism, and optical range sensing are examples of imaging systems that take advantage of sophisticated computer technology.

The real-life problem with manual experimentation is that manual diagnostic procedures are time-consuming, less accurate, and prone to mistakes due to different human variables such as stress, exhaustion, fatigue, and so forth. As a result, many automated techniques have been developed to combat the flaws in manual diagnostic approaches. When compared to manual diagnosis procedures, these computer-aided technologies are faster, more dependable, more efficient, more standardization and more accurate. Computer-aided diagnosis (CAD) aids in the calculation of computational and statistical features that people cannot gather visually or intuitively. Computer-assisted diagnosis also reduces the reliance on the operator in ultrasonic imaging and makes the diagnosis procedure reproducible. Interference testing and 3D animations are simple to accomplish in computer-aided diagnosis [14].

Machine learning has been applied in a variety of fields all over the world and the health industry is no exception. On the other hand, deep learning is part of the family of machine learning algorithms relying on representation and artificial neural networks are being utilized for the analysis of medical data. For quite some time, these algorithms were used to assess patients' status with respect to the image or non-image-based medical data acquired using new generation medical equipment. These developments are attributable to the emergence of new CAD systems known as knowledge-based systems, including expertise or knowledge. As a result, the modern CAD systems include some intelligence [15]. The major job of the software related to these systems nowadays is to automate the analytical phases. To ensure that components and assemblies achieve design standards, CAD software is used to make computer modeling, fit them together, and simulate their performance. Because design reviews, conducted by specialists, evaluate if changes should be made, the analytical phases of the design process are repeated (design synthesis). Design synthesis may be done immediately with AI-based technologies without the need for a separate design review, and they are correctly implemented.

Based on the recent advancements, computer-aided diagnosis is used to diagnose heart abnormalities such as arrhythmias and heart blockages using electrocardiogram (ECG) signal analysis [16]. Although electrocardiography (ECG) is affordable and commonly available, ECG abnormalities are not specific for the diagnosis of congestive heart failure (CHF) which is the inability of the heart to efficiently circulate blood throughout the body without a rise in intracardiac pressure. Based on the ECG, a well-designed computer-aided detection (CAD) system for CHF might possibly eliminate subjectivity and give a quantitative evaluation for better decision-making.

Cardiologists and medical practitioners frequently utilize ECG to assess heart health. The difficulty in identifying and classifying distinct waveforms and morphologies in ECG signals is the major issue with manual analysis. This task is both time-consuming and error-prone for a human. Cardiovascular illnesses are the leading cause of mortality worldwide, accounting for around one-third of all fatalities. Millions of individuals, for example, suffer from irregular heartbeats, which can be fatal in some circumstances. As a result, precise and low-cost arrhythmic heartbeat diagnosis is extremely desirable.

Many research in the literature investigated the utilization of machine learning approaches to reliably detect abnormalities in ECG data to solve the drawbacks present in human analysis. Pre-processing, like passing through bandpass or high pass filter, is used in most of these methods to prepare the signal to be compatible for machine-based analysis. The handcrafted features, which are typically statistical summarizations of signal windows, are then retrieved from these signals and employed in subsequent processing. For the last categorization task, conduct an analysis.

In terms of the conclusion, for ECG, traditional machine learning algorithms [2] like support vector machines, multi-layer perceptrons, decision trees, and other methods of analysis were used previously. Automated feature extraction and representation approaches have been shown to be more scalable and capable of producing more accurate predictions, according to current machine learning research. In this study, we are going to elaborate on a few of the new emerging and compatible technologies and their applications.

The rest of the article has been organized in the following manner. First, Section 2 provides a brief theoretical and mathematical background related to this domain of study which is followed by the problem statement in Section 3. Next, Section 4 discusses about the significance of noise removal with stages of data processing. Section 5 gives a brief survey about the recent state-of-the-art techniques related to automated signal processing of ECG signals that is followed by the promising experimental results reported in the recent literature. Finally, Section 7 concludes this chapter.

2. Theoretical and mathematical background

2.1 Mathematical foundation

In signal processing [17], several mathematical methods like sampling frequency, Nyquist filtering, Fourier analysis series and transform, Z transform, pole zero plot are used for processing signals.

The reduction of a continuous-time signal to a discrete-time signal is known as sampling and the sampling frequency represents the number of samples per second collected from a continuous signal to create a discrete or digital signal. There are few applications of the sampling process. The sampling process is utilized in music recordings to ensure sound quality. The sampling technique is also used to convert analog to discrete data. It is also used in speech recognition systems, radar and radio navigation, sensor data evaluation, modulation and demodulation, and pattern recognition systems.

2.1.1 Sampling frequency or sampling rate

The sampling frequency [18] or sampling rate f_s is defined as the average number of samples acquired in 1 second, therefore $f_s = \frac{1}{T}$ where T is the sampling period and is measured with the unit samples per second or hertz. The sampling theorem indicates the lowest sampling frequency where a continuous-time signal must have been uniformly sampled in order for the original signal to be fully recovered or reconstructed using just these samples.

If a continuous-time signal has no frequency components greater than a sampling rate of W Hz (where W is called the bandwidth), then uniform samples taken at a rate of f_s samples per second can be used to identify it completely [19]. This implies $f_s > = 2W$ and when it comes to the sampling period $T < = \frac{1}{2W}$. Here $2W$ is termed as the Nyquist rate.

2.1.2 Nyquist filter

A Nyquist filter is an electrical filter that equalizes the visual characteristics of TV receivers. In receivers, a Nyquist filter is utilized to equalize the low and high-frequency components of the VF signal. It plays an essential role in the creation of n bandlimited pulses in wired and wireless communication systems to ensure minimal inter symbol interference. Its principal application is as a pulse-shaping filter. Nyquist filters are a form of multi-rate finite impulse response filter that is also known as M^{th} band filters.

The following equation indicates the impulse response of a Nyquist filter $h(n)$:

$$h(Mn + k) = \begin{cases} c & n = 0 \\ 0 & otherwise \end{cases} \tag{1}$$

where, c and k are constants.

The following equation satisfies the z-transform of a Nyquist filter $H(z)$:

$$\sum_{k=0}^{M-1} H\left(zW^k\right) = Mc = 1 \tag{2}$$

where, $W = e^{-\frac{j2\pi}{M}}$ and $c = \frac{1}{M}$.

The frequency responses of all M uniformly shifted versions of $H(z)$ add up to a constant because the frequency response of $H\left(zW^k\right)$ is the shifted version of the frequency response of $H(z)$.

2.1.3 Fourier series and Fourier transform

The Fourier series is a periodic function made up of harmonically compatible sinusoids that are integrated together using a weighted summation. The Fourier series is an infinite series that can be used to solve several forms of differential equations. It's mainly composed of an infinite sum of sines and cosines, and it's valuable for evaluating periodic functions since it's periodic. The Fourier series is widely utilized in telecommunications systems for voice signal modulation and demodulation.

The Fourier transform is a technique for transforming time-domain signals to frequency-domain signals. The Fourier transform is a useful image processing method for decomposing an image into sine and cosine components. The image in the Fourier or frequency domain is represented by the output of the transformation, whereas the spatial domain equivalent is represented by the input image. It's utilized in electrical circuit design, solving differential equations, signal processing, signal analysis, image processing, and filtering, among other things.

The Fourier transform is a mathematical approach for converting a time function, $x(t)$, to a frequency function, $X(\omega)$. It has a lot in common with the Fourier series. The Fourier transform of a function can be determined as a specific instance of the Fourier series when the period is $T \to \infty$.

The Fourier transform of a sequence is represented as:

$$x(t) = \sum_{n=-\infty}^{\infty} c_n e^{jn\omega_o t} \tag{3}$$

where c_n is provided by the Fourier series analysis equation:

$$c_n = \frac{1}{T}\int_T x(t)e^{-jn\omega_o t}dt \tag{4}$$

It can also be written as:

$$X\left(e^{j\omega}\right) = \sum_{n=-\infty} [n]e^{-j\omega n} \tag{5}$$

As $T \to \infty$ the initial frequency, $\omega_0 = \frac{2\pi}{T}$ decreases dramatically and the quantity $n\omega_0$ becomes a continuous quantity that may take on any value (because n has a range of $\pm\infty$). So, we generate a special variable $\omega = n\omega_0$ and set $X(\omega) = Tc_n$. The analytical equation for the Fourier transform is obtained by substituting these values in the previous equation. This transform is also called the forward Fourier transform.

The analysis equation of forward Fourier transform is:

$$X(\omega) = \int_{-\infty}^{+\infty} X(t)e^{-j\omega t}dt \tag{6}$$

On the other hand, the synthesis equation of inverse Fourier transform is:

$$x(t) = \frac{1}{2\pi}\int_{-\infty}^{+\infty} X(\omega)e^{j\omega t}d\omega \tag{7}$$

2.1.4 Z-transform

Z transform is a useful mathematical tool for converting differential equations to algebraic equations. *Z* transform is utilized when converting a discrete-time domain signal to a discrete frequency domain signal. It has a broad range of statistical and digital signal processing applications. It is mostly used to process and evaluate digital data.

The bilateral z-transform of a discrete-time signal $x(n)$ is given as:

$$Z.T[x(n)] = X(Z) = \sum_{n=-\infty}^{\infty} x(n)z^{-n} \tag{8}$$

The unilateral z-transform of a discrete-time signal $x(n)$ is represented by the following equation:

$$Z.T[x(n)] = X(Z) = \sum_{n=0}^{\infty} x(n)z^{-n} \tag{9}$$

Fourier transform and Z transform equations have an operation in an embedded system. If we substitute z with e^{jw} then the z-transform becomes the Fourier transform. On the other hand, when $|z| = 1$, the Fourier transform is simply $X(z)$ with $z = e^{jw}$ and the z-transform correlates to the Fourier transform. If we express z in polar form, we get $z = re^{jw}$.

A system's Fourier transform and z-transform can be written as:

$$H(\omega) = \sum_{k=0}^{M} b_k e^{-j\omega k} \tag{10}$$

$$H(z) = \sum_{k=0}^{M} b_k z^{-k} \tag{11}$$

$$H(\omega) = H\left(e^{j\omega}\right) = H(z)\big|_{z=e^{j\omega}} \tag{12}$$

2.1.5 Pole-zero plot

The pole-zero plot is a valuable tool for relating a system's Frequency domain and Z-domain representations. A pole-zero plot is a graphical depiction of a rational transfer function in the complex plane that aids in the communication of system attributes.

Pole-zero plot can be expressed as the following equation:

$$H(z) = \frac{B(z)}{A(z)} = \frac{\sum_{k=0}^{M} b_k z^{-k}}{1 + \sum_{k=0}^{N} a_k z^{-k}} \tag{13}$$

where the numerator and denominator are both polynomials in z. The zeros of $H(z)$ are the values of z for which $H(z) = 0$, while the poles of $H(z)$ are the values of z for which $H(z)$ is ∞. M and N are the order of the numerator and denominator polynomial, respectively. On the other hand, b_k is the mth coefficient of the numerator polynomial whereas a_k is the nth coefficient of the denominator polynomial.

2.2 ECG signal

The electrocardiogram (ECG) signal is a representation of the electrical impulses of the heart that can be seen from the strategic points of the human body. It can be visually depicted by a quasi-periodic voltage signal. ECG refers to a 12-lead ECG recorded while laying down and electrodes or sticky patches are put on the body surface and often over the chest and limbs to record a standard surface ECG. These electrode wires are linked to a 12-lead ECG machine which records data from 12 distinct locations on the body's surface. The aggregate amplitude of the heart's electrical potential is then monitored and recorded over a period of time from those distinct angles ("leads").

The graphical representation of the heart's electrical activity is formed by analyzing numerous electrodes in **Figure 1(a)**. There are three types of leads: limb augmented limb, and precordial or chest. Three limb leads and three augmented

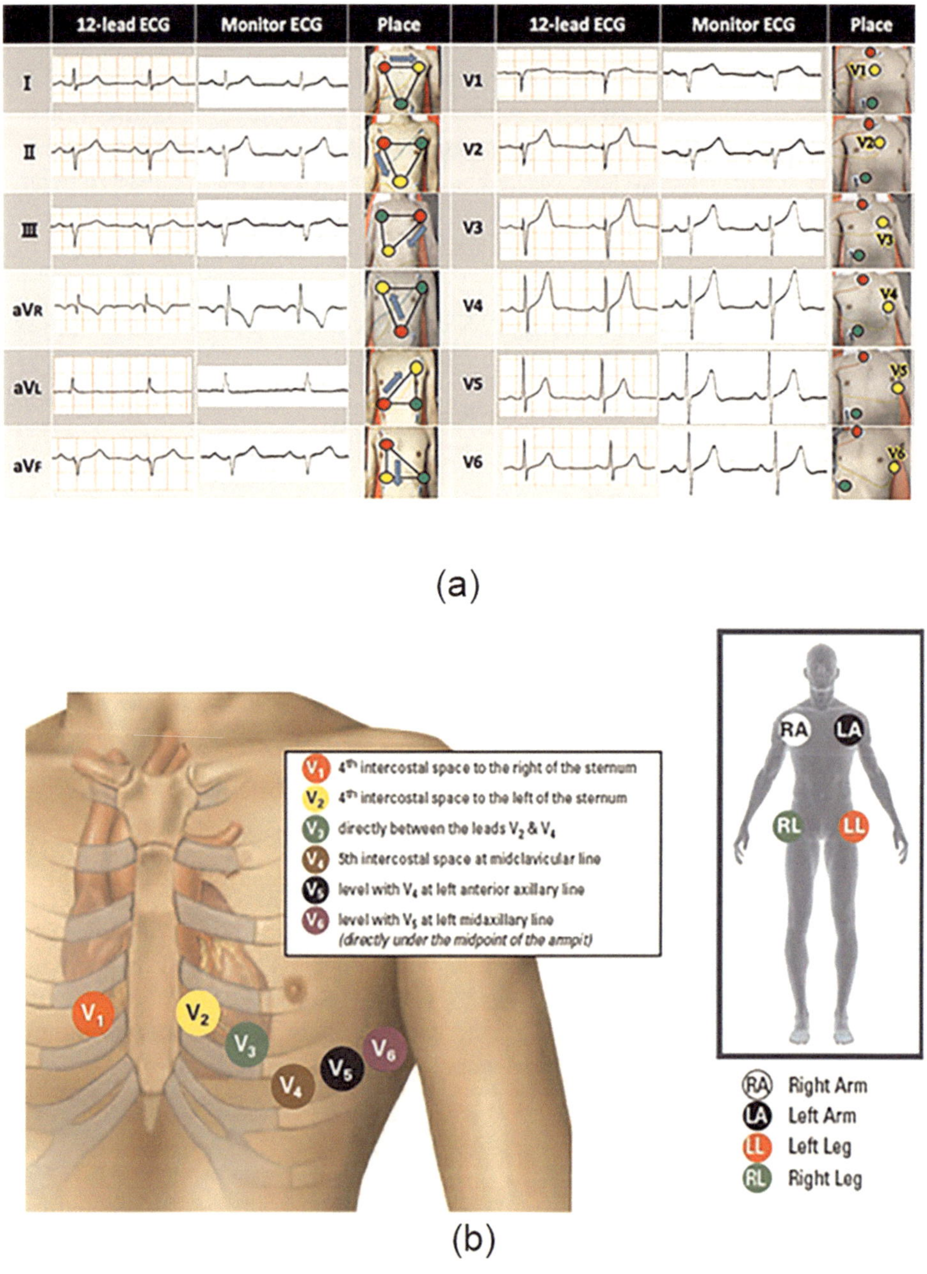

Figure 1.
12 leads ECG. a) Signals from 12 Leads ECG [20]. b) Position of placements of the 12 leads on human body [21].

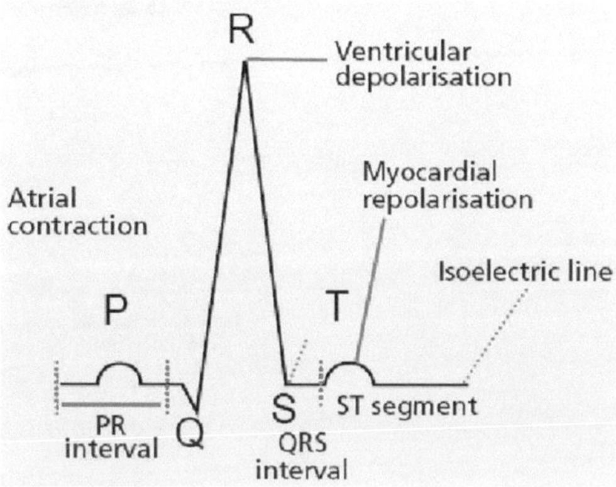

Figure 2.
PQRST waveform [22].

limb leads are organized in the coronal plane like the spokes of a wheel, and six precordial leads or chest leads are organized in the perpendicular transverse plane. In three-dimensional space, each of the 12 ECG leads represents a distinct direction of cardiac activation. The conventional ECG leads are denoted as lead I, II, III, aVF, aVR, aVL, V1, V2, V3, V4, V5, and V6. The limb leads are I, II, III, aVR, aVL, and aVF whereas the precordial leads are V1, V2, V3, V4, V5, and V6.

The 12-lead ECG is typically made up of 10 electrodes linked to the body, each monitoring a distinct electrical potential difference. The 10 electrodes in a 12-lead ECG are RA, RL, LA, LL, V1, V2, V3, V4, V5, and V6. Each of the 10 electrodes has a different placement as shown in **Figure 1(b)**. RA is used to place on the right arm and similarly, LA is used to place on the left arm. RL is located in the lower end of the inner portion of the calf muscle on the right leg, similarly, LL is placed in the same standard position but on the left leg. V1 is placed in the fourth intercostal space (between ribs 4 and 5) immediate right of the sternum. V2 is placed in the fourth intercostal space (between ribs 4 and 5) immediate left of the sternum. V3 is placed between leads V2 and V4 where V4 is placed in the fifth intercostal space (between ribs 5 and 6) in the midclavicular line. On the other hand, V5 and V6 are placed in the left anterior axillary line and midaxillary line, respectively. The electrodes which are located on the limbs are called limb leads which are leads I, II, and III. Lead I refer to the voltage difference between LA and RA, that is, Lead I = LA-RA. Similarly, Lead II denotes the voltage difference between LL and RA, that is, Lead II = LL-RA. And Lead III denotes the voltage between LL and LA, that is, Lead III = LL-LA.

Lastly, a PQRST complex is part of an ECG complex which is shown in **Figure 2**. The P wave is produced by the sinoatrial node which is the heart's pacemaker and implies atrial depolarization in an ECG complex. The atrioventricular node generates the QRS wave. Ventricular depolarization is represented by the QRS, while ventricular repolarization is indicated by the T wave.

2.3 Deep learning

2.3.1 Artificial neural network

In biology, neural networks develop the structure of animal brains, where the phrase "artificial neural networks" comes from. It is widely used in deep learning

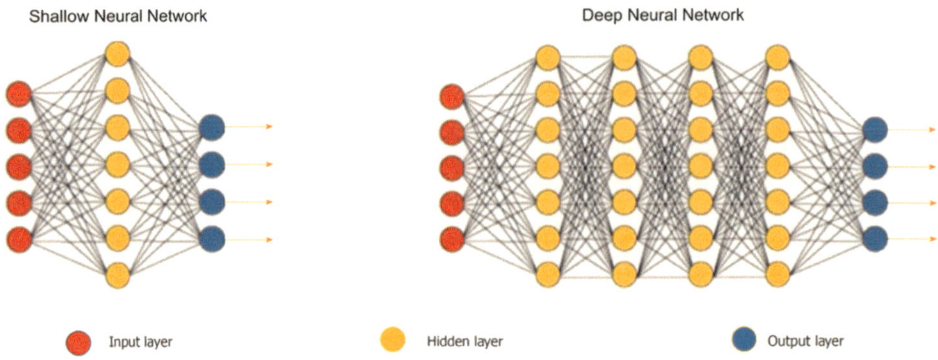

Figure 3.
Architecture of a general ANN [24].

algorithms. An artificial neural network (ANN) [23] generally consists of three layers, namely, the input layer, hidden layer, and output layer. The hidden layers are present in-between input and output layers. It executes all the calculations to find hidden features and patterns. A shallow neural network consists of only one hidden layer and a deep neural network consists of multiple hidden layers. Generally, each node in one layer is linked to every other node in the next layer. By increasing the number of hidden layers, the network becomes deeper. This architecture is demonstrated in **Figure 3**.

2.3.2 Convolutional neural network

Based on the concept of ANNs, a convolutional neural network (CNN) [25] was formulated which is a deep learning method that can take an image as input and learn some filters that can be used to extract essential features from those images. The brain is the source of inspiration for convolutional neural networks. CNN performs a linear mathematical procedure known as a convolution in the several hidden layers between an input and output layer. The general mathematical expression of convolution operation is provided in the following equation:

$$Y = W * X + b \tag{14}$$

where W and X represent the filter and the input, respectively whereas b represents the bias matrix and the * represents the convolution operation between the matrices W and X.

CNN's have the benefit of being able to construct an internal demonstration of a two-dimensional image. This enables the model to learn position and scale in different data formats, which is essential when working with images.

2.3.3 Recurrent neural network

A recurrent neural network (RNN) [26] is a form of artificial neural network which is designed to operate with time series, analyzing temporal and sequential data. It's one of the algorithms responsible for the incredible advances in deep learning over the last few years. RNN can handle inputs/outputs of varying lengths. The idea of "memory" in RNNs is used to store the states or information of earlier inputs in order to generate the sequence's next output. It has the ability to store or memorize historical information.

Long short term memory (LSTM) [27] is a type of recurrent neural network and LSTM networks are well-suited to categorize, processing, and generating predictions based on time series data as there might be delays of undetermined duration between critical occurrences in a time series. LSTMs were designed to explode gradients and solve the problem of vanishing gradients that can occur while training standard RNNs.

LSTM uses the concept of gates. It has three gates which are input gate, forget gate, and output gate. The input gate determines what new information will be stored in the cell state. The forget gate determines what information to throw away from the cell state whereas the output gate is used to activate the LSTM block's final output. In LSTM, output of the gates are operated with sigmoid activation functions, which calculates a value between 0 and 1, which is usually rounded to either 0 or 1 depending upon a predetermined threshold. "0" indicates that the gates are blocking everything and "1" denotes gates that enable everything to pass through it. The LSTM gates have the following equations:

$$\begin{aligned} i_t &= \sigma(w_i[h_{t-1}, x_t] + b_i) \\ f_t &= \sigma(w_f[h_{t-1}, x_t] + b_f) \\ o_t &= \sigma(w_o[h_{t-1}, x_t] + b_o) \end{aligned} \tag{15}$$

where, i_t, f_t, o_t represents input, forget, and output gates, respectively whereas w_x, b_x and x_t represents weights and biases of gate x and input at the current timestamp, respectively. On the other hand, σ is the sigmoid function. Lastly, h_{t-1} indicates the output of the LSTM block at $t-1^{th}$ timestamp.

The cell state, candidate cell state, and final output equations are given as follows:

$$\begin{aligned} \bar{c} &= tanh\ (w_c[h_{t-1}, x_t] + b_c) \\ c_t &= f_t * c_{t-1} + i_t * \bar{c}_t \\ h_t &= o_t * tanh\ (c^t) \end{aligned} \tag{16}$$

where, c_t and $\bar{c}_t$ represents cell state and candidate for cell state at timestamp(t) where the rest of the notations follows from the previous equations.

The architecture of LSTM at any timestamp t is shown in **Figure 4**.

Bidirectional LSTMs [29] are a kind of LSTM that can be used to increase model performance on sequence classification issues. Bidirectional long-short term memory is the process of allowing any neural network to store sequence information in both backward (future to past) and forward (forward to future) directions. BI-LSTM is typically used when sequence to sequence activities are required. Text classification, speech recognition, and forecasting models can all benefit from using this type of network. **Figure 5** shows the architecture of a BI-LSTM.

3. Problem statement

Before the invention of CAD, diagnosis used to be done manually and manual diagnostic procedures were time-consuming, less accurate. In the manual diagnostic

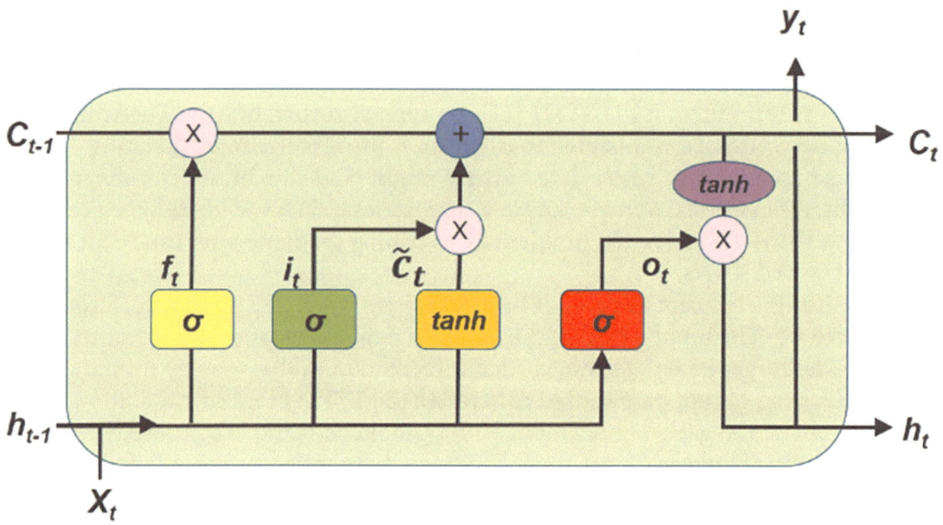

Figure 4.
Graphical representation of LSTM unit [28].

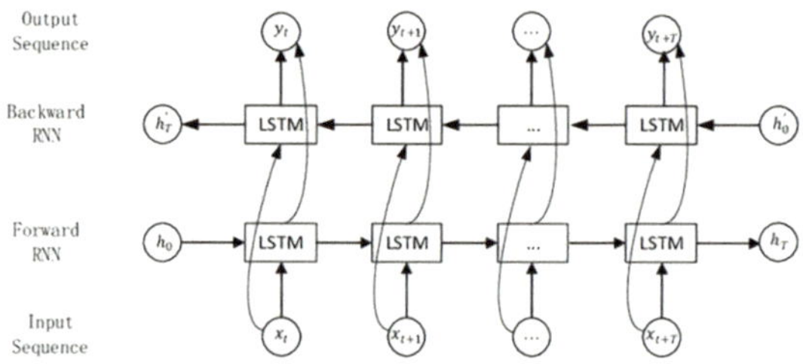

Figure 5.
Graphical representation of bi-directional LSTM unit [30].

procedures, there might be errors in the calculation of computational and statistical features. To counteract the faults in manual diagnostic procedures, deep learning has been introduced to diagnosis. CAD application has heightened the diagnostic performance of non-expert radiologists. Regardless of radiologist expertise, the fundamental benefit of CAD is the minimum false-negative rate and enhanced sensitivity. CAD technologies are faster, more dependable, more accurate and also help to improve in the calculation of computational and statistical features [31]. In this regard, this study focuses on speculating about some of the valuable technologies and trying to approach a conventional solution.

4. Effect of noise in ECG signals and importance of data preprocessing

Noise is an undesirable signal which disrupts the original message signal and causes the message signal's parameters to be altered. Noise distorts the message and hinders it from being understood in an intended manner. When there is loud, distracting noise that disrupts the communication assimilation process, comprehension suffers.

There is no signal without noise. The signal strength may be affected or aided by noise. Noise can cause signal distortion, which is most noticeable in agitated receivers. Both analog and digital systems suffer from noise, which diminishes their performance. Noise degrades the quality of the received signal in analog systems. Noise reduces the overall performance of a digital system because it necessitates retransmission of data packets or additional coding to recover data in the event of an error. The most prevalent and evident issue produced by signal noise is the distortion of the processed signal, which causes inaccurate interpretation or display of a process state by the equipment. Unusual signal noise can cause an apparent signal loss. Noise filtering is incorporated into most current electrical devices. However, in excessively loud circumstances, this filter may not be sufficient, resulting in the device getting no signal and no connection.

The presence of noise can make it difficult or impossible to identify a representative ECG signal. Noises in the ECG signal can lead to incorrect interpretation. In the ECG signal, there are primarily two kinds of noise. Electromyogram noise, additive white Gaussian noise, and power line interference are examples of high-frequency noises. Power line interference distorts the amplitude, duration, and shape of low-amplitude local waves of the ECG signal. Baseline wandering is an example of low-frequency noise. Baseline wandering alters the ECG signal's ST-segment and LF components.

Noise can be reduced by keeping the signal wires as short as possible or by keeping the wires away from electrical machinery. By using differential inputs, noise can be reduced from both wires. Noise also can be reduced by filtering the signal or by using an integrating A-D converter to reduce mains frequency interference.

There are various ECG denoising techniques [32] that are being used to reduce the noise from signals. Some ECG denoising techniques are EMD-based models, deep-learning-based models, wavelet-based models, sparsity-based models, Bayesian-filter-based models, hybrid models, discrete wavelet transform, etc.

The discrete wavelet transform is a digital processing computational technique that allows for electrical noise with a higher signal-to-noise ratio than lock-in amplifier equipment. A discrete wavelet transform decomposes a signal into a number of sets, each set including a time series of coefficients that describe the signal's time evolution in the associated frequency band.

The process of converting raw data into a comprehensible format is known as data preprocessing. Dealing with raw data is not suitable, thus this is a key stage in data mining. Before using machine learning or data mining methods, make sure the data is of high quality. In every brain-computer interface-based application, preprocessing data is a necessary and significant step. It checks the accuracy, completeness, believability, consistency, interpretability, timeliness of the data. It assists with the removal of undesirable artifacts from the data and prepares it for subsequent processing.

5. State-of-the-art techniques

Peimankar et al. [33] proposed a deep learning model for real-time segmentation of heartbeats which might be utilized in real-time telehealth diagnostic systems. The proposed technique integrates a CNN and an LSTM model to predict and analyze the onset, peak, and offset of various heartbeat waveforms such as the P-wave, QRS complex, T-wave, and no wave. The proposed model is also known as DENS-ECG model. Using 5-fold cross-validation, this model is trained and evaluated on a dataset of 105 ECGs with a length of 15 min each. It attains an average sensitivity and accuracy of 97.95 and 95.68%, respectively. In addition, the method is calibrated on an unknown dataset to assess how robust it is at detecting QRS with a sensitivity of 99.61% and accuracy of 99.52%. This model illustrates the combined CNN-LSTM model's adaptability and accuracy in delineating ECG signals. The accuracy of the proposed DENS-ECG model in recognizing ECG waveforms leaves the door open for cardiologists to apply this algorithm in-house to evaluate ECG recordings and diagnose cardiac arrhythmias. This model is provided in **Figure 6**.

In **Figure 6**, noise reduction refers to the filtering of the ECG signals to reduce noise and remove baseline wanders. In the segmentation, the ECG signals are divided into 1000-sample chunks and sent into the model as input. Then the segmented ECG signals are split into two sets to separate the testing set from a non-testing set. This model used a 5-fold cross-validation technique to provide a more trustworthy performance in terms of interpretability. The model consists of eight layers, including an input layer, three 1D convolution layers, two BiLSTM layers, and a dropout layer. And the Adam optimization algorithm is used to validate the algorithm, which is radically different from the steepest gradient descent (SGD) optimization technique and achieved higher performance on the validation. The trained model is tested on 26 unseen test records from the QTDB dataset to assess the classifier's performance. Furthermore, the model is evaluated for QRS detection on the unexplored MITDB dataset.

Jambukia et al. [34] represented an overview of ECG classification into arrhythmia categories and stated that classification of electrocardiogram (ECG) signals plays a crucial role in the monitoring heart diseases as early and precise diagnosis of arrhythmia types is essential for monitoring cardiac disorders and selecting the best treatment option for a patient. The survey outlines the challenges of ECG classification and provides a comprehensive overview of preprocessing approaches, ECG databases, feature extraction techniques, ANN-based classifiers, and performance measures for

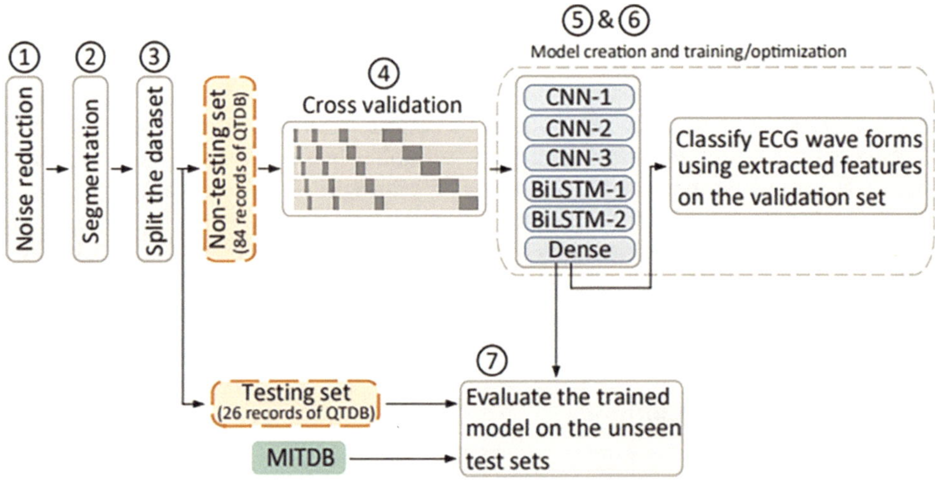

Figure 6.
Flowchart of the proposed DENS-ECG model [33].

evaluating the classifiers' accuracy. According to the survey, many researchers have worked on ECG signal classification. They have used different pre-processing techniques, various feature extraction techniques, and classifiers. For ECG categorization, the majority of the researchers used the MIT-BIH arrhythmia database. A. Dallali et al. used DWT to extract the RR interval and then used Z score to normalize it. They classified ECG beats using FCM. They achieved a 99.05% accuracy rate. RR interval and R point position are two characteristics retrieved using DWT. FCM was used for pre-classification, while 3-layer MLPNN was used for final classification. They were able to reach a 99.99% accuracy rate.

Saadatnejad et al. [35] proposed an ECG classification model, which was suggested for continuous cardiac detection on wearable devices with limited processing resources. This model is demonstrated in **Figure 7** in detail. The model works in such a way that the incoming computerized ECG data were first split into heartbeats and their RR interval while wavelet characteristics were extracted. The ECG signal as well as the extracted characteristics were then put into two RNN-based models that categorized every heartbeat. After that, the two outputs were combined to create the final categorization for every pulse. The suggested method fits the temporal criteria for continuous and real-time execution on wearable devices. Unlike many compute-intensive deep-learning-based techniques, the proposed methodology is accurate and lightweight, allowing wearable devices to have continuous monitoring with accurate LSTM-based ECG categorization having negligible computing expenses while running indefinitely on wearable devices with modest processing capability.

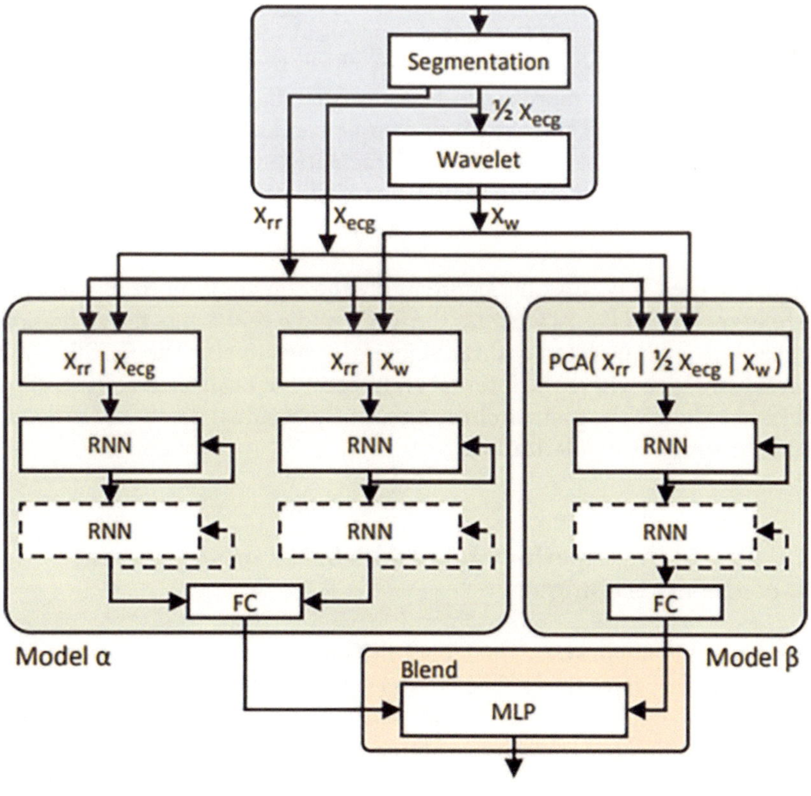

Figure 7.
The proposed algorithm of LSTM-based ECG classification model [35].

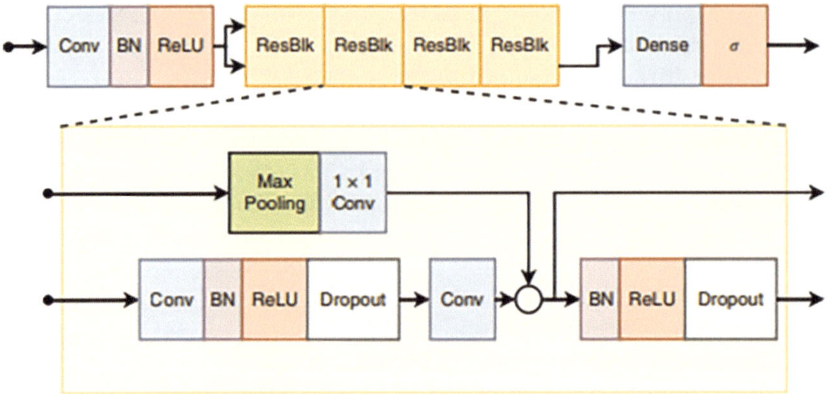

Figure 8.
The DNN architecture used for ECG classification [36].

Ribeiro et al. [36] had proposed an end-to-end DNN competent of accurately identifying six ECG abnormalities in S12L-ECG examinations, with diagnostic performance comparable to that of medical residents and students. This DNN model trained on data from the Clinical Outcomes in Digital Electrocardiology research which included over 2 million labeled tests analyzed by the Telehealth Network of Minas Gerais. The DNN surpassed cardiology resident medical practitioners in detecting six different types of abnormalities in 12-lead ECG recordings with F1 scores over 80% and specificity exceeding 95%. These results suggest that DNN-based ECG analysis, which was previously tested in a single-lead scenario, generalizes well to 12-lead examinations, bringing the technology closer to practical use. This model has the potential to lead to more accurate automated diagnosis and better clinical practice. Even professional assessment of complex and borderline cases appears to be essential in this future scenario, the implementation of such automatic interpretation by a DNN algorithm may increase the population's access to this fundamental and valuable diagnostic test. **Figure 8** shows the deep learning model used in this work.

In **Figure 8**, the Conv, BN, and dense imply the convolution, batch normalization, and the fully connected layers whereas the ReLU and σ represents the activation layers namely the rectified linear unit and the sigmoid, respectively. The ResBlk is nothing but the residual block where the internal architecture of each such block is shown in a detailed fashion below the main architecture. In the residual block, the dropout layer represents the dropout regularization.

6. Discussion on the experimental results based on the current state-of-the-art techniques

Figure 9a and **b** demonstrate the DENS-ECG model's confusion matrices for the 5-fold CV and test set, respectively. The no wave class has the majority of incorrect cases in all three classes which are P-wave, QRS, and T-wave or it can be said that the model does not make significant errors in classifying the three major classes (P-wave, QRS, and T-wave). The minimal discrepancy between the 5-fold CV and test outcomes indicates that the model has been effectively trained and does not have an overfitting problem.

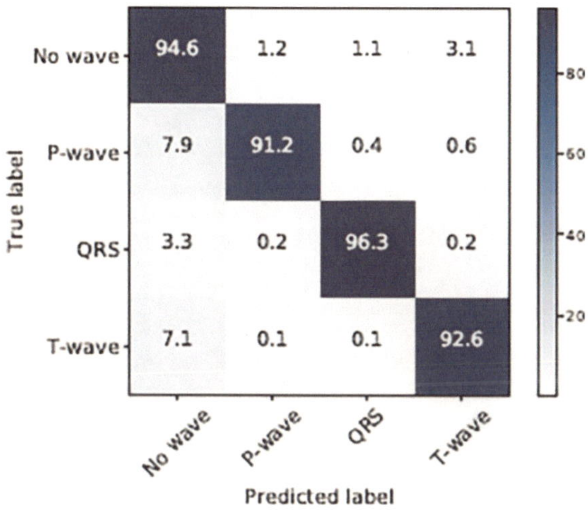

(a)

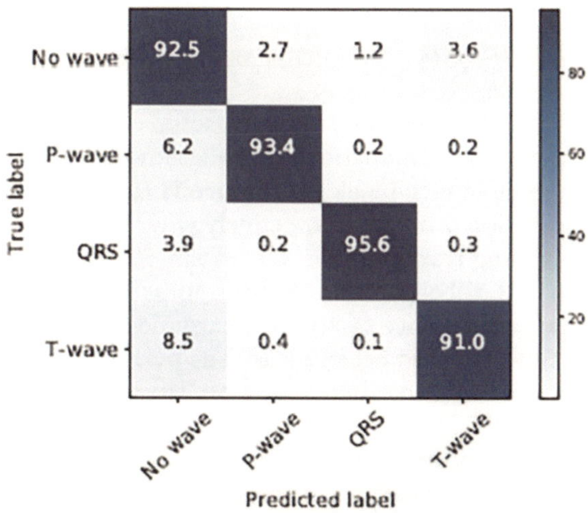

(b)

Figure 9.
Confusion matrix [33]. (a) 5-fold Cross Validation. (b) Test set.

As demonstrated in **Figure 10** the performance plot, the DENS-ECG model performs similarly to other models in QRS detection with 99.61% of sensitivity and 99.52% of precision. The wavelet-based model proposed by Martinez et al. has the best performance in terms of sensitivity and accuracy of 99.8 and 99.86%, respectively followed by Kim and Shin's proposed model. The postulated DENS-ECG model performed similarly to the well-known Pan and Tompkins's QRS detection model but it outperformed the QRS detection methods proposed by Poll et al.

In [35], the classification ECG signals from heartbeat were classified into both 7 and 5 arrhythmia classes, respectively. For 5-classification problems, the heartbeats are divided into five categories by the Association for Advancement of Medical Instrumentation (AAMI). normal (N), supraventricular (S) ectopic, ventricular (V) ectopic, fusion (F), and unknown (Q) beats are the four types of an ectopic heartbeat.

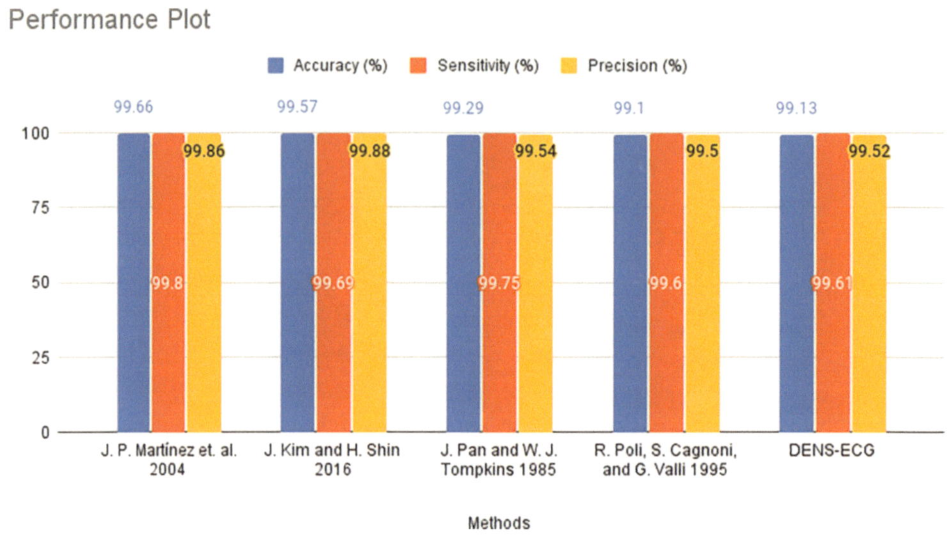

Figure 10.
Comparison of DENS-ECG and various deep model architectures' classification performance on the test set [33].

Further, the class N is divided into three more classes in the 7-classification to improve resolution by isolating the two conduction anomalies known as left bundle branch block (L) and right bundle branch block (R). **Figure 11** represent the confusion matrix of 7 and 5-class classification problem, respectively where the former model is capable of effectively distinguishing L and R from N.

As shown in **Figure 12**, Ribeiro et al. [36] has compared DNN's performance indexes to the average performance of 4th-year cardiology residents, 3rd-year emergency residents, and 5th-year medical students. The performance of the DNN on the test set is demonstrated in the above accuracy plot. The above-shown figure shows that the performance of DNN which exceeds human performance. In most cases, the accuracy of DNN on the data set is more than 95%.

Finally, the work of Jambukia et al. [34] presents a survey on the performance of various works present in the literature which are based on ECG signal categorization utilizing different pre-processing approaches, feature extraction techniques, and classifiers. **Figure 13** presents the plot of the accuracy of different ECG classification techniques which have used the MIT-BIH arrhythmia database over time.

7. Conclusions

Health issues in the human race are increasing day by day and cardiac issues are one of the most common diseases which has been noticed in the past few decades. Therefore, many technologies have been introduced and CAD is the most emerging technology to diagnose cardiac issues or solve heart-related diseases. Furthermore, deep learning has played an important role in the area of computer-aided diagnosis (CAD). From the above discussion, it can be observed that various algorithms or methods have performed pretty well in the field of cardiovascular disease detection. This indicates that deep learning in cardiac signal processing has an unbounded scope in the research field for enhancing CAD and getting more accurate and cost-effective and fast output.

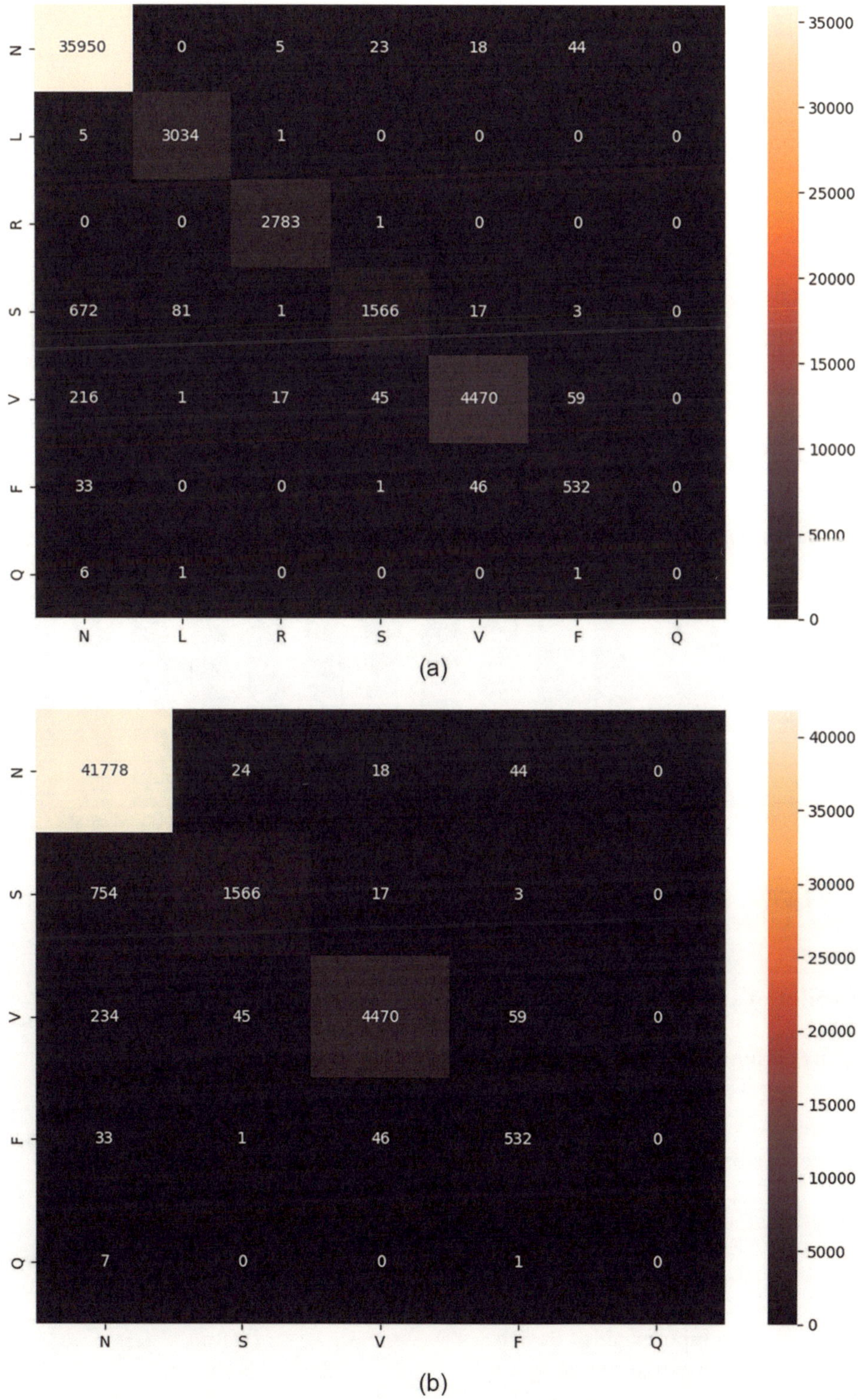

Figure 11.
Confusion matrix [35]. (a) 7 heartbeat classes. (b) 5 heartbeat classes.

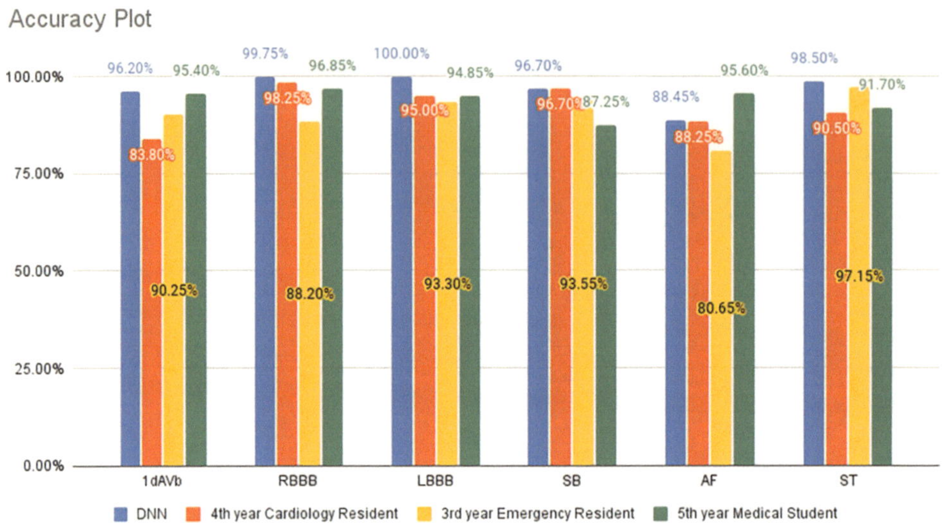

Figure 12.
Comparison of performance indexes of DNN and the average performance of cardiology students on the test set [36].

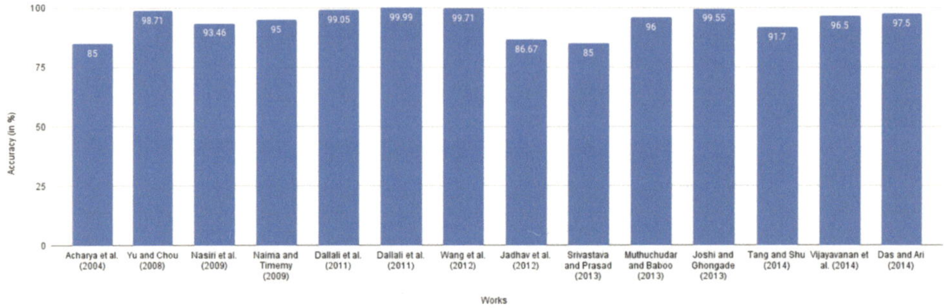

Figure 13.
Comparison of the accuracy of the different ECG classification techniques [34].

Conflict of interest

The authors declare no conflict of interest or delete this entire section.

Abbreviations

ECG	electrocardiogram
CVD	cardiovascular disease
AI	artificial intelligence
ICD	International Classification of Diseases
CAD	computer-aided design
CT	computed tomography
CHF	congestive heart failure
ANN	artificial neural network
CNN	convolutional neural network

RNN	recurrent neural network
LSTM	long short-term memory
BI-LSTM	bi-directional long short-term memory
DNN	deep neural networks

Author details

Sumagna Dey[1*†], Rohan Pal[2†] and Saptarshi Biswas[3†]

1 Meghnad Saha Institute of Technology, Kolkata, India

2 Kalyani Government Engineering College, Kalyani, India

3 Iowa State University, Ames, USA

*Address all correspondence to: sumagna.dey@gmail.com

† These authors have contributed equally to this work.

References

[1] Huffman MD, Prabhakaran D, Osmond C, Fall CHD, Tandon N, Lakshmy R, et al. Incidence of cardiovascular risk factors in an Indian urban cohort results from the New Delhi birth cohort. Journal of the American College of Cardiology. 2011;**57**(17):1765-1774. DOI: 10.1016/j.jacc.2010.09.083

[2] By 2030, Deaths Due to Heart Disease Likely to Increase by 2.3cr: Doctor. Available from: https://www.dnaindia.com/jaipur/report-by-2030-deaths-due-to-heart-disease-likely-to-increase-by-23cr-doctor-2667520 [Accessed: 18 December 2021]

[3] Cardiovascular Diseases (CVDs). Available from: https://www.who.int/news-room/fact-sheets/detail/cardiovascular-diseases-(cvds) [Accessed: 15 December 2021]

[4] Olvera Lopez E, Ballard BD, Jan A. Cardiovascular disease. In: StatPearls. Treasure Island, FL: StatPearls Publishing; 2022

[5] Jordaens L. A clinical approach to arrhythmias revisited in 2018: From ECG over noninvasive and invasive electrophysiology to advanced imaging. Netherlands Heart Journal: Monthly Journal of the Netherlands Society of Cardiology and the Netherlands Heart Foundation. 2018;**26**(4):182-189. DOI: 10.1007/s12471-018-1089-1

[6] Maganti K, Rigolin VH, Sarano ME, Bonow RO. Valvular heart disease: Diagnosis and management. Mayo Clinic Proceedings. 2010;**85**(5):483-500. DOI: 10.4065/mcp.2009.0706

[7] Saleh M, Ambrose JA. Understanding myocardial infarction [version 1; peer review: 2 approved]. F1000Research. 2018;**7**:1378. DOI: 10.12688/f1000.research.15096.1

[8] Seetharam K, Brito D, Farjo PD, Sengupta PP. The role of artificial intelligence in cardiovascular imaging: State of the art review. Frontiers in Cardiovascular Medicine. 2020;**7**:618849. DOI: 10.3389/fcvm.2020.618849

[9] Sherly SI, Mathivanan G. ECG signal noises versus filters for signal quality improvement. In: 2021 International Conference on Advances in Electrical, Computing, Communication and Sustainable Technologies (ICAECT). Piscataway, New Jersey, United States: IEEE; 2021. pp. 1-5. DOI: 10.1109/ICAECT49130.2021.9392621

[10] Bayoumy K, Gaber M, Elshafeey A, Mhaimeed O, Dineen EH, Marvel FA, et al. Smart wearable devices in cardiovascular care: where we are and how to move forward. Nature Reviews Cardiology. 2021;**18**:581-599. DOI: 10.1038/s41569-021-00522-7

[11] Yanase J, Triantaphyllou E. A systematic survey of computer-aided diagnosis in medicine: Past and present developments. Expert Systems with Applications. 2019;**138**:112821. DOI: 10.1016/j.eswa.2019.112821

[12] Karssemeijer N. Computer aided detection in breast imaging: More than perception aid. In: 2010 IEEE International Symposium on Biomedical Imaging: From Nano to Macro. Piscataway, New Jersey, United States: IEEE; 2010. pp. 273-273. DOI: 10.1109/ISBI.2010.5490360

[13] Wang EK, Zhang X, Pan L. Automatic classification of CAD ECG signals with SDAE and bidirectional long short-term network. IEEE Access. 2019;

7:182873-182880. DOI: 10.1109/ACCESS.2019.2936525

[14] Doi K. Computer-aided diagnosis in medical imaging: Historical review, current status and future potential. Computerized Medical Imaging and Graphics: The Official Journal of the Computerized Medical Imaging Society. 2007;**31**(4–5):198-211. DOI: 10.1016/j.compmedimag.2007.02.002

[15] Dey S, Nath P, Biswas S, Nath S, Ganguly A. Malaria detection through digital microscopic imaging using deep greedy network with transfer learning. Journal of Medical Imaging. 2021;**8**(5):054502. DOI: 10.1117/1.JMI.8.5.054502

[16] Saad NM, Abdullah AR, Low YF. Detection of heart blocks in ECG signals by spectrum and time-frequency analysis. In: 2006 4th Student Conference on Research and Development. Piscataway, New Jersey, United States: IEEE; 2006. pp. 61-65. DOI: 10.1109/SCORED.2006.4339309

[17] Signal Processing: A Mathematical Approach, Second Edition. Available from: https://library.oapen.org/bitstream/id/3eb04f39-67d7-4b4d-8569-3185fbefd944/1005624.pdf [Accessed: 20 December 2021]

[18] Discrete-Time/Frequency Analysis. Available from: https://ccrma.stanford.edu/courses/150-2001/time_frequency.html [Accessed: 31 December 2021]

[19] Sampling Theorem. Available from: https://www.sciencedirect.com/topics/engineering/sampling-theorem [Accessed: 28 December 2021]

[20] Yoneyama K, Naka M, Harada T, Akashi Y. Creating 12-lead electrocardiogram waveforms using a three-lead bedside monitor to ensure appropriate monitoring. Journal of Arrhythmia. 2020;**36**(6):1107. DOI: 10.1002/joa3.12441

[21] Demystifying the 12 Lead ECG! Available from: https://nurseyourownway.com/2016/04/20/demystifying-the-12-lead-ecg/ [Accessed: 28 December 2021]

[22] Al-Qazzaz NK. Comparison of the RLS and LMS algorithms to remove power line interference noise from ECG signal. Al-Khwarizmi Engineering Journal. 2021;**6**(2):51-61

[23] Ozyilmaz L, Yildirim T. Artificial neural networks for diagnosis of hepatitis disease. Proceedings of the International Joint Conference on Neural Networks. 2003;**1**:586-589. DOI: 10.1109/IJCNN.2003.1223422

[24] Mao WB, Lyu JY, Vaishnani DK, Lyu YM, Gong W, Xue XL, et al. Application of artificial neural networks in detection and diagnosis of gastrointestinal and liver tumors. World Journal of Clinical Cases (WJCC). 2020;**8**(18):3971-3977. DOI: 10.12998/wjcc.v8.i18.3971

[25] Krizhevsky A, Sutskever I, Hinton GE. ImageNet classification with deep convolutional neural networks. Communications of the ACM. 2017;**60**(6):84-90. DOI: 10.1145/3065386

[26] Takase H, Gouhara K, Uchikawa Y. Time sequential pattern transformation and attractors of recurrent neural networks. In: Proceedings of 1993 International Conference on Neural Networks (IJCNN-93-Nagoya, Japan). Vol. 3. Piscataway, New Jersey, United States: IEEE; 1993. pp. 2319-2322. DOI: 10.1109/IJCNN.1993.714189

[27] Sunny MAI, Maswood MMS, Alharbi AG. Deep learning-based stock price prediction using LSTM and bi-

directional LSTM model. In: 2020 2nd Novel Intelligent and Leading Emerging Sciences Conference (NILES). Piscataway, New Jersey, United States: IEEE; 2020. pp. 87-92. DOI: 10.1109/NILES50944.2020.9257950

[28] LSTM and Its Equations. Available from: https://medium.com/@divyanshu132/lstm-and-its-equations-5ee9246d04af [Accessed: 2 January 2022]

[29] Yu X, He J, Zhang Z. Facial image completion using bi-directional pixel LSTM. IEEE Access. 2020;**8**: 48642-48651. DOI: 10.1109/ACCESS.2020.2975827

[30] Xiang J, Qiu Z, Hao Q, Cao H. Multi-time scale wind speed prediction based on WT-bi-LSTM. MATEC Web Conference. 2020;**309**:05011. DOI: 10.1051/matecconf/202030905011

[31] Dey S, Biswas S, Nandi S, Nath S, Das I. Deep greedy network: A tool for medical diagnosis on exiguous dataset of COVID-19. In: 2020 IEEE 1st International Conference for Convergence in Engineering (ICCE). Piscataway, New Jersey, United States: IEEE; 2020. pp. 340-344. DOI: 10.1109/ICCE50343.2020.9290715

[32] Subashini A, Raghuraman G, Sai Ramesh L. Enhancing the classification accuracy of cardiac diseases using image denoising technique from ECG signal. In: 2019 International Conference on Computational Intelligence in Data Science (ICCIDS). Piscataway, New Jersey, United States: IEEE; 2019. pp. 1-4. DOI: 10.1109/ICCIDS.2019.8862168

[33] Peimankar A, Puthusserypady S. DENS-ECG: A deep learning approach for ECG signal delineation. Expert Systems with Applications. 2020;**165**: 113911

[34] Jambukia SH, Dabhi VK, Prajapati HB. Classification of ECG signals using machine learning techniques: A survey. In: 2015 International Conference on Advances in Computer Engineering and Applications. Piscataway, New Jersey, United States: IEEE; 2015. pp. 714-721. DOI: 10.1109/ICACEA.2015.7164783

[35] Saadatnejad S, Oveisi M, Hashemi M. LSTM-based ECG classification for continuous monitoring on personal wearable devices. IEEE Journal of Biomedical and Health Informatics. 2020;**24**(2):515-523. DOI: 10.1109/JBHI.2019.2911367

[36] Ribeiro AH, Ribeiro MH, Paixão GMM, Oliveira DM, Gomes PR, Canazart JA, et al. Automatic diagnosis of the 12-lead ECG using a deep neural network. Nature Communications. 2020; **11**(1):1760. DOI: 10.1038/s41467-020-15432-4

Chapter 7

EEG Authentication System Using Fuzzy Vault Scheme

Fatima M. Baqer and Salah Albermany

Abstract

Authentication is the process of recognizing a user's identity by determining claimed user identity by checking user-provided evidence, combining cryptographic with biometric can solve many of security issues, including authentication. Our goal is to try to combine cryptography and biometrics to achieve authentication using fuzzy vault scheme. Electroencephalography (EEG) signals will be used as they are unique and also difficult to expose and copy; also they are difficult to be hack, using nine healthy persons' EEGs from the BCI Competition and extracting power features from signals spectrum of beta and alpha band of EEG signal, the extracted features are from three channels (C3, Cz, and C4), then support vector Machine (SVM) is used for classification. In this chapter, two tasks (left hand and right hand) are used from a four tasks in the dataset, and the system achieves 96.98% validation accuracy, using 10-fold cross-validation on the training set and the model is saved, after extract features, these features will used to be evaluated on a polynomial generated from the secret key using reed Solomon code and chaff points generated using tent map are added to hide the data, which create the final result that is the vault, for decoding the system using Lagrange interpolation for polynomial reconstruction and returning the key.

Keywords: fuzzy vault, EEG, brain wave, cognitive biometric, authentication, electroencephalogram

1. Introduction

User authentication is an important phase in security systems. Authentication is the determining process of a person is really, who claimed to be. Authentication technology affords the access to the systems after checking/verifying if a user's certification matches the authorized certification in a database, usually provided with an ID of a user, and authentication is achieved when the user provides a certification. Generally, authentications can be according to their use: password-based, token-based, and biometrics-based. Each of has its advantages and disadvantages [1].

Biometrics systems based on human being's measurements analyze statistic aspects of unique physical and behavioral characteristics, which can be consumed to identify or verify a human [2].

The term biometric is a Greek word, referring to bio means "life" and metric means "measurement." Biometrics is used to achieve reliable authentication and identification that can be expressed as face fingerprints, iris, retina, signatures, gait, voice, etc. Recently, a new biometric field has gained its popularity because of its less drawbacks over other biometrics; it is the brain wave biometric or electroencephalography (EEG) [3].

However, without the drawbacks of both passwords-based and biometric-based, the EEG-based biometric authentication system combines their advantages [1]. EEG signals are dynamic, sensitive, and inexpensive and used to observe mental state that can be used to distinguish persons.

These signals can be bound with a cryptography to empower the security, a scheme that can be used with brain wave signals is called fuzzy vault scheme, key-based cryptographic scheme uses error correction codes to generate polynomials to secure the key.

1.1 Biometric concept

Biometric structure helps to find out the person with the physical-behavioral mechanism using statistics from person. [4], there are two types of biometrics: conventional and cognitive, conventional refers to physical and behavioral characteristics, such as fingerprint, voice, oder, DNA, face, iris, retina. Etc., cognitive refers to mental state signals as electroencephalography (EEG), these biometrics are unique for every individual. Physical biometrics is distinguished by "what the individual is" while behavioral is distinguished by "how individual do," cognitive is "what individual think" [5]. **Figure 1** illustrates biometric types.

1.1.1 Electroencephalogram (EEG)

Electroencephalogram, EEG for short, is the human brain's electrical activity. Nerve system of human, including the brain, consists of neurons, which are nerve cells. The electrical current transmitted signals by neurons to other neurons [6]. The changes in voltage resulting from the electrical current are then measured by electrodes. Patterns form waves used by EEG and are sinusoidal. Based on the frequency bandwidth can be classified into several bands. Each band of waves corresponds to different activities. Most common bands classification [6]: Delta (0.5–4) HZ, Theta (5–7) HZ, Alpha (8–15) HZ, Beta (16–31) HZ, Gamma(32-higher) HZ, the correspondence for each band, **Table 1** describes each band and its activity.

It is the measurement of electrical activity of the brain, sensor used to obtain these signals. Brain consists of millions of neurons, and these neurons express emotions and thoughts as signals [7].

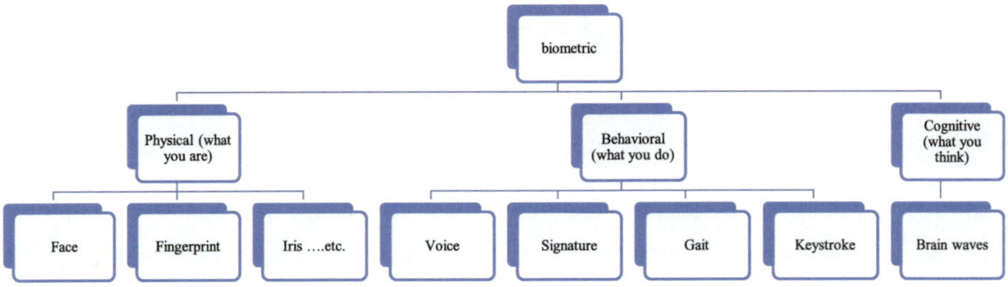

Figure 1.
Biometric types.

Band name	Range in HZ	Activity
Gamma	32–higher	Consciousness, higher processing tasks
Beta	16–31	Awake, active thinking, concentration and arousal states, eyes opened
Alpha	8–15	Relaxation, eyes closed
Theta	5–7	Drowsy, meditating and sleeping
Delta	0.5–4	Deep sleeping

Table 1.
EEG bands description.

"EEG measures the currents that flow during synaptic excitations of the dendrites of many pyramidal neurons in the cerebral cortex. Differences of electrical potentials are caused by summed postsynaptic graded potentials from pyramidal cells that create electrical dipoles between soma (body of neuron) and apical dendrites (neural branches) [5]."

The potentials are measured between two or more points called electrodes or sensors, which are placed on the scalp at different locations. EEG resembles waves, which is why the term brain waves is used when referring EEG signals. Padfield et al. [8], these EEG signals are unique for every individual and less exposed because it is under the scalp, which is hard to obtain and cannot be copied or manipulated [2].

Universality, uniqueness, permanency, performance, collectability, acceptability, and robustness satisfy the requirements of EEG-based biometric authentication method [7].

1.1.2 Motor imagery (MI)

MI is imagining a motor action without any efferent information to neuromuscular system. Thoughts and actions are intimately linked. A confirmation of this prediction is found in the spatial patterning of activated cortical areas seen with functional brain imaging techniques such as PET and fMRI [9]. MI is widespread in BCI systems because it has naturally occurred discriminative properties and also because signal acquisition is not expensive [8]. It is widely used in sport training as mental practice of action, neurological rehabilitation, and has also been employed as a research paradigm in cognitive neuroscience and cognitive psychology to investigate the content and the structure of covert processes (i.e., unconscious) that precede the execution of action. The effectiveness of motor imagery has been demonstrated in musicians. There have also been conducted multiple studies on its uses in neurological rehabilitation in patients after stroke [10].

1.2 Literature survey

1.2.1 EEG person authentication

Marcel and Millan [11] investigate the use of brain activity for person authentication, using a statistical framework based on Gaussian Mixture Models and Maximum a posteriori model adaptation. Intensive experimental simulations are performed using strict train/test protocols to show the potential of method [11].

Fladby [12] performs an experiment with 12 participants for eight different tasks in three sessions. They extract features from time and frequency domain by analyzing EEG and then the proposed algorithm is applied as dynamic time warping as well as a feature-based distance metric [12].

He [7] proposes an EEG feature hashing approach for person authentication, by extracting the coefficients of the autoregression model from multiple EEG channels, Fast Johnson-Lindenstrauss transform that is based dimension reduction algorithm to hash vectors. For person authentication, a Naive Bayes probabilistic model is applied [7].

Nguyen et al. [13] investigated the person verification based on brain wave features extracted from EEG signals of motor imagery tasks. For each subject, left, right, and best motor imagery tasks were used. As for modeling, the Gaussian mixture model (GMM) and support vector data description (SVDD) methods were used [13].

Nieves and Manian [14] proposed a system use an effective time-frequency-based feature extraction method using the short-time Fourier transform (STFT) or spectrogram. Computed features on the spectrogram were energy, variance, and skewness. These features were used to train a SVM and neural network classifier. Using cross-validation for testing data for person authentication the classifiers are tested. Results using a different number of channels with optimum features presented [14].

Soni et al. [2] "design a system and implement it, so that users set patterns as an unlock pattern to obtain the access's permission. This pattern can be any combination of eye blink, attention and various brain rhythms like Alpha, Beta, Theta and Delta. Provided two-level authentication. First level of which is brain waves. Once the correct pattern of brain signal is provided the system will ask for a pass key as a second level of authentication [2]."

Sjamsudin [15] "investigates the aspects of performance and time-invariance of EEG-based authentication. Two sets of experiments are done to record EEG of different individuals. The system implemented the use of machine learning such as SVM and deep neural network to classify EEG of subjects [16]."

1.2.2 Fuzzy vault

Juels and Sudan [16] propose a novel cryptographic construction scheme defined as a fuzzy vault. Alice is a player lock a secret value in a fuzzy vault and "lock" it, using a set of element A. using set B of the same length Bob will try to "unlock" the vault, he gets the secret only, if A and B overlap substantially [16].

Uludag et al. [17] explore the combination of fuzzy vault with the fingerprint minutiae data, which try to secure the important data using the fingerprint data, such that only the authorized user can access the secret by providing the valid fingerprint [17].

Nandakumar and Jain [18] use the fuzzy vault to secure a multi-biometric template derived from a person's templates. Exhibiting that a multi-biometric vault provides better recognition performance and higher security compared with a uni-biometric vault [18].

Khalil-Hani et al. [19] "propose a new chaff generation algorithm which is computationally fast and viable for hardware acceleration by employing simple arithmetic operations" [19].

You et al. [20] proposed cancelable fuzzy vault algorithm based on the user's transformed fingerprint features, which are used to generate a fuzzy vault [20].

1.2.3 Combining cryptography with EEG signals

Damaševilius et al. [21] "combine an EEG based biometric with the fuzzy commitment scheme and BCH error correcting for person. Evaluating features that are covariance matrix of EEG data using EEG recorded from 42 subjects. The experimental results present that the system can generate up to 400 bits of cryptographic key from the EEG codes, while tolerating up to 87 bits of error [21]."

2. The proposed system

2.1 Problem statement

With the rapid development of technology, large institutions and government institutions, which have sensitive information and also applications, need systems with high security and reliable authentication way that is hard to/or possible to copy or manipulate brain wave biometric has these proprieties, in authentication it is very important that people accept the system (acceptability). With this in mind it is safe to say that a noninvasive method of capturing brain wave signals is the best way for biometric acquisition as for securing these biometrics.

2.2 EEG dataset

In this chapter, the winning BCI competition Graz IV2a Dataset (2008) by burner is used [22], which is consists of nine subjects each performing four MI tasks randomly (this process called trial), each task is a class (left hand, right hand, foot, and tongue) corresponding to (1,2,3,4) respectively, the experiment is done by experts, with no feedback. For our system we use only left and right classes [22].

Each subject sat on comfortable armed chair in front of a computer screen at time ($t = 0$) a fixation cross appeared on the screen and a beep tone to alarm the subject, at ($t = 2$) a cue appear for 1.25 s in form of arrow that refers to one of classes (left, right, down, up) to inform the subject of the beginning of MI tasks this last until $t = 6$ the cue disappears and a break is followed [22].

The dataset is divided into two sessions each in separate day, one for training and other for evaluation, each subject performs 48 trial (each class 12 trial) for 6 runs, yielding in total 288 trial [22]. The sampling rate of the signal is 250 Hz, a bandpass filter was applied between 0.5 Hz and 100 Hz. The sensitivity of the amplifier set to 100 μV, to suppress line noise, a 50 HZ notch filter was applied, and artifact trials were marked. The signals were recorded from 25 channels, 22 EEG, 3EOG [22].

2.3 Extraction of EEG trials

Extraction of EEG trials means the process of finding trial of interest of EEG signals by segment the signal according to the event associated with the dataset.

Events gives the time that the MI trail starts and ends to facilitate extraction of the task and the segment number, also the dataset that gives the artifact in each trial to eliminate it if need, in our case we need a clear signal so we eliminate these artifacts for the subjects. The proposed system segments the signals of each channel (C3, C4, Cz), these channels are the most effected by MI tasks. Also, because we use two classes only (left and right hand) the other two classes (feet and tongue) eliminated and their corresponding trials also eliminated. **Figure 2** shows the signal of C3 channel before and after segmentation for three trials.

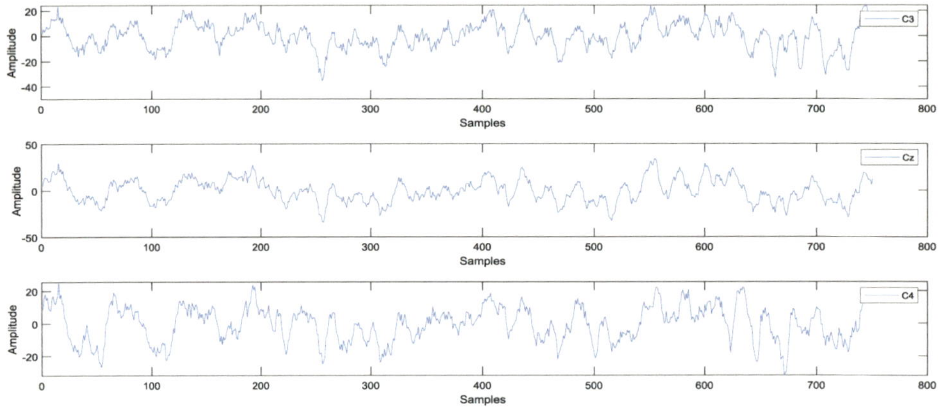

(a)

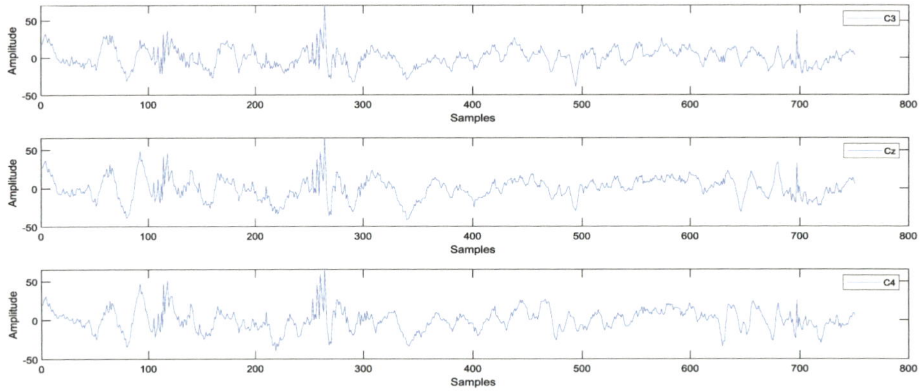

(b)

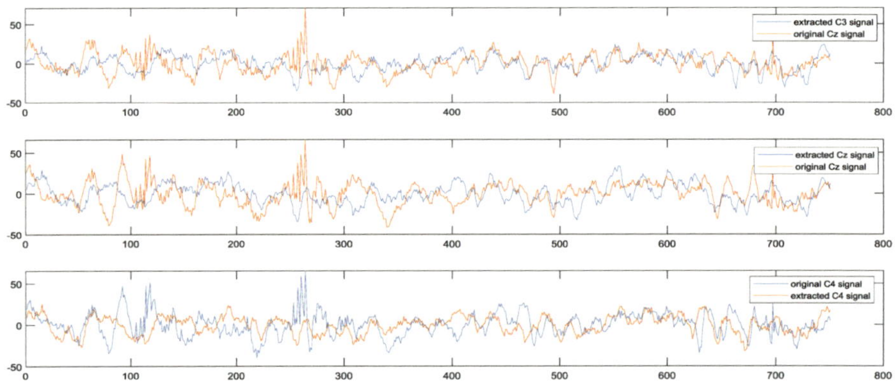

(c)

Figure 2.
(a) Signal three channels before trials extraction; (b) signal after trials extraction (c) show the deference between original signal and extracted signal for three trial.

2.4 Artifact's reduction

Artifacts can be defining as the unwanted signals that appear in EEG signals, they can be caused from various origins including body or eye movement, heart beating blinking, or frequency from utility, which is (50 Hz in Europe or 60 Hz in the United States) [23]. The utility frequency was removed already by applying notch filter while eye artifacts are left due to possibility of artifacts removal algorithms testing [22].

To handle eye artifact, there are three main approaches: avoidance, rejection, and removal [23].

For artifacts avoidance can be by asking the user to avoid movement during the recording that causes EEG artifact, which decreases the artifact's number, but eye movement and blinks cannot be avoided.

Another way is to reject all corrupted trials by artifacts, which can automatically have done or manually. Manually can be done through visual examination, as the corrupted trials marked if they are corrupted or not by an expert. An algorithm is implemented in automatic artifact rejection, that can determine if artifacts corrupt a trial or not, and artifact rejection reduces the size of the training set. Last, is artifact removal, in order to remove the EEG signal artifact, some algorithms are used that leave the desired brain-originated signal intact.

2.5 Bandpass filtering

After applying segmentation algorithm to segment signals of each channel into 3 s sub signal according to the event associated with the data set then remove all marked artifact trials, **Figure 3** shows EEG signal for three trials after applying bandpass filter, the signal is filtered using a bandpass filter designed for a given frequency band. Using, for each channel, a 4th order Butterworth infinite impulse response (IIR) filter, IIRs are used to change the frequency component of a time signal by reducing or amplifying a particular frequency. This filter is used to pass only the band-limited portion of frequency content.

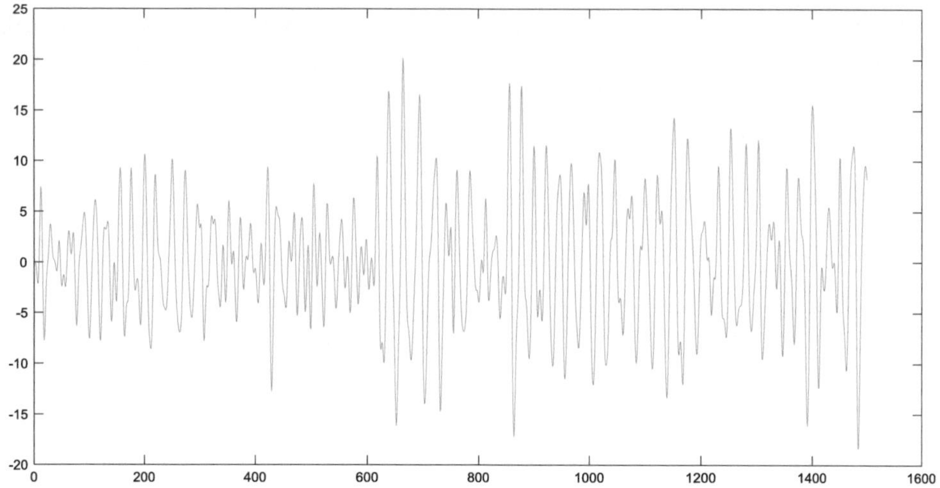

Figure 3.
Signal of C3 channel after applying bandpass filter between (8–30 HZ).

2.6 Feature extraction

The filtered signals are used to calculate spectrum PSD, in detail, estimate the PSD in the band between 8 and 30 Hz, this is based on the fact that the beta rhythm has distinct topographies and responses to the limb movements, compared with the alpha rhythm, the oscillatory power of the mu rhythm in the sensorimotor cortex ipsilateral to the tasks increased, while that of the beta rhythm in the contralateral sensorimotor cortex decreased simultaneously. The Welch's averaged used for spectral estimation that is a modified periodogram method. With 1 s Hamming window and 50% overlap, Welch's method can reduce noise. Each trial is divided into five bands and then the power and variance of each band are calculated, and energy of the whole trial is calculated.

2.7 Model building

The SVM method was used to train person EEG models using 10-fold cross-validation training and was used to train models on the whole training set and test on a separate test set.

SVM developed by Cortes and Vapnik [24] is a practical implementation of statistical learning theory capable of processing difficult problems of supervised learning, SVM is nonprobabilistic classifier; the two limitations of SVM are linear and binary features [25].

A decision boundary (plane) in SVM is used to separate the feature vectors. SVM classifier finds during training into two classes. The problem is to find the decision boundary (a linear hyperplane) that has the maximum separation (margin) between the two classes. The margin of a hyperplane is the distance between parallel equidistant hyperplanes on either side of the hyperplane such that the gap is void of data objects. The optimization during training finds a hyperplane that has the maximum margin. The SVM then uses that hyperplane to predict the class of a new data object once presented with its feature vector. See **Figure 4** [26].

2.8 Fuzzy vault

It is an updated version of the ideas of the fuzzy commitment scheme [27]. In this scheme, a message M is encoded as coefficients of a k-degree polynomial (p) using Reed Solomon code RS, in x (data points evaluated on polynomial(p)) over a finite

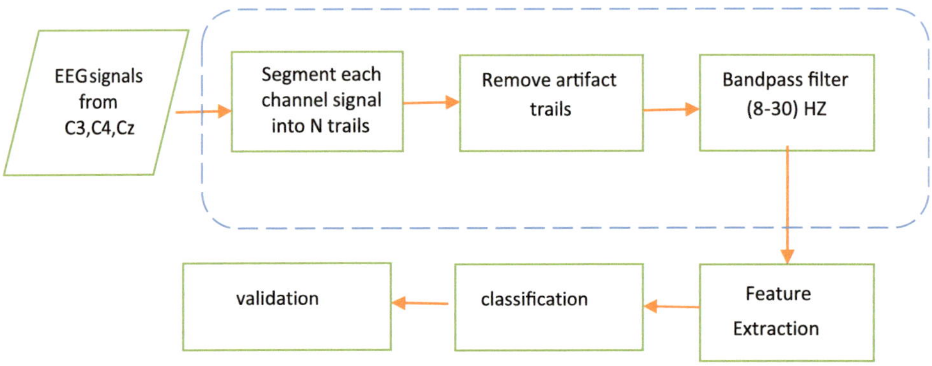

Figure 4.
Model building.

field F_q. Then the polynomial p is evaluated at the input data points (X) to calculate p (X) = Y. These (X, Y) pairs, known as genuine points, constructing the locking set, which become the vault later. False points (called chaff) are used to hide the identity of the genuine points, and then, they are added to the genuine points set. This is called vault, which is then stored. The difficulty of the fuzzy vault scheme is shown in polynomial reconstruction problem, which is to make it secure [28].

2.9 Lock the vault

Polynomial is generated by using the code results from encoding a polynomial coefficient called secret that is a secret value using RS. Every EEG feature is projected onto the polynomial. Then it creates the chaff points using the proposed tent chaff points. Then shuffling the two point sets, to produce the vault. As the following algorithm:

Input: Parameters k, t, and r where $k \leq n \leq r \leq q$. A Pre-select Secret $S \in \mathcal{F}$. A locking set A=$\{a_i\}_{i=1}^{n}$ where a_i $\mathcal{F}$.
Output: A set R of points $\{(x_i, y_i)\}_{i=1}^{r}$ such that $x_i, y_i \in \mathcal{F}$
Variables :CH chaff points

$X,R \leftarrow \phi$
$poly\ (x) \leftarrow$ **RSENCODE**(S,k)
for i=1 to n do
$(\mathbf{x}_i; \mathbf{y}_i) \leftarrow (\mathbf{a}_i; \boldsymbol{poly}\ (\mathbf{a}_i))$;
CH $(\mathbf{x}_i; \mathbf{y}_i) \leftarrow$ chaff$(\mathbf{x}_i; \mathbf{y}_i)$;
$X \leftarrow sort \boldsymbol{x_i}$
$\boldsymbol{R} \leftarrow$ CH$(\mathbf{x}_i; \mathbf{y}_i) \cup (x_i, y_i)$
output $\boldsymbol{R}$

S: a secret key intended to protect.
poly (x): a polynomial of degree less than k.
$A = \{a_i\}_{i=1}^{n}$: a locking set containing n elements.
$\mathcal{F}$: finite field.
q: the number of finite field F *elements*.
n: the number of real points.
r: the total number of real points and chaff points.

Figure 5 illustrates feature projection on polynomial produced by encoding the secret s using RS, x_i is the featurea_i, and y_i is the projection on polynomial poly(a_i).

2.10 Tent-chaff points

After projection of the feature onto the polynomial p using features as:

$$p\left(f_q\right) = c_{d+1} \cdot f_q^{\ d+1} + c_d \cdot f_q^{\ d} + \ldots + c_1 \cdot f_q. \tag{1}$$

The genuine point list is comprised of:

$$\text{Genuine Points} = \begin{bmatrix} f_{q_1} & p\left(f_{q_1}\right) \\ \vdots & \vdots \\ f_{q_m} & p\left(f_{q_m}\right) \end{bmatrix} \tag{2}$$

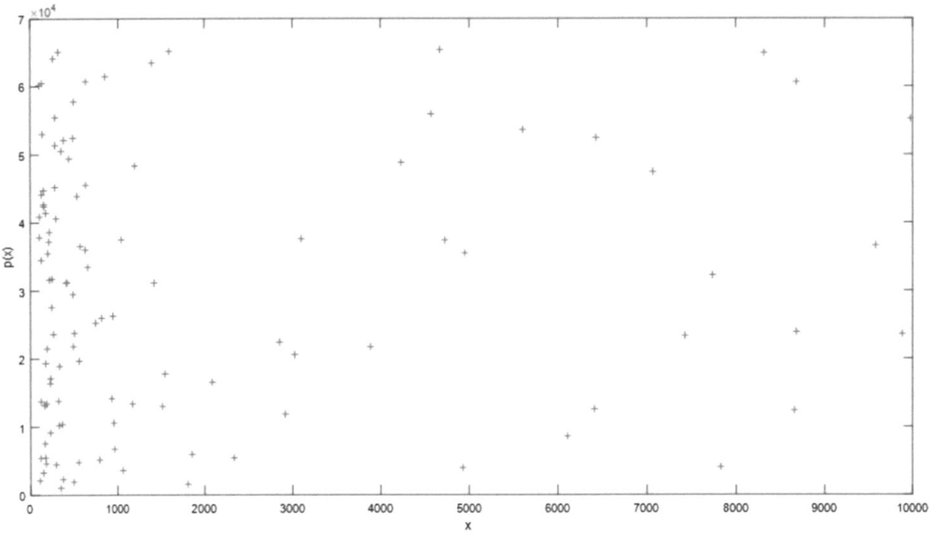

Figure 5.
Features projection on polynomial poly.

To mask the identity of true points, chaff points are added using chaotic tent map. Let μ be the seed, X_n = initial

$$x_{n+1} = \begin{cases} \mu x_n x_n \in [0, 0.5) \\ \mu(1 - x_n), x_n \in [0.5, 1] \end{cases} \tag{3}$$

Each chaff point and other genuine points do not need to put distance between them. The reason is that the chaff points are known for the two sides.

$$\text{Chaff Points} = \begin{bmatrix} Ch_{x_1} & Ch_{y_1} \\ \vdots & \vdots \\ Ch_{x_n} & pCh_{x_n} \end{bmatrix} \tag{4}$$

Finally, genuine Points and Chaff Points are combined, and the new matrix is shuffled. That represents fuzzy vault final matrix.

Figure 6 shows how chaff points hide genuine points; red circles in (a) are chaff points, (b) showing how attacker sees the final points projection.

2.11 Unlock the vault

The message vault is received and is attempted to decrypted it using input features produced from evaluation dataset. (X') are evaluated in the model build to identify the person in the vault pairs. If predicted person is the same as the original, then regenerate the chaff point set using the agreed seed and initial state for both parties and then remove the chaff points, after that from (x_i, y_i) pairs recover the message through polynomial reconstruction; otherwise reject;

Input: A fuzzy vault R,
Output: A value $S' \in \mathcal{F}^k$ $\{null\}$.
Variables : CH :chaff points,R :the vault ,Q:is the reconstructed polynomial
$Q \leftarrow \phi$
regenerate chaff points CH
for i = 1 to n do
Temp= CH(x_i, y_i)==R(x_i, y_i)
R(Temp)= []
Q=R
$Q \leftarrow Q\ (x_i, y_i)$
$S' \leftarrow$ **RSDECODE**(Q, k)
Output S' or null

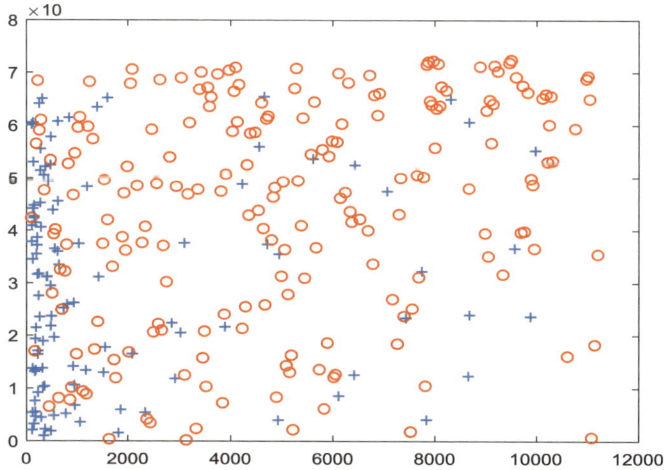

(a)

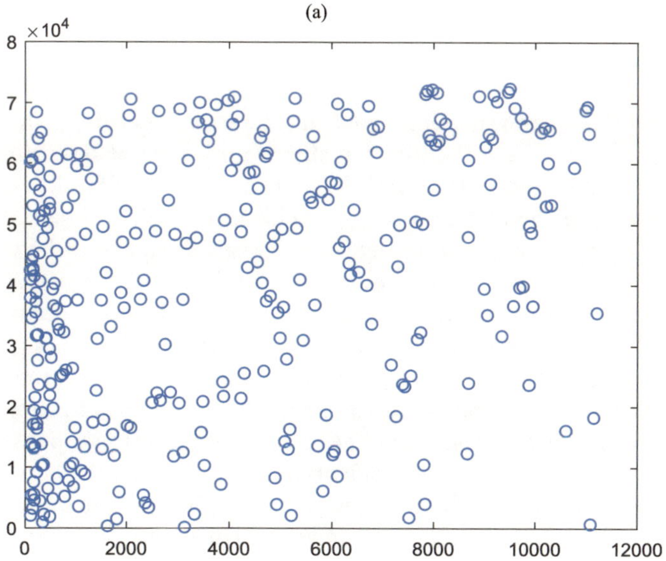

(b)

Figure 6.
How chaff points hide the polynomial.

2.12 Lagrange interpolation

It is a method used to reconstruct polynomials; it is a method that computes the interpolation polynomial to form the system:

$$Ax = b_i, \text{ where } bi = y, \ i = 0, \dots, n, \tag{5}$$

"The A entries can be defined by $a_{ij} = p_j(xi)$, where $i, j = 0, \dots, n$, and $x_i = x_0, x_1, \dots, x_n$ are the points at which the data $y_0, y_1, \dots, y_n$ are obtained, and $p_j(x) = x^j, j = 0, 1, \dots, n$. The basis $\{1, x, \dots, x^n\}$ of the polynomials'
space of degree $n + 1$ is called the monomial basis, and the corresponding matrix A is called the Vandermonde matrix for the points $x_0, x_1, \dots, x_n$, In Lagrange interpolation, the matrix A is simply the identity matrix, by virtue of the fact that the interpolating polynomial is written in the form:"

$$p_n(x) = \sum_{j=0}^{n} y_i \mathcal{L}_{n,j}(x) \tag{6}$$

where the polynomials $\{\mathcal{L}_{n,j}\}, {}^{n}_{j=0}=0$ have the property that

$$\mathcal{L}_{n,j}(x_i) = \begin{cases} 1 & if\ i = j \\ 0 & if\ i \neq j \end{cases} \tag{7}$$

The Lagrange polynomials for interpolation is: $\{\mathcal{L}_{n,j}\}$ where $j = 0, \dots, n, x_0, x_1 \dots,$ x_n. are the interpolation points, they are defined by:

$$\mathcal{L}_{n,j}(x) = \prod_{k=0, k \neq j}^{n} \frac{x - x_k}{x_j - x_k} \tag{8}$$

3. Conclusion

After testing the system, it gives a good accuracy of classifying, which is 96%, but the run time of fuzzy vault authentication algorithm is kind of slow regarding that authentication must be fast to be practical for using it in real life; the reason of its slowness is because of the high number of EEG features, which result of many of multiple operations to compute Lagrange's interpolation that slow the work of the algorithm that make the algorithm impractical, on the other hand, using the tent chaff points gives the system an advantage because it reduces the error occurrence when separating chaff points from the genuine points, which are the EEG signal features because the initial seeds are known by both sender and receiver so, the system can regenerate the chaff points again and rise them without or less effecting the genuine points, and in the traditional chaff point generation, it needs to keep distance from the genuine point, which requires more calculation, which this method does not. Also we have difficulties in converting the features that are float numbers into integers so they can be used in Galois field, which needs integers to deal with, another problem is the repeated numbers produced from the conversion into integers because the features' values are close so they result in a repetition. The repeated values cannot use when reconstructing the polynomial because it results in division on zero, which is not acceptable because we need a unique number.

The system used nine healthy persons' EEGs from the BCI Competition and extracted features from signals spectrum of beta and alpha band of EEG signal, then extracted features from three channels and used support vector Machine (SVM) to classify two tasks left hand and right hand that achieve 96.98% validation accuracy, using 10-fold cross-validation on the training set and then saved the model, these features are evaluated on a polynomial generated from the secret key, then chaff points using tent map are added, which reduce the error; for decoding, we use Lagrange interpolation for polynomial reconstruction and returning the key.

To measure performance, a confusion matrix was calculated from which its precision and recall are calculated, a part from using the confusion matric to find precision and recall, it is important to analyze the result by the help of the confusion matrix to analyze the results as it also gives a very strong, it gives the evidence where your

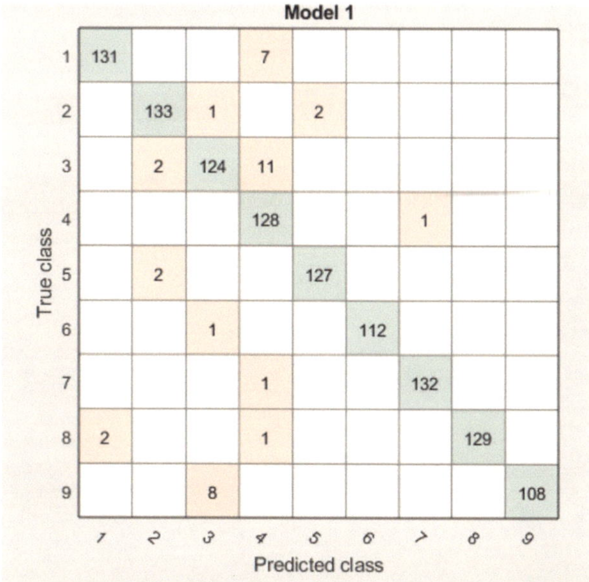

Figure 7.
Confusion matrix for the classification model.

Subject	TPR (%)	FNR (%)
1	95	5
2	98	2
3	91	9
4	99	1
5	98	2
6	99	1
7	99	1
8	98	2
9	93	7

Table 2.
TPR and FNR.

classifier is going wrong. So for our model, we can see that our classifier goes in the right direction, which means the classifier can distinguish between subjects' labels; **Figure 7** illustrates confusion matrix for nine subjects.

The total validation accuracy is 96.98%, from confusion matrix; also, one can calculate the true positive rate (TPR) and the false negative rate (FNR) as shown below, by observing the table; TPR is high and FNR is low, which means the performance at its best. See **Table 2**.

Author details

Fatima M. Baqer* and Salah Albermany
University of Kufa, Najaf, Iraq

*Address all correspondence to: fatimam.alkhersan@student.uokufa.edu.iq

References

[1] Pham T Ma W, Tran D, Tran DS, Phung DQ. A study on the stability of EEG signals for user authentication. In: 2015 7th International IEEE/EMBS Conference on Neural Engineering (NER). New Jersey: IEEE; 2015. pp. 122–125

[2] Soni YS, Somani SB, Shete VV. Biometric user authentication using brain waves. In: 2016 International Conference on Inventive Computation Technologies (ICICT). New Jersey: IEEE; 2016. pp. 1–6

[3] Story R. Using machine learning to improve motor imagery neurofeedback [master thesis[. Halifax, Canada: Dalhousie University; 2015

[4] Sujitha V, Chitra DR. A novel technique for multi biometric cryptosystem using fuzzy vault. Journal of Medical Systems. 2019;**43**:1-9

[5] Reshmi K, Muhammed PI, Priya VV, Akhila V. A novel approach to brain biometric user recognition. Procedia Technology. 2016;**25**:240-247

[6] Sharma M, Atri ES. A review on cryptography mechanisms. International Journal of Computer Technology and Applications. 2011;**2**(4):1048-1050

[7] He C. Person authentication using EEG brainwave signals [unpublished master's thesis]. 2009

[8] Padfield N, Zabalza J, Zhao H, Masero V, Ren J. EEG-based brain-computer interfaces using motor-imagery: Techniques and challenges. Sensors. 2019;**19**(6):1423

[9] Yüksel A. Classification Methods for Motor Imagery Based Brain Computer Interfaces [thesis]. Istanbul Technical University; 2016. p. 21

[10] Hlinka M. Motor Imagery Based Brain-Computer Interface Used in a Simple Computer Game. Brno, Czechia: Masaryk University Faculty of Informatics; 2017

[11] Marcel S, Millán JDR. Person authentication using brainwaves (EEG) and maximum a posteriori model adaptation. IEEE Transactions on Pattern Analysis and Machine Intelligence. 2012;**29**(4):743–752. DOI: 10.1109/TPAMI.2007.1012

[12] Fladby K. Brain wave based authentication [master thesis]. Gjøvik, Norway: Gjøvik University College; 2008

[13] Nguyen P, Tran D, Le T, Huang X, Ma W. EEG-based person verification using multi-sphere SVDD and UBM. In: Pacific-Asia Conference on Knowledge Discovery and Data Mining. Berlin, Heidelberg: Springer; 2013. pp. 289-300

[14] Nieves O, Manian V. Automatic person authentication using fewer channel EEG motor imagery. In: 2016 World Automation Congress (WAC). New Jersey: IEEE; 2016. pp. 1-6

[15] Sjamsudin FP. EEG-based authentication with machine learning. 2017

[16] Juels A, Sudan M. A fuzzy vault scheme. Designs, Codes and Cryptography. 2006;**38**:237-257. DOI: 10.1007/s10623-005-6343-z

[17] Uludag U, Pankanti S, Jain AK. Fuzzy vault for fingerprints. In: International Conference on Audio-and Video-Based Biometric Person

Authentication. Berlin, Heidelberg: Springer; 2005. pp. 310-319

[18] Nagar A, Nandakumar K, Jain AK. Securing fingerprint template: Fuzzy vault with minutiae descriptors. In: 2008 19th International Conference on Pattern Recognition. New Jersey: IEEE; 2008. pp. 1-4

[19] Khalil-Hani M, Marsono MN, Bakhteri R. Biometric encryption based on a fuzzy vault scheme with a fast chaff generation algorithm. Future Generation Computer Systems. 2013;**29**(3):800-810

[20] You L, Wang Y, Chen Y, Deng Q, Zhang H. A novel key sharing fuzzy vault scheme. KSII Transactions on Internet and Information Systems. 2016; **10**:4585-4602

[21] Damaševičius R, Maskeliūnas R, Kazanavičius E, Woźniak M. Combining cryptography with EEG biometrics. Computational Intelligence and Neuroscience. 2018;**2018**:1-11

[22] Brunner C, Leeb R, Müller-Putz G, Schlögl A, Pfurtscheller G. BCI Competition 2008–Graz data set A. Institute for Knowledge Discovery (Laboratory of Brain-Computer Interfaces), Graz University of Technology. 2008;**16**:1-6. Available from: http://www.bbci.de/competition/iv/desc_2a.pdf

[23] Fatourechi M, Bashashati A, Ward RK, Birch GE. EMG and EOG artifacts in brain computer interface systems: A survey. Clinical Neurophysiology. 2007;**118**(3):480-494

[24] Cortes C, Vapnik V. Support-vector networks. Machine Learning. 1995; **20**(3):273-297

[25] Hetal B, Ganatra AMIT. Variations of support vector machine classification technique: A survey. International Journal of Advanced Computer Research. 2012;**2**(6):230-236

[26] Bridgelall RPHD. Introduction to Support Vector Machines. Lecture. 2017. p. 1

[27] Jain AK, Ross AA, Nandakumar K. Introduction to Biometrics. Berlin: Springer Science & Business Media; 2008. pp. 1–22

[28] Gui Q, Jin Z, Xu W. Exploring EEG-based biometrics for user identification and authentication. In: 2014 IEEE Signal Processing in Medicine and Biology Symposium (SPMB). Philadelphia, PA, USA: IEEE; 2014. pp. 1–6

Chapter 8

Automatic Noise Reduction in Ultrasonic Computed Tomography Image for Adult Bone Fracture Detection

Marwa Fradi, Kais Bouallegue, Philippe Lasaygues and Mohsen Machhout

Abstract

Noise reduction in medical image analysis is still an interesting hot topic, especially in the field of ultrasonic images. Actually, a big concern has been given to automatically reducing noise in human-bone ultrasonic computed tomography (USCT) images. In this chapter, a new hardware prototype, called USCT, is used but images given by this device are noisy and difficult to interpret. Our approach aims to reinforce the peak signal-to-noise ratio (PSNR) in these images to perform an automatic segmentation for bone structures and pathology detection. First, we propose to improve USCT image quality by implementing the discrete wavelet transform algorithm. Second, we focus on a hybrid algorithm combining the k-means with the Otsu method, hence improving the PSNR. Our assessment of the performance shows that the algorithmic approach is comparable with recent methods. It outperforms most of them with its ability to enhance the PSNR to detect edges and pathologies in the USCT images. Our proposed algorithm can be generalized to any medical image to carry out automatic image diagnosis due to noise reduction, and then we have to overcome classical medical image analysis by achieving a short-time process.

Keywords: USCT, image processing, PSNR, automatic segmentation, K-means, Haar wavelet

1. Introduction

Bone disease exploration is assured by a variety of modalities of medical imaging. Bone mineral density is determined by standard scanners and x-rays. Although this technique delineates the bone structure, it remains an invasive method with qualitative information on bone structures. Ultrasound computed tomography (USCT) is the best to give us more details and a very interesting procedure for bone imaging associated with signal and image processing methods [1, 2]. A variety of medical imaging techniques such as x-rays and standard scanners determine bone mineral density.

However, these modalities represent an ionizing method without giving quantitative results. USCT hardware has been propounded to solve this issue [1, 2]. USCT presents an important radiological technique because of its non-ionizing properties. However, it has been the subject of several studies due to the complexity of its visualization and the noisy USCT image quality [3]. In the light of this issue, noise reduction should be the first step to be interested in, to enhance the USCT image resolution and to detect bone diagnosis. Hence, many researchers have studied different techniques for ultrasound image noise reduction, and obtained results achieved the terms of quality improvement (37.14 dB of peak signal-to-noise ratio [PSNR]) [3]. But, these methods cannot be applied to USCT bone images due to its complexity. Actually, USCT bone imaging is a very difficult method that encounters many problems mainly related to high bone echogenicity. Noise reduction is one of the crucial topics in digital image processing and has been conducted in various fields such as ultrasound imaging [4]. Many obstacles still exist, but several results have been successful [5, 6]. Accordingly, we will try here to propose optimizations for image processing by implementing discrete Haar wavelet algorithm and a proposed hybrid algorithm combining k-means with the Otsu method. It is an important process for removing noise, as it produces promising results in terms of image resolution, noise removal and diagnosis detection. In this work, our objective aims to automatically remove noise levels generated during the rebound of ultrasonic waves against bony structures, from USCT images, improving the PSNR.

In this chapter, we divide the work into seven sections: Section 2 presents an overview of the medical history in this area, some physical considerations and the description of existing algorithms. Section 3 presents fundamental mathematical theorems that will be implemented in the next section. Section 4 describes the proposed hardware and software method to segment USCT. Section 5 shows the obtained results, the comparison of our work with previous work and the discussions. Section 6 concludes this chapter.

2. State of the art

In 2019, a Ram-Lak filter is implemented in the Radon domain to reduce the noise levels in the USCT images and facilitate their observation giving a PSNR with a value of 13.07 [3]. In 2018, different filters such as median and a high pass filter have been used to reduce noise in Magnetic Resonance Imaging (MRI) images as a pre-processing step and the first results are promising [7]. In addition, bilateral filter and trilateral filter are used for noise removal in [8] by considering the small structure as noise to be removed and conserving the large structure. Moreover, in [9] adaptive filter of Kuan, Frost or maximum medium median (MMM) have been produced to enhance ultrasound images resolution giving promising results. However, these methods fail to give encouraging results when applied to USCT images [3, 9].

The Fourier transform with its decomposition of a trigonometric series has been widely introduced in the field of signal processing as well as in medical image processing, but it is insufficient for giving a piece of complete information in both time and frequency areas simultaneously. Indeed, using the classical Born approximation and the spatial Fourier transform, the result is a poor contrast-to-noise ratio (CNR) image. Some previous work to improve the CNR has been introduced while handling signal and image processing [2, 5]. Although image analysis is an important process for noise removal, it cannot produce the intended result in some digital image processing [4]. Actually, a flow of image processing should be applied to improve the USCT image quality and to achieve automatic diagnosis detection. The active contour method was introduced in the process of USCT image segmentation. Its use avoided the issue of noise in USCT images [10]. In [11], authors appended this algorithm on USCT paired-bone images. However, the results were not good enough and the detection of the distances between the two bone forms (tibia and fibula) was not possible.

The method, called the "Wavelet-based Coded Excitation" (WCE) method [5] is based on the wavelet decomposition of the signal and on a suitable transmitted incident wave correlated with the experimental set-up. Indeed, the contrast with reports of noise was improved, but the detection of edges and areas of child-matched bone by ultrasound with USCT was impossible [5, 11]. However, this method has remained very interesting. During the last two decades, a lot of research has involved the use of the transformed wavelet for removing noise through its energy compaction and its multiresolution parameter proprieties [12, 13]. Thanks to these parameters, we can obtain different versions (dilated or compressed, and translated or shifted) from the same mother wavelet.

The k-means algorithm is known for its simplicity in clustering a database into clusters. Nevertheless, this number of clusters has to be identified. It has been used for resolving the issue of data clustering. k-means followed by fuzzy c-means were introduced by Alan Jose et al. in [14, 15] to detect a brain tumor, and the result of the segmented image remained for the feature extraction and the image resolution was improved. Image segmentation using the k-means algorithm is a process of separating images into different regions with high resolution. The purpose of such segmentation is the detection of regions of interest simultaneously with noise removal in an image. Moreover, image segmentation has been an increasingly expanded issue especially in the area of medical imaging and more specifically in USCT considering the inhomogeneity of pixels and complex anatomical topology [6].

Otsu method has been used for a long time to medical image analysis for image resolution enhancement [16] obtaining the right diagnostic. In [7], a proposed Otsu method has been used for MRI images for tumor brain detection.

3. Mathematical theoretical

3.1 Wavelet transform

The wavelet transform is a mathematical function that allows image compression and signal processing. It resolves the problem of the Fourier analyses. It is defined by the following equation:

$$\Psi(a,b) = \frac{1}{\sqrt{\mathrm{a}}}\Psi\left(t - \frac{\mathrm{b}}{\mathrm{a}}\right) \tag{1}$$

where a is the scale parameter or the expansion factor, and b is the translation or proposition parameter. The bigger a is, the more the wavelet is dilated.

3.1.1 Principle of wavelet transform

The wavelet transform is a multiresolution analysis tool able to transfer accurate temporal and spatial information. In the literature, various noise reduction techniques concerning wavelet approaches have been put forward [14]. From an original image, low frequencies are analyzed by the application of a low-pass filter. Then, high frequencies are analyzed by the application of a high-pass filter. It allows dividing the information of the image in an approximation and detail as depicted in **Figure 1**. We will use the Haar wavelet to keep the edge detection of an image as follows:

- On the lines, estimate the medium of each pixel of paired data.
- On the lines, calculate the variance between each datum and its respective average.
- Point the averages in the first half of the matrix data which corresponds to the L approximation image.
- Point the average in one-half of the data corresponding to the H detailed image matrix.
- Rehearse the process on the first half of the L data, but on columns so we get two images corresponding to the approximation of LL (means of dimension matrix) and LH (matrix of differences in dimension) image details.
- Renew the process on the LL image approximation to have a decomposition level greater than 1.
- A low-pass filter application remains to get an L image which is compressed and the application of a high-pass filter leads to obtain an H image which introduces image details. This process is done by Eqs. (2) and (3) as follows:

$$YH[k] = \sum_{n} x[n]\, G[2k - n] \tag{2}$$

$$Yl[k] = \sum_{n} x[n] H[2k - n] \tag{3}$$

3.2 k-means algorithm

It is based on grouping similar data points into clusters. There is no prediction involved. Its algorithm is illustrated by these steps [18].

- Fix the k number of cluster values.
- Identify the k cluster centers.

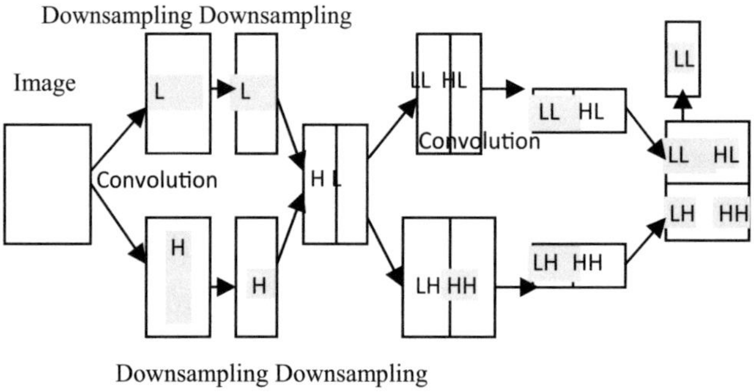

Figure 1.
Principle of wavelet application.

- Determine the cluster center.
- Determine the pixel distance for each cluster center.
- If the distance is close to the center value, budge to that cluster.
- Otherwise, move to the next cluster.
- Re-identify the center.

3.3 k-means algorithm combined with Otsu algorithm + morphologic algorithm

The proposed hybrid algorithm uses the combination of k-means with the Otsu method and the morphologic algorithm. The k-means algorithm implementation is important. It works well in a large number of cases and it is a powerful tool to have in the closet point. Unfortunately, in medical image processing, it is not sufficient for region detection and edge detection. k-Means combined with the morphologic and Otsu algorithms give us sufficient results.

3.3.1 Morphologic algorithm

Morphological filters are a valuable aid in the segmentation and noise removal process. Morphological filtering is based on mathematical morphological operations, well applied to binary images as well as monochrome (grayscaled) images. To be limited to binary image morphological filtering, morphological operations aim to perfect the improper structure of an image [17]. The morphological erosion of X by B is defined by the principle of duality where X is the set of points described in the space and B is the structuring element. Its equation is written under the following form:

$$\varepsilon\, B\overline{(x)} = \overline{\delta B\ (x)} \tag{4}$$

$$\varepsilon\, B(x) = \overline{\delta\ B\ \overline{(x)}} = \overline{\overline{x} \oplus \overline{B}} = x \ominus \overline{B} \tag{5}$$

3.3.2 Otsu algorithm

The Otsu method of the threshold is the most powerful and global threshold method. It performs image binarization based on the histogram image shape. It assumes that the image for binarization contains the only foreground and background pixels [19, 20]. Using the simple formula in the Otsu algorithm, we get:

$$\sigma^2 = \Psi A\ (u\ A - u)^2 + \Psi B\ (u\ B - u)^2 \tag{6}$$

where σ^2 is the variance between both clusters, Ψ_A is the probability of class A, Ψ_B is the probability of class A, u_A is the average gray of class A, u_B is the average gray of class B, and u is the threshold value which divides the image into two classes A and B. The best threshold u maximizes the variance between both clusters. It computes the optimal threshold by minimizing the intra-class variance that separates the foreground pixels from background pixels [21]. The main purpose of the Otsu method is to find the threshold values where the sum of the values of the foreground and background pixels has to be minimal [22].

3.4 Peak-signal -to noise ratio (PSNR)

The PSNR is defined by the ratio of the power of the signal and the corrupting noise presented in the image.

4. Materials and methods

4.1 Materials

The used hardware device is illustrated in Ref. [5] in section material and method.

4.2 Methods

Our approach is based on a hardware and software co-design to enhance the signal-to-noise ratio (SNR), to automatically segment the USCT images and finally to detect fractures in bones. It is described in **Figure 2.**

4.3 Hardware method

The acquisition of the signal is done in retro diffusion, transmission and diffraction. The frequencies of measurements are performed at 1 MHz. Each transducer plays the role of a transmitter and a receiver. A transmitted signal is sent and

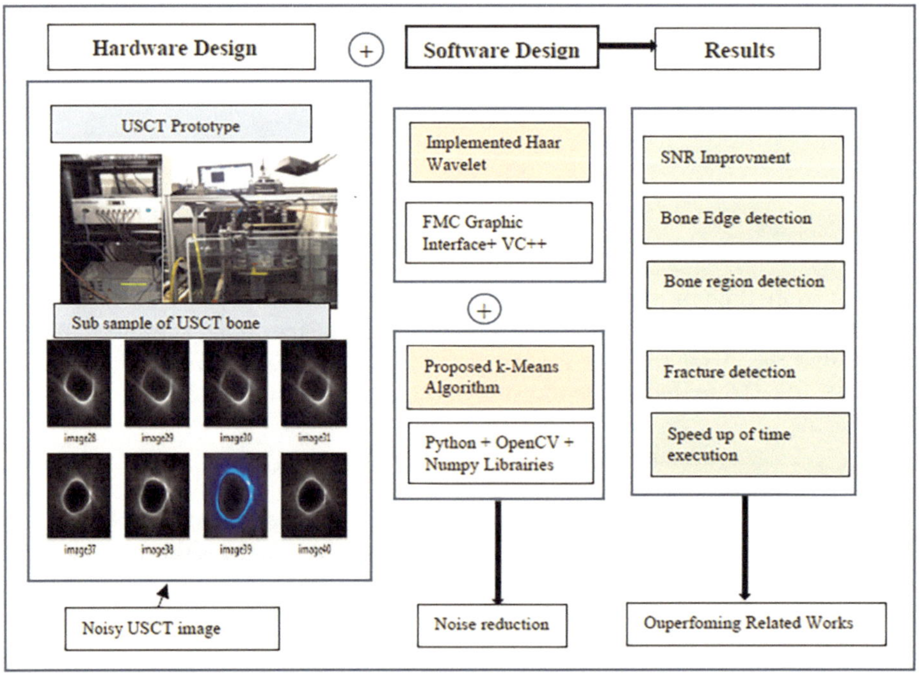

Figure 2.
Synoptic flow of our approach.

diffracted on the object to be imaged, reaching the other seven receivers. There are three configurations per zone. The wave is transmitted, or back-propagated or diffracted as illustrated in Ref. [2].

4.4 Software method

Using an adult bone defect as depicted in **Figure 3 (a)**. We have a USCT noisy bone image in **Figure 3 (b)**. USCT image processing recognition is kept by the application of some algorithms such as the Haar wavelet transformation and the improved k-means, as depicted by the synoptic flow in **Figure 4**.

4.4.1 Implemented Haar wavelet algorithm

Algorithm 1: Direct Haar wavelets transform

1: Download the source which contains the converted binary image
2: Download f-L and f-H filter file.
3: Treatment following lines.
4: Treatment following columns.
5: //Sgl is the converted binary image.
6: while.
7: {
8: Bf [0] and Bf [1] take the sgl values.
9: CVh = 0 compute the mean CVh $= \frac{Bf(0)+Bf(1)}{2.}$
10: CVl = 0 compute the difference CVl $= (Bf(0) - CVh)$
11: }
12: Display the values of CVh, CVl
13: Display LL, HL, LH and HH image values

4.4.1.1 Proposed k-means algorithm

Our proposed k-means algorithm is described in **Figure 4**.

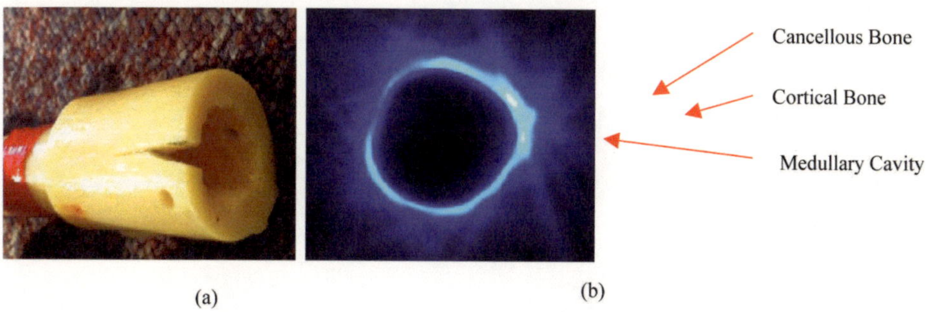

Figure 3.
Ultrasonic bone tomography with USCT: (a) adult cortical bone defect (copyright/rights reserved, CNRS-LMA-Marseille), (b) USCT image defect.

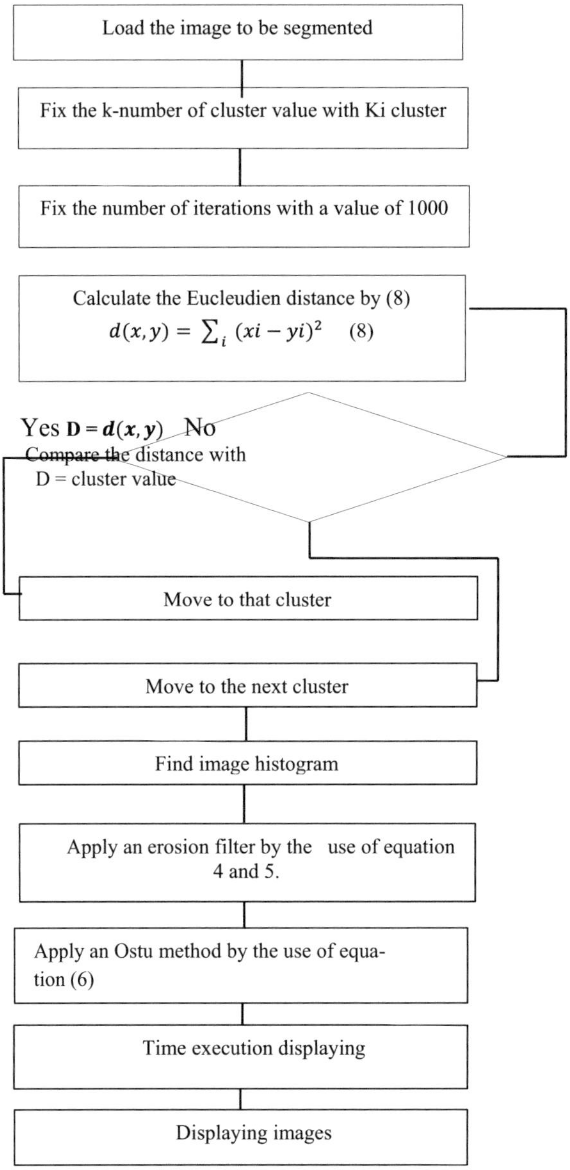

Figure 4.
Hybrid algorithm combining k-means with Otsu method.

5. Results

5.1 Fracture detection

Figure 5 shows an example of how to identify an artificial defect on a human femur. The defect is through an incision at the end of the sample whose width is reduced in depth. Three heights are analyzed: one (H1) in the very fine portion of the crack, a second (H2) in the intermediate zone, and the third (H3) in the very open

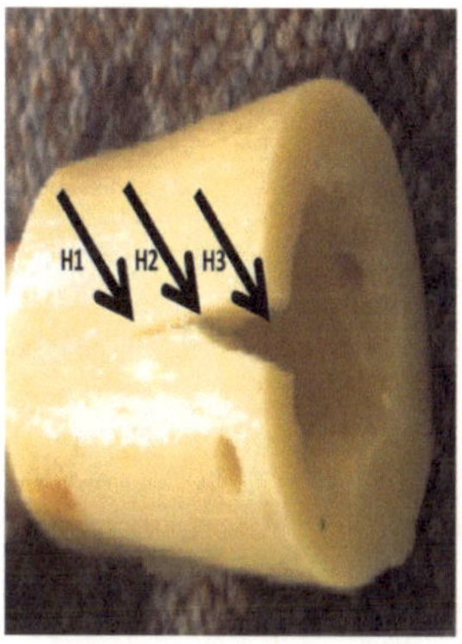

Figure 5.
Adult bone defect.

upper zone. We can see in **Figures 6** and 7 that the implemented Haar wavelet detects the external edge. Hence, it is very clear, but the fracture is not detected and the problem still exists. It is because of the noise, the inhomogeneity of pixel intensities and the difficulty of separating anatomic regions. We do not have any idea about the intensity of the three regions. The problem is how to detect the fracture and how to obtain the different regions of interest. For this fact, a hybrid algorithm is proposed in the second step.

An example of the application of the k-means algorithm in the identification of a bone defect is discussed as an interesting breakthrough work of USCT bone imaging. Despite the ability of automatic fracture detection with k-means, as shown in **Figure 8** (a), (b) and (c), the results are not sufficient because we need to have an excellent quality of images and to extract the background that noises the ultrasonic image. With k-means, we detect regions and fractures. We need to extract the background and detect the edges. For this fact, we apply the morphologic algorithm. As shown in **Figure 9** (d), (e) and (f), with the morphologic algorithm, edges are well detected and we can calculate the distances with more precision. We can clearly distinguish the different zones, especially in the H1 part where the rack is not very open. The PSNRs

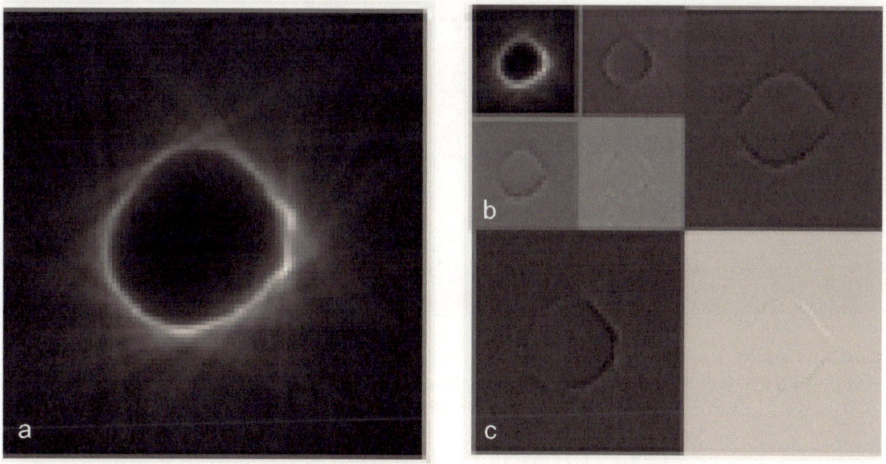

Figure 6.
External edge detection by wavelet transform with FMC interface, (a1): LH1, (b1): HL, (c1): HH1.

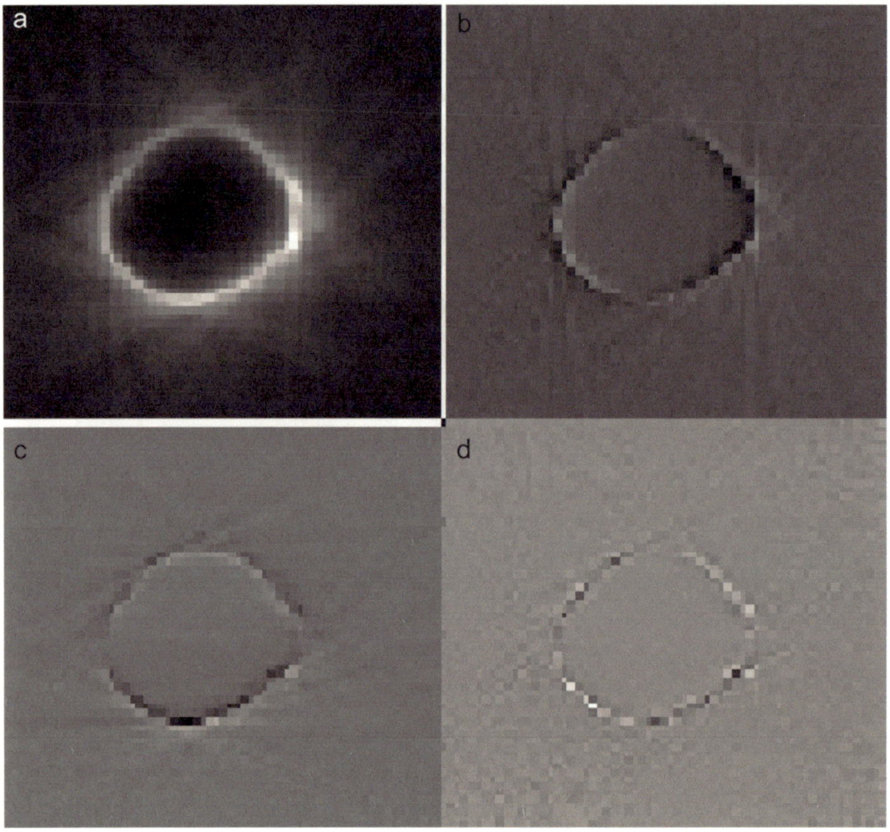

Figure 7.
External edge detection by wavelet transformation: (a) LL: PSNR = 16.18, (b) LH: PSNR = 24.65, (c) HL: PSNR = ***25.15****, (d) HH: PSNR = 22.98.*

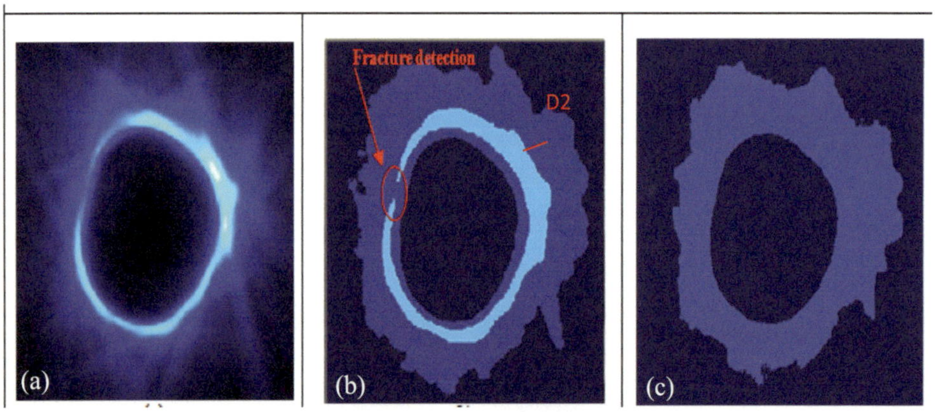

Figure 8.
Denoised USCT image with k-means algorithm: (a) adult bone USCT image, (b) segmented USCT adult bone image with the k-means algorithm, k = 3, (c) segmented USCT adult bone image with the k-means algorithm, k = 2.

are (H1) 13.08, (H2) 13.11 and (H3) 13.14, respectively. As seen in **Figure 10 (g)**, **(h)** and **(i)**, due to the application of the Otsu method, we obtain the image histogram value. After that, we extract the background. Finally, we obtain every region

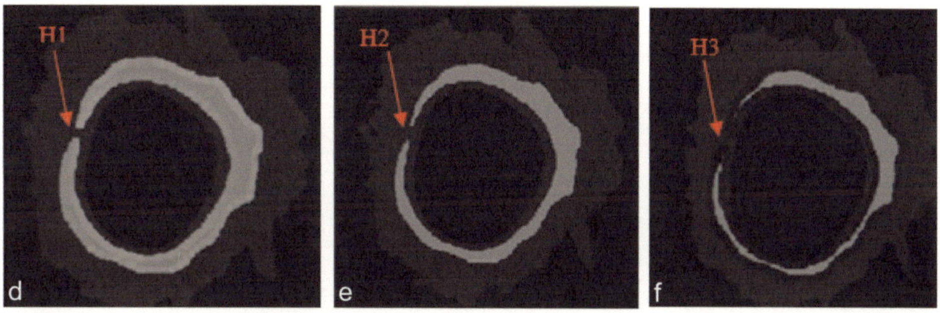

Figure 9.
Denoised USCT with k-means algorithm combined with the morphologic algorithm: (d) H1 fracture defect detection in USCT image, (e) H2 fracture defect detection in USCT image, (f) H3 fracture defect detection in USCT image.

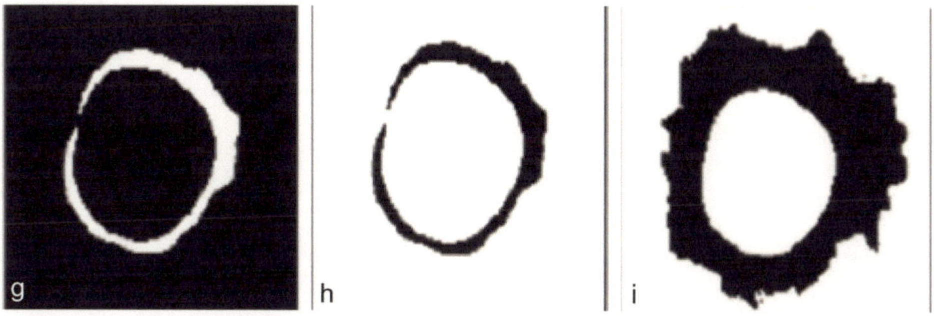

Figure 10.
Denoised USCT with k-means algorithm combined with morphologic algorithm and Otsu algorithms: (g) cortical bone detection, (h) cortical bone detection with enhanced PSNR, (i) medullary cavity detection.

independent of the other. We are interested in the internal region which is the medullary cavity with a diameter of 0.8 cm. These results are similar to the reality measures where the cortical bone width D2 is about 3 mm, as given in **Figure 8 (b)** and the cancellous bone represents a D3 width of 1 mm as depicted in **Figure 9(d)**.

5.2 PSNR results

The PSNR results provided in **Table 1** demonstrate the best result with a value of 25.15 with an implemented Haar wavelet. However, a value of 13.08 is recorded with k-means combined with the morphologic algorithms and Otsu method. In general, image areas with higher PSNR and CNR estimates indicate having better contrast resolution [23]. The PSNR is important as it is a good measure of image quality. In detecting lesions in the body, however, a high PSNR alone will not guarantee that sufficient contrast exists to make the lesion detectable. The CNR between the lesion and background is important as it serves as a quantitative metric for low-contrast lesion detection: The higher the CNR between the lesion and the background, the more likely the lesion detection [24, 25].

5.3 Time process

As shown in **Figure 11**, the time execution process is about 33 s while time execution with k-means combined with the Otsu and morphologic algorithms is about 1.8 s.

Algorithm	Image	Size	PSNR
—	Source	256*256	17.87
Haar Wavelet (**Figures 6**, and 7)	Image LL	64*64	16.18
Proposed Algorithm (**Figures 8–10**)	Image LH	64*64	**24.65**
	Image HL	64*64	**25.15**
	Image HH	64*64	22.98
	Image LH1	128*128	22.04
	Image HL1	128*128	21.38
	Image HH1	128*128	19.15
	Image (a)	256*256	10.62
	Image (b)	256*256	10.94
	Image (c)	256*256	11.32
	Image (d)	256*256	**13.08**
	Image (e)	256*256	13.11
	Image (f)	256*256	13.14
	Image (g)	256*256	11.36
	Image (h)	256*256	11.42

Table 1.
PSNR results.

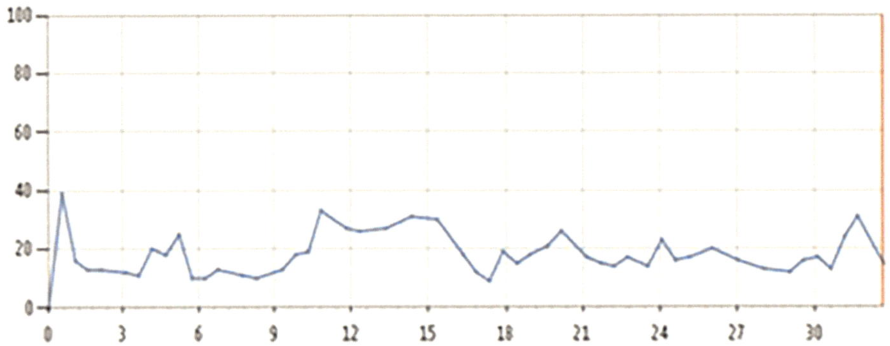

Figure 11.
Time process.

6. Discussions

6.1 Comparative study with related work

A comparative study with the state of the art is depicted in **Table 2**. Our implemented Haar wavelet shows a PSNR enhancement of 7.27 dB compared to the original image. Compared to that found by [2, 5], we have gained an enhancement with a result of 43%, outperforming the related work. In the discrete wavelet transform, one approximation can be further split, as it will remove the noise from images, but for higher noise, it will lose the details and create irregularities in the edges [26, 27]. In this context, we have used the 2D Haar wavelet decomposition to detect osteopathologies, we have to detect edges for distance measurements between bones. As a result, we have improved the PSNR and we have detected external edges, but the

Parameters	Our Work	[5] 2017	[3] 2019
PSNR	25.15	low	21.17
Edge detection	++++	———	+++ +
Region detection	++++	———	+++
Diagnostic detection	+ ++++	——	++
		———	++

Table 2.
Comparative study with related works.

fracture has not been detected. With our hybrid proposed algorithms, we have detected it from the bone image. Consequently, we have outperformed [2, 5] detecting pathologies from USCT images. In 2019 [3], the authors achieved a USCT PSNR value of 21.17 dB. We outperform them with a PSNR enhancement value of 4 dB. In addition, our denoised images represent a high USCT image quality and we have produced a free USCT database, given the difficulty to have a big data of USCT images.

6.1.1 Edge detection

If we assimilate the method of the Haar wavelet transform with visual C++ with the sliding window algorithm using MATLB [11, 12], we can say that we have made a net automatic edge detection and we have improved the resolution. The increase in the USCT imaging process utilizing only signal processing cannot be isolated. The way to enhance the resolution of the image [5], we can detect some bone abnormalities. First, the associated signals are treated before processing the image reconstruction. Afterward, the automatic image processing tool and precision are used. This will be the right way for the method perspective.

6.1.2 Time execution with visual C++ and python

We can say that we have reduced the time of execution of the image to 1.8 seconds. The implemented Haar wavelet algorithm is faster than the one proposed by Lasaygues in 2006. Comparing our time execution with the run time using Matlab. We have saved and gained with about 5.45 times. However, with k-means, Python runtime is about 1.8 seconds. Thus, our proposed k-means algorithm is the best method to save time compared to that found with the algorithm of the Haar wavelet. On the other hand, we must think of a deep learning algorithm that combines the neural network and the genetic algorithm to help accelerate the time execution by its implementation on a Graphic Processor Unit (GPU) system.

6.1.3 Region detection

Comparing our work done with the suggested algorithm and the method of classification with the Laboratory of Mechanic and Acousttics (LMA) work [5, 12] done with the sliding window, the present error to determine the bone cortical area is roughly between 4% and 20%. It is very high. However, our proposed algorithm aims to detect different regions of interest, as depicted in **Figures 9** and **10**.

6.1.4 Results validations

A comparative study with ground truth: To validate our results, a comparative study has been done with an echographic image of human bones. As illustrated in **Figure 12**, multiple structures of an ultrasonic bone have not been detected because of the issue of echographic frequencies to perforate bones.

In the ground truth, the used bone to be imaged is a real adult Padilla bone with a fracture of three levels (H1, H2 and H3) as depicted in **Figure 5**. The lengths of these fracture diameters are approximately similar to those lengths found with our proposed algorithm. Moreover, the width of the cancellous and cortical bone as well as the diameter of the medullary cavity is similar to the ground truth width with an error of + − 1 mm. Indeed, this similarity of diameter measurements indicates the performance of our used method.

Our implemented Haar wavelet using the FMC interface and Visual C++ can be applied to various tomographic images, such as cerebral computed tomography (CT) and retinal vessel computed tomography for edge and pathology detection. **Figure 13** shows the performance of our implemented Haar wavelet algorithm.

Our k-means combined with the morphologic and the Otsu algorithms have resolved the problem of adult bone region detection and outperformed the wavelet

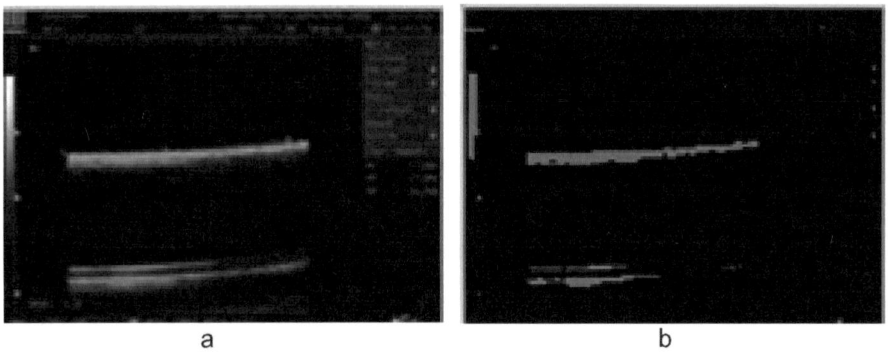

Figure 12.
Echographic bone image segmentation results: (a) Echographic bone image, (b) segmented image.

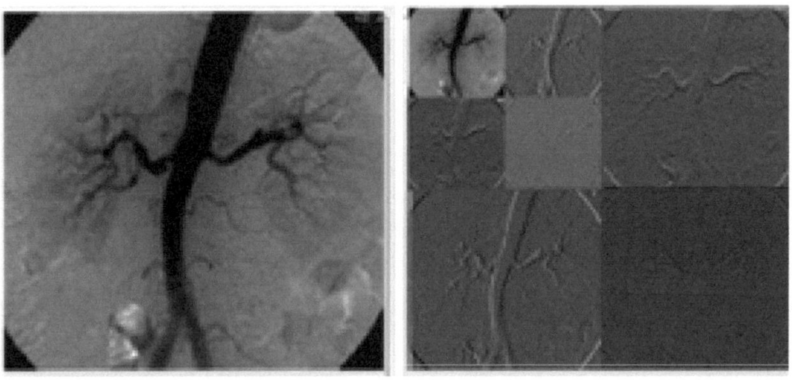

Figure 13.
Vessels retinal detection in CT image.

signal processing method [2, 5]. Furthermore, it has detected osteopathologies such as fractures with its highest ability to remove noise and save time.

7. Conclusion

In this chapter, an improved hardware/software design has been used. In the beginning, we have presented the USCT prototype to avoid any x-ray exposure to human beings. Thus, we have had USCT noisy images. As a solution, we have implemented the Haar wavelet and improved k-means combined with the morphologic and Otsu algorithms. It is a very crucial method that has solved the problem of noise in USCT images. Therefore, with this approach, the resolution has been improved, the time execution has been reduced, the noise has been removed and we have gained automatic diagnosis detection. In fact, we have to say that compared to what has been already published, the method presents more resolved results. With unsupervised developed k-means, the USCT image is segmented into three anatomic regions of interest, namely, the cortical and cancellous bone and the medullary cavity. These regions will be the labeled features of bone tomographic images. The next step will be devoted to the combination of unsupervised deep learning and supervised deep learning to automatically classify our image data into two classes (pathologic bone images and healthy bone images) and for the extraction of the region of interest from big data of bone tomographic images. Besides, interest will be given to the reconstruction of 3D images.

Funding

This study was funded by the Ministry of High Education and Scientific Research in Tunisia and the Laboratory of Mechanics and Acoustics in Marseille.

Conflict of interest

Authors declare that they have no conflict of interest.

Ethical Approval

This chapter does not contain any studies with human participants performed by any of the authors.

Informed consent

This chapter does not contain patient data.

Author details

Marwa Fradi[1], Kais Bouallegue[2], Philippe Lasaygues[3]* and Mohsen Machhout[1]

1 Physic Department of Faculty of Sciences of Monastir, Laboratory of Electronics and Microelectronics, Monastir University, Tunisia

2 Department of Electrical Engineering, Higher Institute of Applied Sciences and Technology of Sousse, Sousse University, Tunisia

3 CNRS Marseille Central Station, LMA, Aix Marseille University, Marseille, France

*Address all correspondence to: marwa.fradi@gmail.com

References

[1] Lasaygues P, Lefebvre J. Bone imaging by low frequency ultrasonic reflection tomography. In: Hallowell M, Wells PNT, editors. Acoustical Imaging. Vol. 25. Boston: Kluwer Academic Publishers; 2002

[2] Lasaygues P. Assessing the cortical thickness of long bone shafts in children, using two-dimensional ultrasonic. Ultrasound in Medicine & Biology. 2006;**32**(8):1215-1227

[3] Torres JSM et al. Linear filtering method for bone structures in computerized ultrasonic tomography images. In: 2019 XXII Symposium on Image, Signal Processing and Artificial Vision (STSIVA). Colombia: IEEE. 2019: 1-4

[4] Cronan JJ. Ultrasound: is there a future in diagnostic imaging. Journal of the American College of Radiology. 2006;**3**:645-646

[5] Lasaygues P, Guillermin R, Metwally K, Fernandez S, Balasse L, Petit P, et al. Contrast resolution enhancement of Ultrasonic Computed Tomography using a wavelet-based method – Preliminary results in bone imaging. Speyer, Germany modified: International Workshop on Medical Ultrasound Tomography; 2017 Avril 2018

[6] Dera D, Bouaynaya N, Hassan M. Fathallah-Shaykh automated, "Robust Image Segmentation: Level Set Method Using Nonnegative Matrix Factorization with Application to Brain MRI". Society for Mathematic al Biology, Springer; 2016

[7] Mittal K, Shekhar A, Singh P, Kumar M. Brain tumour extraction using otsu based threshold segmentation. International Journal of Advanced Research in Computer Science and Software Engineering. 2017;7(4)

[8] Vaishali S, Kishan Rao K and Subba Rao GV. A review on noise reduction methods for brain MRI images. 2015 International Conference on Signal Processing and Communication Engineering Systems. IEEE. 2015

[9] Krithiga R. Reduction of speckle-noise in ultrasound images using MMM filter. International Journal of Pure and Applied Mathematics. 2017;**113**:84-95

[10] Dahdouh S. Filtrage, segmentation et suivi d'images échographiques applications cliniques [thèse]. Orsay, France: université Paris Sud; 2011

[11] Lasaygues P, Lefbvre JP, Guillermin R, Kaftandjian V, Berteau JP, Pithroux M, et al. "Advanced Ultrasonic tomography of children's bones", Acoustical Imaging. Vol. 31. Springer Science + media B.V; 2012

[12] Mallat S, Hwang WL. Singularity detection and processing with wavelets. IEEE Transactions on Information Theory. 1992;**38**(2):617-643

[13] Bruni V, Piccoli B, Vitulano D. A fast computation method for time scale signal denoising. Signal, image and video processing. 2009;**3**(1):63-83

[14] Alan Jose, Ravi S, Sambath M. Brain tumour segmentation using k-means clustering and fuzzy c-means algorithm and its area calculation. International Journal of Scientific Engineering And Technology Research. 2015;**4**(10): 1805-1808

[15] Dhanachandra N, Manglem K, Chanu YJ. Image Segmentation using

K-means Clustering Algorithm and Subtractive Clustering Algorithm. The Eleventh International Multi-Conference on Information Processing, (IMCIP-2015). Elsevier. 2015;**54**:764-771

[16] Kalavathi P. Brain tissue segmentation in MR brain images using multiple Otsu's thresholding technique. In: 2013 8th International Conference on Computer Science Education. IEEE; 2013. pp. 639-642

[17] Mahendran SK, Baboo S. Enhanced Automatic X Ray Bone Image Segmentation using Wavelets and Morphological Operators. Vol. 6. 2011 International Conference on Information and Electronics Engineering (IPCSIT); 2011. pp. 125-129

[18] Dubey AK, Gupta U, Jain S. Analysis of k-means clustering approach on the breast cancer Wisconsin dataset. International Journal of Computer Assisted Radiology and Surgery. 2016; **11**(11):2033-2047

[19] Divya BNG, Sowjanya K. Otsu's Method Of Image Segmentation Using Particle Swarm Optimization Technique. International Journal Of Scientific Engineering And Technology Research. 2015;**4**(10):1805-1808

[20] Liu S. Image Segmentation Technology of the Ostu Method for Image Materials Based on Binary PSO Algorithm. Advances in Computer Science, Intelligent System and Environment, Springer, CSISE 2011, AISC. 2011;**104**:415-419

[21] Kalpana Chauhan ML, Dewal RKC, Rohit M. Regurgitation Area Segmentation Using the Particle Swarm Optimization and Multilevel Threshold Selection. International Journal of Computer and Communication Engineering. 2015;**4**(4):282-289

[22] Zahara E, Fan SS, Tsai D. Optimal multithresholding using a hybrid optimization approach. Pattern Recognition Letters. 2005;**26**:1082-1095

[23] Habib W, Siddiqui AM, Touqir I. Wavelet based despeckling of multiframe optical coherence tomography data using similarity measure and anisotropic diffusion filtering. Shanghai: 2013 IEEE International Conference on Bioinformatics and Biomedicine (BIBM); 2013. pp. 330-333

[24] Liao Y-Y, Jui-Chen WU, Li C-H, Yeh C-K. Texture feature analysis for breast ultrasound image enhancement. Ultrasonic Imaging. 2011;**33**:264-278

[25] Hendrick RE. Signal, Noise, Signal-to-Noise, and Contrast-to-Noise Ratio, Breast MRI. Springer; 2008. pp. 93-111

[26] Diwaar M, Kumar M. CT image denoising using NLM and correlation-based wavelet packet thresholding. IET Image Processing; 2018

[27] Borsdorf A, Raupach R, Hornegger J. Multiple CT-reconstructions for locally adaptive anisotropic wavelet denoising. International Journal of Computer Assisted Radiology and Surgery. 2008; **2**(5):255-264

Chapter 9

Soft Tissue Image Reconstruction Using Diffuse Optical Tomography

Umamaheswari K, Shrichandran G.V. and Jeba Derwin D.

Abstract

Diffuse optical tomography (DOT) is favorable to analyze physical records in organic tissue with a specific purpose by means of a method related to the forward problem and the inverse solution. This study develops morphological soft tissue realization using an image reconstruction algorithm constructed on multifrequency DOT in Near-Infra-Red (NIR) wavelength. Forward problem solves the Diffusion Equation to compute the optical flux distributed in the phantom geometrical model. Inverse solution, the image is reconstructed using the absorption and reduced scattered coefficients under different boundary conditions. The inverse image reconstruction algorithm is tested for several simulation, with variation in background contrast ratios for different frequencies are simulated. The image reconstruction in DOT eliminates spatial resolution by optimizing source-detector separation and modulation intensities of the source.

Keywords: diffuse optical tomography, near infrared wavelength, forward model, inverse model, soft tissue, image reconstruction

1. Introduction

Forward problems are used to explain the propagation of photons within a tissue and to calculate the optical flux at the tissue boundary. The reconstruction of the tissue image is the inverse problem, from light measurements at the boundary phantom surface, tissue absorption, scattering factors, and optical flow [1]. The inverse problem is difficult to solve due to the issue of fairness. This indicates that the problem is not properly configured. Appropriate problem characteristics include the existence of a solution, the uniqueness of the solution, and the constant reliance on the data [2]. The third property determines the stability of the solution and is important for determining the inverse problem. The ill-posedness problem occurs when the problem solution does not depend on the data indefinitely. Small changes to the data can make a big difference in the solution in this case. Regularization method is used to solve this problem, which is a regularization method that introduces additional information in order to create well-posed data [3, 4]. Diffuse optical imaging [5–8] is a technique that uses an MRI scan and X-rays generate spatially decomposed images and uses high-resolution complementary structural information to improve low-resolution functional images. A set of fiber optics has been connected the object's boundary in experimental systems. The light source was a near-infrared (NIR) laser source that was diffused on the phantom, the scattered rays were measured with a photodetector [9]. Regularization method [10] is used to remove the ill-posedness, with the Levenberg–Marquardt method (LM) being one of the most commonly used methods. Following the regularization process, the Split Bregman reconstruction method [10–12] is used to reconstruct a soft tissue image. The sparsity regularization technique for image reconstruction in DOT is described by Bo Bi et al. [9]. Gehre et al. [13] investigates the possibility of sparsity constraints in the inverse problem of deriving distributed conductivity from critical potential measurements in electrical impedance tomography (EIT). Chamorro et al. [14] proposed an Algebraic reconstruction technique—Split Bregman (ART-SB) algorithm solved the L1-regularized problem. Wang et al. evaluated the Split Bregman iteration algorithm for the L1 norm regularization inverse problem in electrical impedance tomography. Figueiredo et al. [15] investigated the use of Split Bregman iterative algorithms for the L1-norm regularized inverse problem of electrical impedance constrained quadratic programming ill-tomography formulation.

2. Inverse model solution

In most cases, the measurement data in DOT reconstruction is derived from the numerical solution of the forward problem. Regularization techniques are used to eliminate the obtrusive inverse problem variables. The measurement technology of optical devices is so limited that their existence cannot be accurately determined from all angles. Instead, it gets the average contact angle data for the phantom. The purpose is to reconstruct the image from known scattering and absorption coefficients, which are assumed to be known. The reconstructed result is obtained by comparing the true value to the measured value. A variety of practical reconstruction algorithms have been developed in tomography to implement the process of reconstructing a 3D object from a projection [16]. These algorithms are mainly based on the mathematics of statistical knowledge of the data acquisition process and the geometry of the data imaging system [17].

2.1 Levenburg-Marquardt method

The inverse problem is used to reconstruct an image in the following ways by estimating the scattering coefficient, absorption coefficient, and optical flux [18, 19]. The noise level is present in the actual measurement; both actual measurement data and actual data are shown here [9]. The following nonlinear equation is used to solve the inverse problem of DOT for i = 1, … …,s. Assume you know the total attenuation coefficient.

$$F_i(\mu_t, \mu_s) = M_i^{\delta}, (\mu_t, \mu_s) \in D \quad (1)$$

The inverse problem of DOT is inappropriate and uses regularization techniques to reconstruct the image [8], i.e. the Tikhonov functional feature that is minimized for the coefficient. R (μ_S) is a penalty function for regularization [4]. By analyzing the minimization problem,

$$J(\mu_s) = \frac{1}{2}\sum_{i=1}^{s} \|F_i(\mu_s) - M_i\|^2_{L^2(\partial X)} + \alpha R(\mu_s) \quad (2)$$

Over the set,

$$Q_{ad} = \{\mu_s \in L^\infty(X)\} \tag{3}$$

$$\inf_{\mu_s \in Q_{ad}} J(\mu_s) \tag{4}$$

The standard reconstruction method is considered using Eqs. (3) and (4).

2.1.1 Standard reconstruction

Traditional norm-squared penalties are believed to reduce the following functions,

$$R(\mu_s) = \frac{1}{2}\|\nabla\mu_s\|^2_{L^2(X)} \tag{5}$$

$$J(\mu_s) = \frac{1}{2}\sum_{i=1}^{s}\|F_i(\mu_s) - M_i^\delta\|^2_{L^2(\partial x)} + \frac{\alpha}{2}\|\mu_s - \mu_s^*\|^2_{L^2(X)} \tag{6}$$

In the inverse problem of DOT, the Levenberg–Marquardt regularization method [20] is used. The forward operator is linearized around the initial estimation for each;

$$F_i(\mu_s) = F_i\left(\mu_s^0\right)\left(\mu_s - \mu_s^0\right) + R\left(\mu_s^0; i\right) \tag{7}$$

where Eq. (7) denotes the Taylor remainder for the linearization around and the Frechet derivative is obtained by substituting the above equation and ignoring the higher-order remainder [13].

$$\inf_{\mu_s \in D} \frac{1}{2}\sum_{i=1}^{s}\|F_i\left(\mu_s^0\right) + F_i'\left(\mu_s^0\right)\left(\mu_s - \mu_s^0\right) - M_i^\delta\|^2_{L^2(\partial x)} \tag{8}$$

The Euler equation for discrete problems is

$$\sum_{i=1}^{s} F_i'\left(\mu_s^0\right)^*\left(F_i\left(\mu_s^0\right) + F_i'\left(\mu_s - \mu_s^0\right) - M_i^\delta\right) + \alpha\left(\mu_s - \mu_s^0\right) = 0 \tag{9}$$

Solving this (9) yields the final Equation [16].
That is,

$$\left(\sum_{i=1}^{s} F_i'\left(\mu_s^0\right)^* F_i'\left(\mu_s^0\right) + \alpha I\right)\left(\mu_s - \mu_s^0\right) = -\sum_{i=1}^{s} F_i'\left(\mu_s^0\right)^*\left(F_i\left(\mu_s^0\right) - M_i^\delta\right) \tag{10}$$

where I is the identity matrix to solve the new estimate of μ_s based on the initial guess μ_s^0.

2.2 Sparsity reconstruction

Sparsity reconstruction function can be minimized as

$$J(\mu_s) = \frac{1}{2}\sum_{i=1}^{s}\|F_i(\mu_s) - M_i^\delta\|^2_{L^2(\partial x)} + \frac{\alpha}{2}\|\mu_s\|_{l_1} \tag{11}$$

Such that d= $\boldsymbol{\mu_s}$. Decouple the L1 and L2 portion in (11). The constrained problem [10].

where $\beta > 0$ is a split parameter, and iteratively, the next subproblem can be solved as [3, 4].

$$\left(\mu_s^k, d^k\right) = argmin \frac{1}{2}\sum_{i=1}^{s} \|F_i(\mu_s) - M_i^\delta\|^2_{L^2(\partial x)} + \alpha\|d\|_{l_1} + \frac{\beta}{2}\left\|d - \mu_s - b_d^{k-1}\right\|_2^2, \quad (12)$$

$$b_d^k = b_d^{k-1} + \mu_s^k - d^k$$

By dividing the minimization of (12) and d separately, the sub-problem can be minimized.

1. Consider

$$\mu_s^k = argmin \frac{1}{2}\sum_{i=1}^{s} \|F_i(\mu_s) - M_i^\delta\|^2_{L^2(\partial x)} + \frac{\beta}{2}\left\|d^{k-1} - \mu_s - b_d^{k-1}\right\|_2^2 \quad (13)$$

2. Consider

$$d^k = \underset{d}{argmin}\|d\|_{l_1} + \frac{\beta}{2}\left\|d - \mu_s^k - b_d^{k-1}\right\|_2^2 \quad (14)$$

3. Consider

$$b_d^k = b_d^{k-1} + \mu_s^k - d^k \quad (15)$$

Minimize $\boldsymbol{\mu_s^k}, \boldsymbol{d^k}$ as

$$\mu_s^k = \underset{\mu_s}{argmin} \frac{1}{2}\sum_{i=1}^{s} \|F_i(\mu_s^{k-1}) + F_i'(\mu_s^{k-1})(\mu_s - \mu_s^{k-1}) - M_i^\delta\|_2^2 + \frac{\beta}{2}\left\|d^{k-1} - \mu_s - b_d^{k-1}\right\|_2^2 \quad (16)$$

The variational equation is given as

$$\left(\sum_{i=1}^{s} F_i'(\mu_s^{k-1})^* F_i'(\mu_s^{k-1}) + \beta I\right)(\mu_s - \mu_s^{k-1})$$
$$= \beta\left(d^{k-1} - \mu_s^{k-1} - b_d^{k-1}\right) + \sum_{i=1}^{s} F_i'(\mu_s^{k-1})^* (F_i(\mu_s^{k-1}) - M_i^\delta) \quad (17)$$

L1 is solved efficiently by the contraction operator; that is

$$d^k = shrink\left(\mu_s^k + b_d^{k-\mathbf{1}}, \frac{\alpha}{\beta}\right) \quad (18)$$

Where the shrinkage operator is defined as

$$Shrink(x,t) = \text{sign}(x)\max(|x|-\text{t},0) = \begin{cases} x-t, x \geq t, \\ 0, |x| < t, \\ x+t, x \leq -t \end{cases} \tag{19}$$

The rate of spilt Bregman is highly dependent on the rate of dissolution $\boldsymbol{F}'_i(\boldsymbol{\mu}_s)$.

3. Levenberg: Marquardt algorithm

Because the DOT image has poor spatial resolution due to severe ill-posedness, the regularization technique is used in conjunction with reconstruction algorithms to reconstruct the images.

Algorithm

Input: Set the initial estimation μ_s^0; The regularization parameter α,β.
Output: Approximate minimizer μ_s.
for k = 1, … … … .k do.
for i = 1, … … … .s do.
i. Compute the Frechet derivative $F'_i(\mu_s^k)$, and $F'_i(\mu_s^k)^*$.
end for.
i. Compute $\sum_{i=1}^{s} F'_i(\mu_s^k)^* F'_i(\mu_s^k)$ + αI, and $-\sum_{i=1}^{s} F'_i(\mu_s^k)^*(F'_i(\mu_s^k)\text{-}M_i^\delta)$.
ii. Update μ_s^{k+1} by solving the linearization problem

$$\left(\sum_{i=1}^{s} F'_i(\mu_s^k)^* F'_i(\mu_s^k) + \alpha\text{I}\right)(\mu_s - \mu_s^k) = -\sum_{i=1}^{s} F'_i(\mu_s^k)^* \left(F'_i(\mu_s^k) - M_i^\delta\right)$$

iii. Check the stopping criterion.
end for.

---

4. Spilt Bregman algorithm

Input: set the initial guess $\boldsymbol{\mu}_0^s$;
Regularization parameters $\boldsymbol{\alpha} > \mathbf{0}, \boldsymbol{\beta} > \mathbf{0}; \boldsymbol{d}^0 = \boldsymbol{b}_d^0 = \mathbf{0}$ and margins of error $\boldsymbol{\varepsilon}$.
Output: Outputs an approximate value $\boldsymbol{\mu}_s = \boldsymbol{\mu}_s^k$.
While $\|\boldsymbol{\mu}_s^k - \boldsymbol{\mu}_s^{k-1}\| > \boldsymbol{\varepsilon}$ do

i. For each **1** $\boldsymbol{i}$ $\boldsymbol{s}$, calculate (17) to be acquired $\boldsymbol{\mu}_s^k$;

ii. $d^k = \boldsymbol{shrink}\left(\mu_s^k + b_d^{k-1}, \alpha/\beta\right)$;

iii. Calculate $b_d^k = b_d^{k-1} + \mu_s^k - d^k$

iv. $\mu_s = \mu_s^k$

end while.

The split Bregman method entails locating the Fréchet derivative, which is nothing more than the first order derivative function. The algorithm is built with regularization parameters in mind.

5. Simulation result of image reconstruction

The reconstructed image can be obtained using the Levenberg–Marquardt algorithm by providing optical flux, scattering coefficient, and absorption coefficient values, which are then compared to distinguish between normal soft tissue and cancer-affected tissue. The forward mesh has more nodes to extract all of the optical parameters of the tissue, whereas the inverse mesh has fewer nodes for reconstruction. As shown in **Figure 1**, the forward mesh has 1097 nodes and 2095 elements, and the reverse mesh has 286 nodes and 522 elements.

Figure 2 depicts the reconstruction based on absorption and scattering coefficient measurements. The image is reconstructed using optical properties of human tissue such as absorption coefficient and scattering coefficient (and (r) = 2). The reconstructed image is based on the absorption and scattering coefficient values. It is possible to predict normal tissue and cancer-affected tissue by examining the reconstructed image with absorption and scattering coefficients. When the absorption and scattering coefficients are higher, the tumor is classified as malignant or benign soft tissue tumor.

The split Bregman algorithm with sparsity regularization efficiently solves the DOT image reconstruction problem. **Figure 3** depicts a Spilt Bregman reconstruction from scattering coefficients. The scattering coefficient value distinguishes the variation of abnormal tissue to normal tissue. According to **Figure 3**, the abnormal tissue scattering coefficient ranges from 150 to 210, whereas the normal tissue scattering coefficient ranges from 0 to 20. When compared to other reconstruction algorithms, the Bregman algorithm produces more accurate results. The reconstructed image's

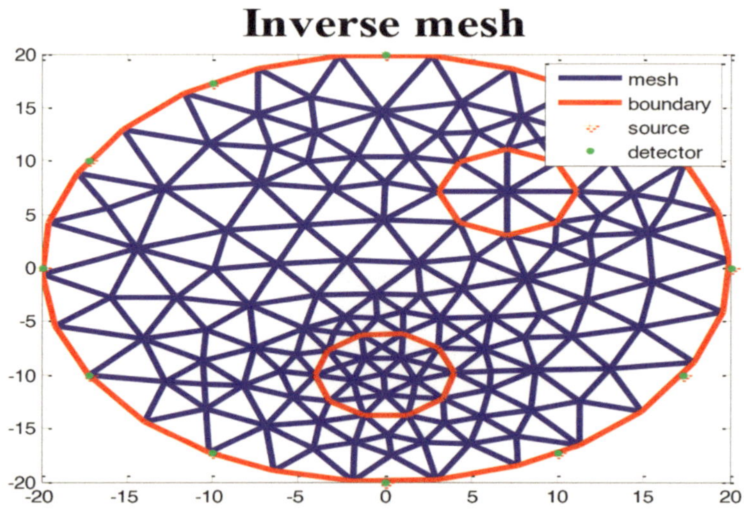

Figure 1.
Mesh diagram of inverse problem.

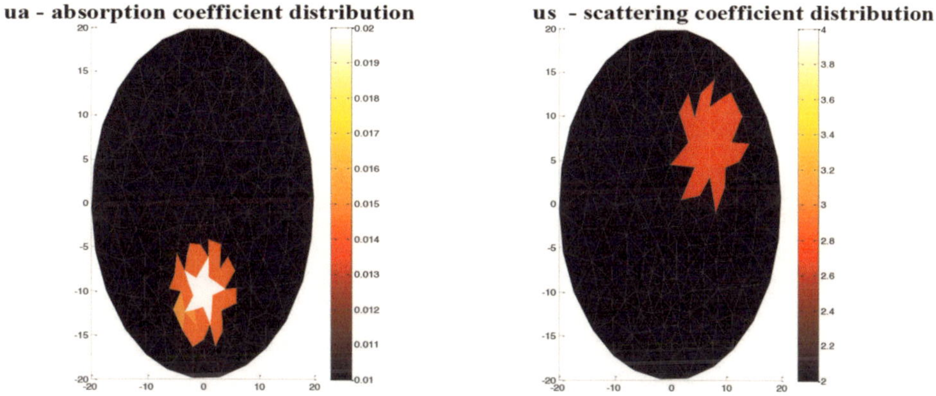

Figure 2.
Levenberg–Marquardt regularization and standard reconstruction.

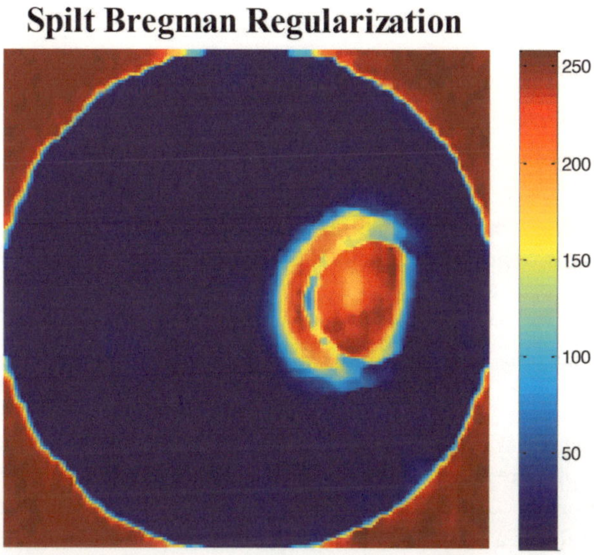

Figure 3.
Spilt Bregman regularization with sparsity reconstruction.

resolution is determined by calculating the signal-to-noise ratio (SNR), contrast-to-noise ratio (CNR), relative solution error norm (RE), and CPU time. SNR is calculated as follows:

$$SNR = 10\,log_{10}\left(\frac{P_{signal}}{P_{noise}}\right) \tag{20}$$

The CNR is a metric used to assess image quality. The mean and standard deviation values are used to calculate it. CNR is calculated as follows:

$$CNR = \frac{S_A - S_B}{\sigma_0} \tag{21}$$

Parameters	Split Bregman method	Gauss Newton
SNR	9.2327	4.3402
CNR	66.947	39.743
RE	0.0508	0.2141
CPU time (s)	72.231	75.197

Table 1.
Performance analysis of reconstruction algorithms.

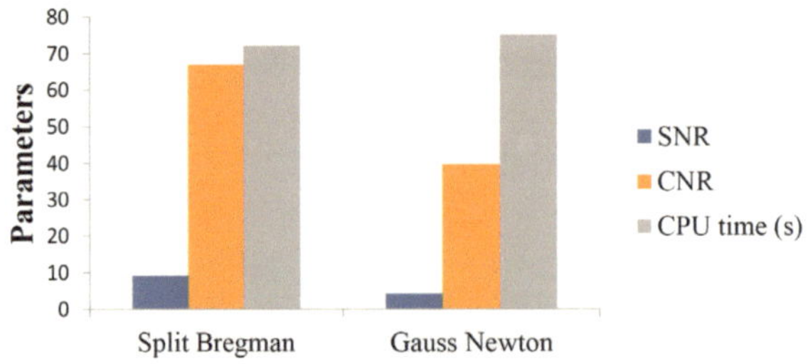

Figure 4.
Performance analysis of reconstruction algorithms.

where are the image signal intensities and is the standard deviation of pure image noise. The Relative solution error norm is computed as follows:

$$E = \frac{\left\| \mu_S - \mu_S^{true} \right\|_2}{\left\| \mu_s^{true} \right\|_2} \tag{22}$$

Table 1 compares parameters used to evaluate the performance of reconstruction algorithms. The Split Bregman method has a higher SNR than the Gauss Newton algorithm and improves CNR more than the Gauss Newton method. To achieve better performance, the RE of a reconstructed image should be low. Because the Gauss Newton method has a high RE value, it is not an optimal solution for image reconstruction. Finally, when compared to the Gauss Newton method, the Split Bregman method requires less CPU time to execute. The graph of the performance analysis of the Split Bregman and Gauss Newton algorithms is shown in **Figure 4**.

6. Conclusion

The solution to diffuse light transport through tissues is provided by iterative nonlinear reconstruction of diffuse optical tomography using a finite element forward model. The efficiency of the forward solver has a significant impact on reconstruction performance and reconstruction time, which is critical in making optical tomography a viable imaging modality in clinical diagnosis. Standard regularization (Levenburg-Marquadt) with a small anisotropy factor identifies the scattering coefficient better than sparsity regularization in the inverse model. Sparsity regularization (Split Bregman) localizes the inclusion position and has high anisotropy factor g while forward-peaking region. The absorption and scattering coefficient values of the reconstructed it is analyzed to determine the difference between normal soft tissue and cancerous tissue. Increasing the number of measurements by adding more photo detectors is one way to improve the quality of a reconstructed image. Finally, a regularization technique is used to remove the ill-posedness problem, and a Split Bregman reconstruction algorithm is used to achieve a high-resolution image.

Author details

Umamaheswari K[1]*, Shrichandran G.V.[2] and Jeba Derwin D.[1]

1 Department of Electronics and Communication Engineering, SRM TRP Engineering College, Trichy, Tamil Nadu, India

2 Department of Computer Science Engineering, SRM Institute of Science and Technology, Chennai, Tamil Nadu, India

*Address all correspondence to: umaragsug@gmail.com

References

[1] Arridge SR. Optical tomography in medical imaging. Inverse Problems. 1999;**15**(2):R41-R93

[2] Nocedal J, Wright SJ. Numerical Optimization. Springer Series in Operations Research. New York, NY, USA: Springer; 1999

[3] Bush J. Bregman Algorithms [M. S. thesis]. Santa Barbara, Calif, USA: University of California; 2011

[4] Wang J, Ma J, Han B, Li Q. Split Bregman iterative algorithm for sparse reconstruction of electrical impedance tomography. Signal Processing. 2012; **92**(12):2952-2961

[5] Uma Maheswari K, Sathiyamoorthy S. Soft tissue optical property extraction for carcinoma cell detection in diffuse optical tomography system under boundary element condition. Optik-International Journal for Light and Electron Optics. 2016;**127**(3):1281-1290

[6] Uma Maheswari K, Sathiyamoorthy S. Stein's unbiased risk estimate regularization (SURE) for diffuse optical tomography (DOT) system enhances image reconstruction with high contrast to noise ratio (CNR). International Journal of Applied Engineering Research. 2015;**10**(24): 21186-21191

[7] Brigade S, Powell S, Cooper RJ, et al. Evaluating real-time image reconstruction in diffuse optical tomography using physiologically realistic test data. Biomedical Optical Express. 2015;**6**(12):4719-4737

[8] Cai JF, Osher S, Shen ZW. Linearized Bregman iterations for compressed sensing. Mathematics of Computation. 2009;**78**(267):1515-1536

[9] Bi B, Han B, Han W, Tang J, Li L. Image reconstruction for diffuse optical tomography based on radiative transfer equation. Computational and Mathematical Methods in Medicine. 2015;**2015**:286161

[10] Goldstein T, Osher S. The Split Bregman method for L1 regularized problems. SIAM Journal on Imaging Sciences. 2009;**2**(2):323-343

[11] Tyin W, Osher S, Durban J, Goldfarb D. Bregman iterative algorithms for l1 minimization with applications to compressed sensing. SIAM Journal on Imaging Science. 2008; **1**(1):143-168

[12] Yin WT. Analysis and generalization of the linearized Bregman model. SIAM Journal on Imaging Science. 2010;**3**(4): 856-877

[13] Gehre M, Kluth T, Lipponen A, et al. Sparsity reconstruction in electrical impedance tomography: An experimental evaluation. Journal of Computational and Applied Mathematics. 2012;**236**(8):2126-2136

[14] Chamorro-servent J, Abascal JFPJ, Aguirre J, Arridge S, Correia T, Ripoll J, et al. Use of split Bergman denoising for iterative reconstruction in fluorescence diffuse optical tomography. Journal of Biomedical Optics. 2013;**18**(7):076016

[15] Figueiredo MAT, Nowak RD, Wright SJ. Gradient projection for sparse reconstruction: Application to compressed sensing and other inverse problems. IEEE Journal of Selected Topics in Signal Processing. 2007;**1**(4):586-597

[16] Kaipio J, Somersalo E. Statistical and Computational Inverse Problems. New York, NY, USA: Springer; 2005

[17] Mudeng V, Nisa W, Suprapto SS. Computational image reconstruction for multi-frequency diffuse optical tomography. Journal of King Saud University-Computer and Information Sciences. 2021. DOI: 10.1016/j.jksuci.2020.12.015. In Press

[18] Gibson AP, Hebden JC, Arridge SR. Recent advances in diffuse optical imaging. Physics in Medicine and Biology. 2005;**50**(4):R1

[19] Tang J, Han W, Han B. A theoretical study for RTE-based parameter identification problems. Inverse Problems. 2013;**29**(9):ID095002

[20] Hanke M. The regularizing Levenberg-Marquardt scheme is of optimal order. Journal of Integral Equations and Applications. 2010;**22**(2): 259-283

Chapter 10

Effective EEG Artifact Removal from EEG Signal

Vandana Roy

Abstract

An EEG (electroencephalography) provides insight into the status of the brain's electrical activity. EEG is based on the electrical activity measured in voltage at various sites in the brain. Generally speaking, these signals are non-stationery and time-varying. Various signal processing techniques can be used to examine these signals. Several statistical approaches to EEG data analysis are discussed in this chapter. In this Chapter, Electroencephalograph Signals and their generation process have been discussed; the EEG signal has been compared with fMRI and PET signals. The classification of the EEG signals on the amplitude, frequency, and shape have been elaborated in wave analysis of EEG, and applications of these components are presented. The artifacts of EEG have been explained in detail.

Keywords: EEG, artifacts, wavelet transform, BSS, EEMD

1. Introduction

One of the most complex structures on this earth is the human brain with an estimated approximately weight of 3lbs. The human brain is so much sophisticated that it has given so many brilliant research works which seem superficial at first look likewise ultra-modern supercomputer, aircraft and one of the missile technologies LGM-30G Minuteman-III, etc. [1]. It controls one's whole human body and consists of approximately 100 billion cells, known as a neuron, a part of the human nervous system. These neurons communicate with each other by sending an electrical potential (charge) down the axon and across the synapse to the very next neuron. Since neurons are not connected physically, it uses a chemical messenger entitled neurotransmitters, which crosses the synaptic gap to carry-forward messages to the next neuron [2]. This chemical messenger (neurotransmitters) then activates receptors corresponding to it in the postsynaptic neuron, this action generates postsynaptic currents this process keeps going on for the next synapse. As this communication passes current (electrical potential) using neurotransmitter, a chemical messenger, it can be considered as communication is a process that is electrical and chemical both.

As shown in **Figure 1**, the neurons are activated using an electrochemical concentration gradient, local current flows are produced.

IntechOpen

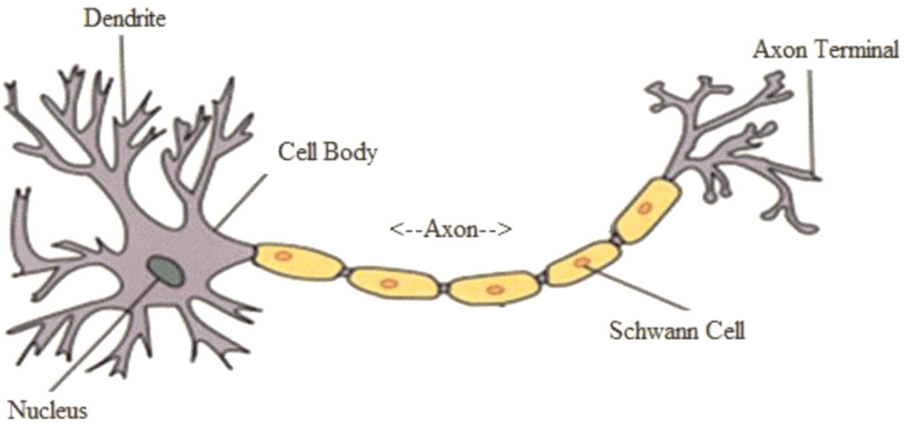

Figure 1.
Typical neurons structure.

1.1 Importance of EEG over fMRI and PET

EEG works as a good tool to explore brain activity and can detect changes within milliseconds. Depending upon the type of neuron, an action potential takes 0.5–130 milliseconds approximately to propagate across a single neuron. Whereas, other methods likewise fMRI and PET has time resolution in terms of seconds and minutes and makes these methods less efficient.

Moreover, EEG directly measures the brain's electrical activity, whilst other methods such as SPECT, fMRI record changes in blood flow, or PET record changes in metabolic activity, which are indirect markers of electrical activity belonging to the brain. The electrical activity is a superposition of the huge number of electrical charges arising from multiple sources likewise brain cells i.e. neurons and artifacts. It is possible to place electrodes inside the human head via surgery for direct measurement from different centers in the human brain, but this is a painful and risky procedure for the subject [3, 4]. However, the desirable technique is to calculate electrical signals of interest invaded on the scalp as shown in the following **Figure 2**.

Signals obtained by an above-maintained process are weighted sums of neuron activity, whose weights depend on the signal path from a specific brain cell to the connected electrodes. Since the same electrical potential is being recorded from more than one electrode, signals being occurred from those electrodes are supposed to be highly correlated [4]. Henceforth, Scientists and Researchers collect these recordings by attachment of tens or hundreds of electrodes, which are positioned in pairs, at various locations on the surface of the subject's head. These electrical potentials (Charges) are tested simultaneously via individuals' channels or amplifiers. Recording for each channel represents the difference in electrical potential between two areas under each electrode's pair [5] as represented in **Figure 3**. In **Figure 3**, the differences between the two electrodes are measured through an operational amplifier for generating EEG signal recording. A machine that is used for this purpose is known as an electroencephalograph, and recordings collected through these amplifiers are known as electroencephalogram (EEG) signals.

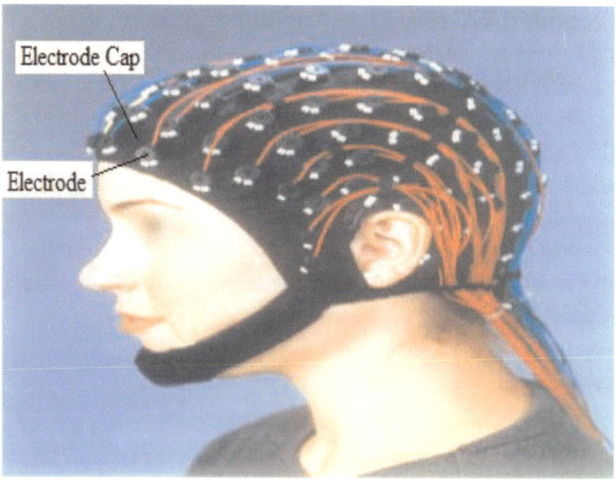

Figure 2.
EEG electrodes placement on a subject, monitoring various sectors of the brain for activities.

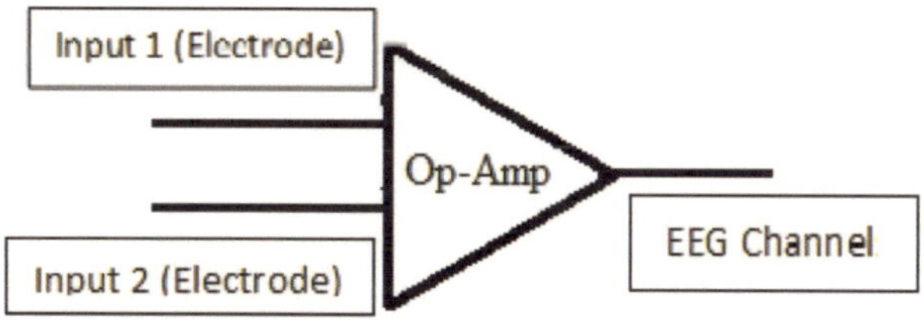

Figure 3.
Differential amplifier for EEG recording/signal.

1.2 Electroencephalograph measuring system

Currently, so many different types of electroencephalographs are available; over which 10–20 system is the internationally standardized method for describing the location of scalp electrodes and is based upon the relationship between an electrode's location and cerebral cortex underlying area and usually employs 21 electrodes. Its positions are determined by dividing the skull into the perimeters by connection of a few reference points lying on the human head.

In this, every perimeter has a letter, that helps in the identification of the lobe, and either a number or another letter for identification of the hemisphere location. Letters that are used are as follows:

1. "F"-Frontal lobe

2. "T"-Temporal lobe

3. "C"-Central lobe

4. "P"-Parietal lobe

5. "O"-Occipital lobe.

Furthermore, numbers (2, 4, 6, 8) refer to the right hemisphere, whereas odd numbers (1, 3, 5, 7) refer to the left hemisphere.

In the below-shown **Figure 4**, the "Z" refers to an electrode placed on the midline; the position of the electrode can be determined by the magnitude of the number, the smaller magnitude represents that electrode is much closer to the midline. The figure given below presents the actual electrode placement on the head and from these points, skull perimeters are measured in the transverse and the median planes [4].

Figure 3.4 presents the system "10" and "20" shows the fact that the actual distances between two adjacent electrodes are in percentage of either 10% or 20% of the three main measurements:

1. nasion, is the delve at the upper portion of the nose, and in level with the eyes.

2. inion, is the bony lump at the base of the skull on the midline of the back of the head.

3. pre-auricular points and circumference of the head.

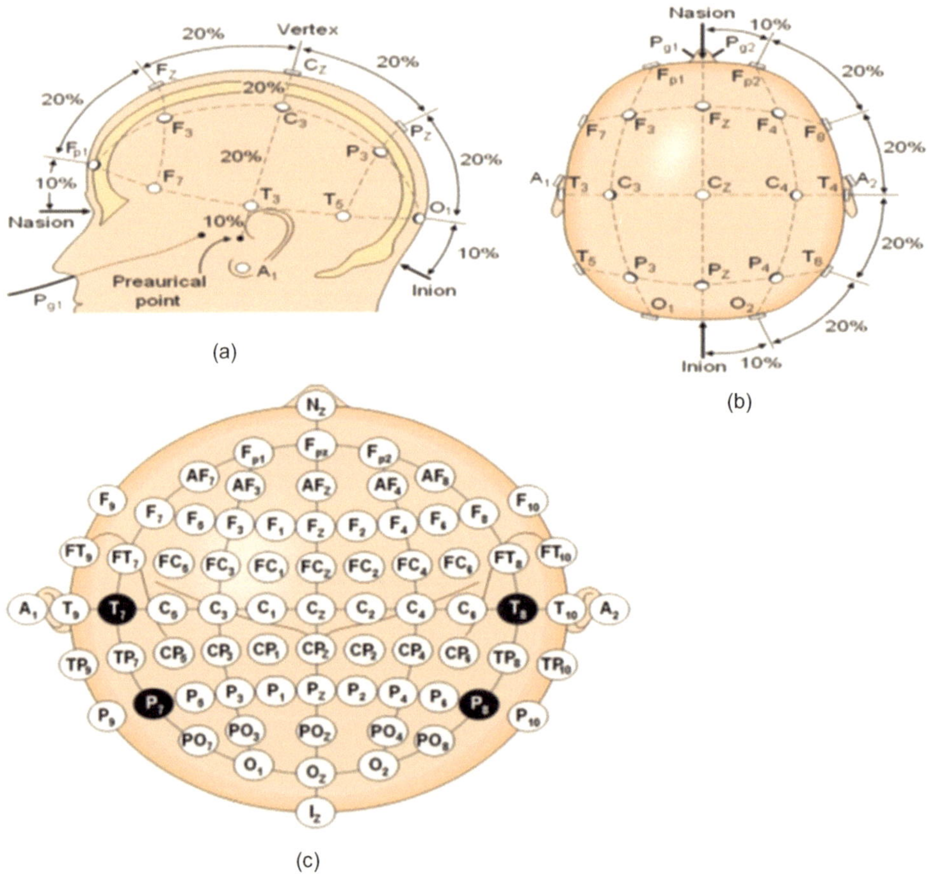

Figure 4.
The international 10–20 system seen from (a) left and (b) top (c) standard location and nomenclature of the intermediate 10% electrodes.

1.3 Wave analysis of the EEG

In the human brain, most of the neurons, which work in synchrony, possess common characteristics, that as much larger the amplitude (potential) of the electrical oscillations in microvolt (mV), will have much faster the neurons work together, and also much higher the frequency of the oscillations in Hertz (Hz). Hence, amplitude and frequency, and shape are important primary characteristics of human brain waves. EEGs are the recordings of these tiny electrical charges (potentials or waves) that are generally less than 300 μV [6]. EEG frequency bands or the brain rhythms arranged according to increased frequencies are shown in **Figure 5**.

The most common classification is based on the frequency of EEG signals (i.e. alpha, beta, theta, and delta). The brain waves with their frequency band and the corresponding brain activities are revealed in **Table 1**.

The EEG signals have been broadly categorized into six classical categories as shown in **Figure 5**. They cause a high level of difficulty to interpret the huge amount of data/information being received from one single EEG recordings. Subsequently, it is highly required to understand every aspect of these categories, which have been explained below in brief:

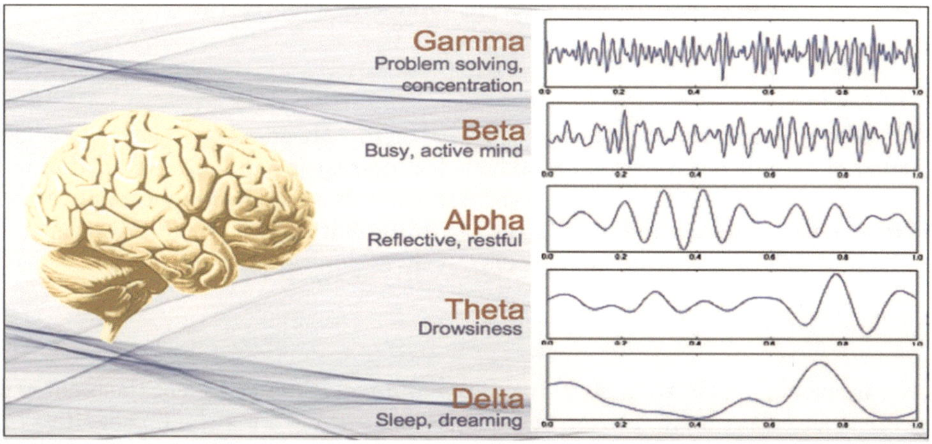

Figure 5.
Fundamental EEG bands classification.

Name	Frequency band (Hz)	Predominantly brain activity
Delta	0.5–4	Sleeping
Theta	4–8	Dreaming, Meditation
Alpha	8–13	Relaxation
Beta	13–36	Alert/Working Problem Solving
Gamma	36–100	Multisensory semantic matching Perceptual function

Table 1.
Electroencephalography (EEG) signal frequency bands.

1.3.1 Alpha (α) waves

The Alpha waves have been discovered around 1908 by Hans Berger. Its frequency ranges from 8 to 13 Hz and is usually seen in the posterior regions of the head on each side of an adult when the patient is relaxing [7]. It appears when closing the eyes and relaxing, and tends to attenuate with open eyes or alerting by any mental exertion.

1.3.2 Beta (β) waves

Its frequency ranges from 14 Hz to about 30 Hz. Beta activity is a "fast" activity and is also called normal rhythm activity. It is usually seen on both sides of the hemisphere in symmetrical distribution and is most evident in the frontal areas. Sedative-hypnotic drugs affect this activity [7]. It may be missing or reduced in regions of cortical damage. It is accentuated in patients who are very anxious or have their eyes open.

1.3.3 Theta (θ) waves

It has a frequency range from 4 to 7 Hz and is classified as "slow" activity. It is found in every person during sleep and in meditation. It can be seen in the state of arousal for adults [7]. Excess theta in adults represents abnormal activity.

1.3.4 Delta (δ) waves

The Delta Waves have a frequency range of up to 4 Hz or below. It is likely to have a higher amplitude but has a low frequency. It is normal as the dominant rhythm in infants of up to one year and stages 3 and 4 of sleep. It is usually more prominent in the frontal part in adults and the posterior part in children [7].

Theta and delta waves are known collectively as slow waves.

1.3.5 Gamma (γ) waves

Its frequency ranges from 30 to 100 Hz. Gamma rhythms represent the binding of an enormous collection of neurons assimilated for carrying out a certain cognitive or motor function [8].

1.3.6 The flow of EEG Waves

The amplitude of EEG signals is very closely related to the level of consciousness of a person [9]. An example of these waves is shown below in **Figure 6**.

From **Figure 6**, the conclusion is drawn that the slow waves Theta and Delta occur in the third and fourth stages of human sleep. The awake condition presents a high level of consciousness with Beta waves. This 90 minutes of the cycle is repeated the whole night with repeated EEG wave activity.

1.4 Artifacts in EEG

The EEG signal is one of those signals which are most widely used for studying brain functions and for the diagnosis of neurological disorders by physicians, researchers, and scientists. A single misinterpretation can become a cause of

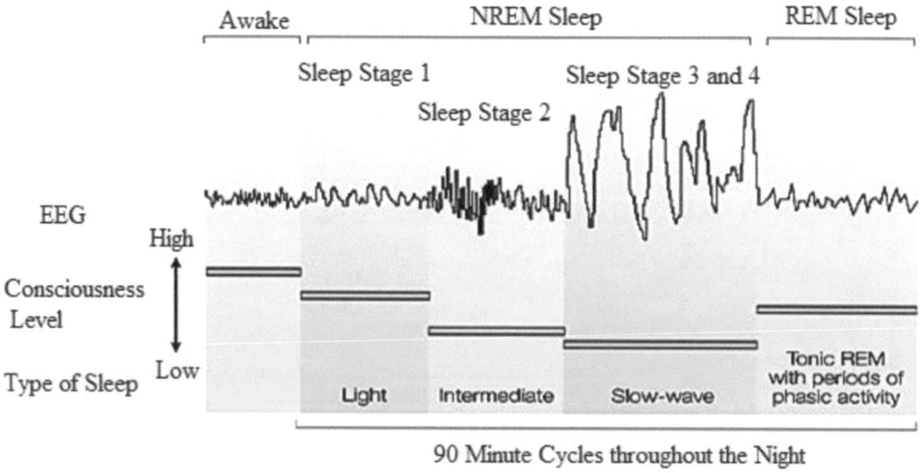

Figure 6.
EEG activity is solely dependent on the level of the subject's consciousness.

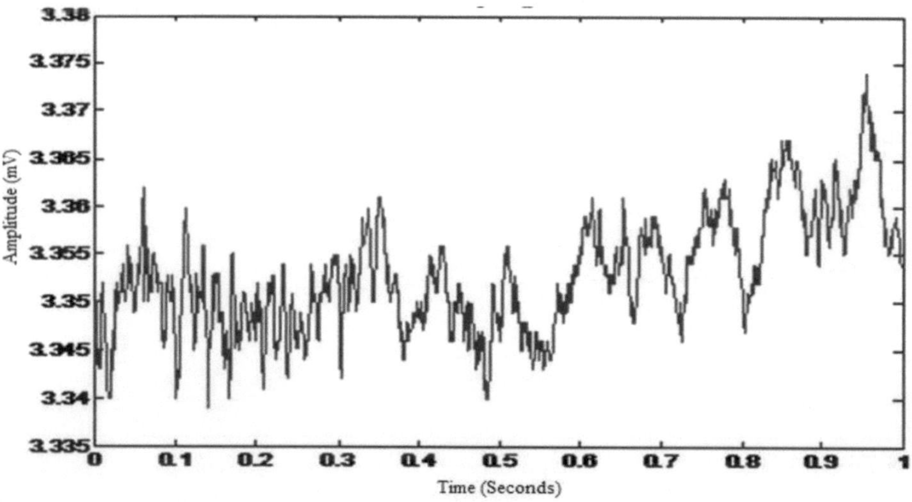

Figure 7.
One second recording of clean pure EEG signal.

misdiagnosis. Henceforth, it is imperative to have a very right and clear image about brain activities being represented by EEG signals shown in **Figure 7**. Skull's low conductivity is the main reason for the poor spatial resolution of scalp EEG.

Furthermore, scalp EEG signals are highly sensitive to the movement of the subject and noises being introduced due to externally likewise human head activation, eye movements, musculature, nearby electrical device interference and because of one's movement conductivity in the electrodes get varies or physicochemical reactions occurred at the electrode sites [6]. Some of the EEG artifacts distributions are displayed in **Figure 8**. All these additional activities are indirectly associated with the subject's current cerebral process and are collectively referred to as background activities. Henceforth, EEG signals are highly enervated and mixed with these non-cerebral

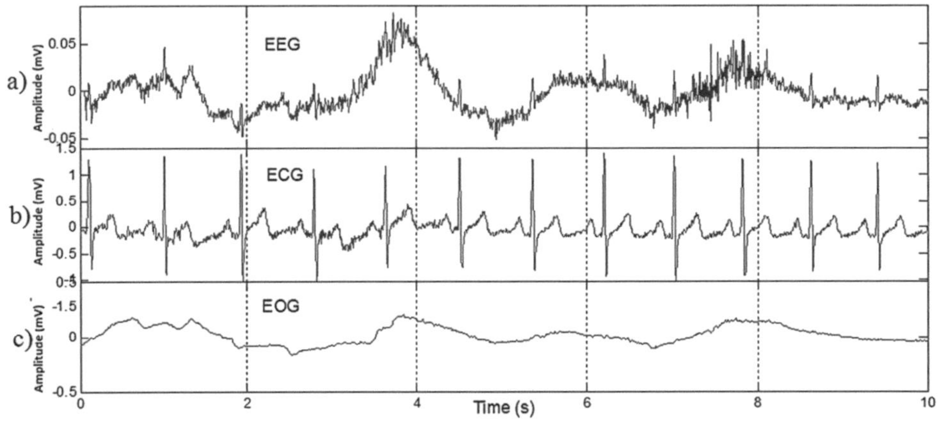

Figure 8.
ECG and EOG artifacts.

impulses known as artifacts or noise. These artifacts or noise fall into two major categories being considered as physiologic and extra-physiologic [5]. Only after removing these artifacts, a true diagnosis can be achieved. Physiologic Artifacts can be produced by any of any sources present in the human body that has an electric dipole or which can generate an electrical or magnetic field that can become a cause of physiologic artifacts.

The following are the types of physiologic artifacts:

- Muscle artifacts
- Glossokinetic artifacts
- Eye blink artifacts
- Eye movement artifacts
- ECG artifacts
- Pulse artifacts
- Respiration artifacts
- Skin artifacts

The following are the types of extra-physiologic artifacts:

- Electrode popping artifacts
- Alternating current artifacts
- Artifacts due to movements in the environment

Some of the most EEG corrupting artifacts are discussed as follows:

1.4.1 Electrooculogram (EOG)

This is mainly used to measure the eye artifacts. Since these measurements are contaminants of EEG signal and so it is not possible to remove this kind of artifacts from the subtraction process only when the exact model of EOG diffusion across the scalp is available [2]. These artifacts are of two types:

I. Eye Blinking.

It is an artifact that is very common in EEG data. This artifact possesses a very high amplitude signal sometimes much greater than the EEG signals of interest. Further, it can corrupt data availed on all electrodes, even those signals too, that are at the back of the head [2].

II. Eye Movement.

It is occurring because of the reorientation of the retained corneal dipole [4]. Eye movement's diffusion across the scalp is greater than that being produced by the eye blink artifact.

EOG artifact can be given in the following form:

$$\beta = \frac{\sum (X_i - \widehat{X}_i)(Y_i - \widehat{Y}_i)}{\sum (X_i - \widehat{X}_i)\text{^}2} \tag{1}$$

where,

β = Estimated EOG present in EEG analysis; X = EOG signal; Y = EEG signal; n = Number of iterations.

1.4.2 Cardiograph (ECG/EKG)

Cardiograph is generally used to measure pulse or heartbeat, which occurs by an electrode on or near a blood vessel as shown in **Figure 8**. The voltage recording changes due to the expansion and contraction of the vessel [2]. The artifact signal generally has frequency proximity to 1.2 Hz and appears as a sharp spike or smooth wave but it can have a variation that solely depends on the state of the patient. An example has been illustrated below where an EEG signal mixed with ECG/EKG signal and got corrupted due to line interference.

Electrocardiogram signal artifacts can represent by using the following equation:

$$\mathrm{ECG}(t) = R \cdot s_m(t) + R \cdot s_f(t) + N(t) \tag{2}$$

Where R is a random unit vector, $s_m(t)$ and $s_f(t)$ are the three components of the dipole model for the maternal and fetal cardiac vectors, respectively and $N(t)$ is the noise in each ECG channel at time t.

1.4.3 Electromyogram (EMG)

Electromyogram (EMG) artifacts could be produced because of some movement disorders. Essential tremor and Parkinson's disease could also be responsible for rhythmic 4–6 Hz sinusoidal artifacts which may be mimicked cerebral activity [2].

Following equation shows the EMG signal:

$$x(n) = \sum_{r=0}^{N-1} h(r)e(n-r) + w(n) \tag{3}$$

Where.

$x(n)$ represents EMG signal;

$e(n)$ point processed, that represent the firing impulse;

$h(r)$ represents the MUAP (Motor Unit Action Potential);

$w(n)$ represents zero-mean additive white Gaussian noise;

and N represents the number of motor unit firings.

Extra-physiologic Artifacts

These include interference due to electrical equipment, kinesiology artifacts because of the human body or movements of electrodes, and mechanical artifact because of human body movement.

1.4.4 Motion artifact

The movement of the patient or even disturbance just during the electrodes settling could become the cause of electrode pops variations of the conduction between electrodes and the skin. Linguistically these signals appear either in the form of single or multiple sharp waveforms due to abrupt variations in the impedance. It can be easily identified by its characteristic appearance and its usual distribution, which is restricted to a single electrode [4]. In usual manners, sharp transients which occur at a single electrode should be considered artifacts, until it has not been proven. **Figure 9a** and **Figure 9b** present the pure EEG signal and motion artifact contaminated EEG signal. **Figure 9b** shows the high amplitude broad spectrum distribution because of motion artifact in the EEG signal.

Figure 9a shows the original EGG signal and (b) represents the motion artifact contaminated EEG signal. **Figure 9b** presented the motion artifacts contamination on the EEG signal.

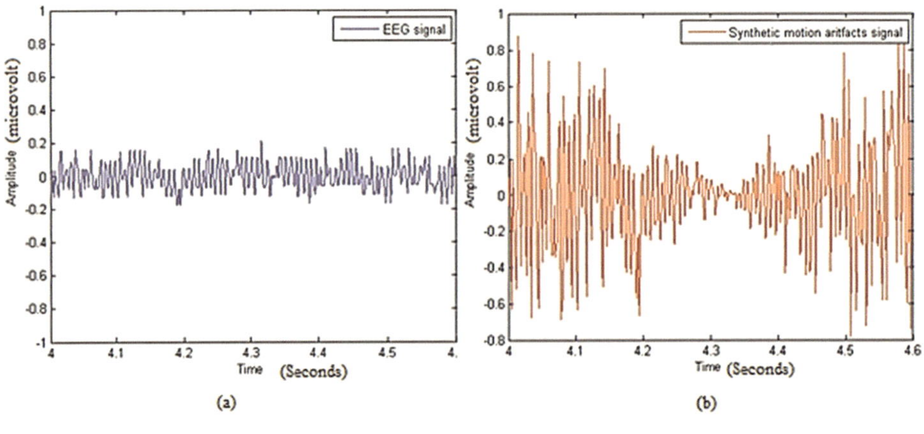

Figure 9.
(a) Original EEG signal (b) EEG signal contaminated with motion artifact.

1.4.5 Power lines

Alternating Currents, ranging from 50 to 60 Hz, that is strong signals from Alternating Current (A/C) power supplies could also corrupt EEG data since it gets transferred to a recording device from the scalp electrodes. Issues co-related to power lines-based artifacts come into the picture when an active electrode has a higher impedance than impedance between the electrodes and the amplifier's ground. In such kinds of scenarios, the amplifier's ground starts to work as an active electrode which solely depends upon its location and implements/generates 50–60-Hz artifact. Usually for removal of these artifact notch filters are used, but still, it could produce a problem of useful information removal, furthermore lower frequency line noise and harmonics are undesirable [10]. If the line noise or harmonics produce in frequency bands of interest it interferes with EEG signals which occur in the same frequency band [9].

Power line noise as shown in **Figure 10** can be presented mathematically as:

$$P(t) = \beta_0 \sin(2\pi * 60 * t) \tag{4}$$

In the above equation β_0 represents power line noise weight.

1.5 De-noising EEG signals

During the recording process, there is always a possibility of occurrence of contamination in EEG data at multiple points. Over which most of the artifacts that occurred here belong biologically generated by sources and are external to the brain. By significant improvement in existing technology, these externally generated artifacts could be removed, thus it is important to study efficient de-noising (a process for noise removal) procedures that would be able to remove these biological overlays from EEG signals. Actual EEG recordings are the summation of artifacts with the pure EEG signal, and can be defined mathematically:

$$E(t) = S(t) + N(t) \tag{5}$$

Where:-.

$S(t)$ is a pure EEG signal,

$N(t)$ is the artifact,

$E(t)$ represents the recorded signal and t is the time when recording has been taken.

The presence of these artifacts introduces spikes that can create issues while reading neurological rhythms. So many methods have been proposed and presented by scientists and researchers to perform the artifacts removal process in EEG.

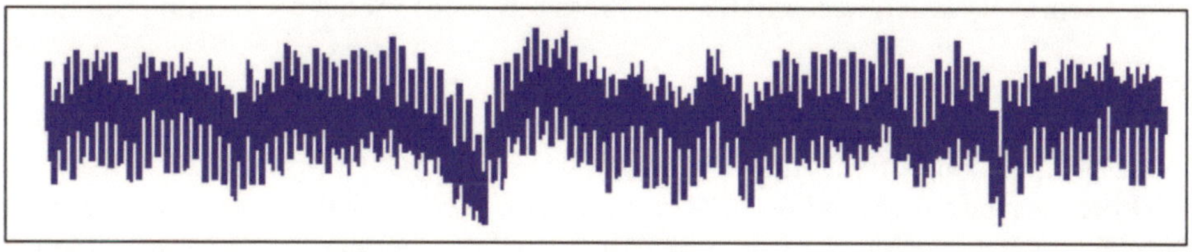

Figure 10.
Line interference of 50 Hz.

1.6 Methods for artifacts removal

To remove artifacts from an EEG recording can be classified into two groups, which are following:

i. Artifact rejection—This method is used for removal of EEG signal that comprises the artifact and

ii. Artifact correction—This method is used for the removal of artifacts from EEG signals while keeping and maintaining the pure EEG signal.

1.6.1 Artifact rejection

1. Basic Artifact Rejection.

The most commonly used de-noising techniques for eliminating all EEG epochs which comprise artifacts larger than some pre-defined threshold EEG voltage level, known as artifact rejection. This method is most commonly and widely used when a limited amount of data or artifacts such as EOG is available. These artifacts occur too frequently in nature that raises elimination of those epochs which are contaminated with the artifacts, which becomes the cause of considerable loss of information and which makes this process impractical for being used in clinical data. As EEG and some artifacts occupy the same frequency band, this method is not that effective [7].

2. Regression Method.

Conventionally artifacts correction processes used a regression-based approach which is based on either time domain or frequency domain [3]. In this method, after a clear measure of artifact signals, it is subtracted from EEG signals and has been recorded. The major issue that comes into existence is bi-directional contamination. As if artifacts potentials are capable of contaminating EEG recordings, then the electrical activity of the brain is also capable of contaminating the artifacts recordings. Henceforth, diminishing a linear combination of the recorded artifacts from the EEG recordings may not only abolish artifacts but also the cerebral activity of interest. Review work for these techniques is discussed in [4, 8].

3. Filtering Method

Low-pass filtering of the artifacts eliminates all high-frequency activity from EOG signal, from both cerebral and ocular origins [7]. Adaptive filtering usage before applying regression correction can substantially reduce issues produced due to bidirectional contamination [3]. However, it is imperative to use adaptive digital filters for artifact removal, which necessitates a suitable reference model for training the filter.

1.6.2 Artifact correction

1. Principal Component Analysis (PCA).

These methods are based on EEG and artifacts decomposition into spatial components, which is inclusive of recognizing artifactual components and reassembling the EEG without those artifactual components that have been recognized, but it is problematic in the case of PCA. The PCA algorithm first decomposes the EEG signals into uncorrelated, but it is not required that these must be independent of each other which are spatially orthogonal and that's why it cannot deal with higher-order statistical dependencies. Furthermore, it is not practically possible to completely separate artifacts from interested brain signals specifically when both of these signals have comparable amplitudes.

The following expression describes principal component decomposition:

$$\beta_1 = \phi_1 X_0' \tag{6}$$

where,

β_1 is set of first principal component scores whose mean equals to zero;

ϕ_1 represents the first principal component;

$\phi_1 X_0'$ could be considered as a vector or matrix transposition.

By maximizing the variance of$\phi_1 X_0'$, $\phi_1$can be simply calculated as:

$$\phi_1 = \arg\max \text{Var}\left(\phi_1 X_0'\right); \text{where } ||\phi_1|| = 1 \tag{7}$$

$$\phi_1 = \arg\max \phi_1 X_0' X_1 \phi_1'; \text{where } ||\phi_1|| = 1 \tag{8}$$

Successive principal components can easily be obtained iteratively by demising the first k principal components from X_0, presented as below:

$$X_k = X_{k-1} - X_{k-1}\phi_k'\phi_k \tag{9}$$

Now to find ϕ_{k+1}, X_k has been treated as a data matrix that can be done by maximizing the variance of $\phi_{k+1}X_k'$ using following equation:

$$\phi_{k+1} = \arg\max \text{Var}\left(\phi_{k+1}X_k'\right) \tag{10}$$

Subject to $||\phi_{k+1}|| = \text{sqrt}\left(\sum_{j=1}^{p}\phi_{k+1j}^2\right) = 1$ and $\phi_{k+1}\perp\phi_k$for $j = 1, 2 \ldots k$.

Alternatively, Singular Value Decomposition (SVD) is the simplest and efficient way that can be applied to find a centered data-matrix X_0, that can be expressed as:

$$X_0 = \text{UDV}' \tag{11}$$

Where $K \leq \min(n, p)$; $U'U = V'V = I_k$;

D is a diagonal matrix with $d_1 > \ldots d_2 > d_k$ on the diagonal.

UD matrix constitutes principal component scores, which are variable coordinates in the case of principal components [3].

2. Independent component analysis (ICA)

This method was developed to handle issues that occurred due to Blind Source Separation, abbreviated as BSS to form the components which must be as independent as possible [8] and can be represented mathematically:

$$X = A\,s + n \tag{12}$$

Where X is the observed signal, n is the noise, A is the mixing matrix, and s is the independent components (ICs) or sources. To find linear transformation W of X, for determining the independent outputs as:

$$u = W\,X = W\,As \tag{13}$$

Where u is the estimated ICs and it is highly required that components must be statistically independent instead of a mixture.

After a thorough investigation and deep analysis and research work conclusion has been drawn that ICA provides much better results for de-noising [6]. A whole chapter has been devoted to describing ICA, which belongs to existing work in Single-Stage Artifact Removal Algorithm.

3. Canonical correlation analysis (CCA)

This algorithm has been developed by *H.* Hotelling and is considered as a way to measure the linear relationship between two multidimensional variables. It detects two bases with the correlation matrix between the variables of interest that are in diagonal form and the correlations on the diagonal get maximized, in such a way that the dimensionality of these new bases is either less than or equal to the smallest dimension of the two variables [5].

Canonical correlation analysis (CCA) is first proposed by Hotelling. CCA is an algorithm for the determination of the linear association between two set variables. This is done with the help of the variance and covariance matrix of the data [6].

A set of linear combinations named A and B are considered as:

$$A_P = [a_{11}, a_{12}, \ldots ..a_{1m}]^T \tag{14}$$

$$B_Q = [b_{11}, b_{12}, \ldots ..b_{1n}]^T \tag{15}$$

Let C_{pp} and C_{qq} be the variance of the A_p and B_Q respectively and C_{pq} is the covariance between A_P and B_Q. Then the above equation can be rewritten as:

$$P^* = \frac{A_p^T C_{pp} B_Q}{\sqrt{A_p^T C_{pp} A_p}\sqrt{B_q^T C_{qq} B_q}} \tag{16}$$

This P^* should be maximum to achieve the best self-correlation. Therefore, this optimization can be solved by

$$C_{pp}^{-1} C_{pq} C_{qq}^{-1} C_{qp} A_P = \rho A_P \tag{17}$$

$$C_{qq}^{-1} C_{qp} C_{pp}^{-1} C_{pq} B_Q = \rho B_Q \tag{18}$$

This ρrepresents the Eigenvalue which is equal to the square of P^*.

$$\rho = \sqrt{P^*} \tag{19}$$

This canonical pair will be calculated and separated by calculating self-correlation and a mutual decorrelation between input sources.

4. Wavelet transform

Wavelet Transform (WT) has good localization properties in the time and frequency domain [6], and so it is a widely accepted and successful method being used for de-noising [11]. Currently, so many approaches are available at the algorithmic level to de-noise using Wavelet Transform, which is mainly based on shrinkage, where the EEG signals get decomposed in the form of wavelets and then noise removal is performed using shrinkage and thresholding. The quality of Wavelet Transform in transforming a time-domain signal into time and frequency localization assists in comprehending the signal's behavior in a much better way.

The Wavelet Transform could be defined as the following equation, which is the inner product or cross-correlation of $\{x_n[m]\}$ signal with scaled and time-shifted wavelet $\Psi a,b[m]$, that is:

$$WT_{x_n}[a,b] = (x_n, \psi_{a,b}) \tag{20}$$

where,

$$\psi_{a,b}[m] = |a|^{-\frac{1}{2}} \psi^{\frac{m-b}{a}}$$

a—Scale parameters.
b—Translation parameters.
$\psi_{a,b}[m]$ - Appropriate wavelet function.

5. Empirical mode decomposition

Empirical mode decomposition is a non-linear method to represent a non-stationary signal into the sum of zero-mean sub-components. This method decomposes a signal into several intrinsic mode functions through an iterative method known as sifting. At the first level, the Intrinsic Mode function (IMF1) is the mean of the upper and lower envelop of the original EEG signal x(t). Then the residual signal is obtained by subtracting IMF1 from x(t). This process is iterated till the stopping criterion is fulfilled (Residual signal energy content is close to zero). The remaining residual signal is

$$P_n(t) = P_{n-1}(t) - IMF_n(t) \tag{21}$$

where, $P_n(t) = x(t)$.
Finally, the signal is reconstructed by adding all IMFs and residual signals as

$$x(t) = P_n(t) + \sum_{i=1}^{N} \mathrm{IMF}_i(t) \tag{22}$$

The method of detecting IMFs is sensitive to the amalgam of undesired signal components present in surroundings. These noises affect the EMD process. Thus, mode mixing is used to overcome the disparate scale oscillations with amplitude in the near range of the IMFs peaks which can be available randomly in the whole dataset. Consequently, a more powerful and noise-assisted version of the EMD algorithm was presented termed as Ensemble Empirical Mode Decomposition (EEMD), which solves this mode mixing quandary and employs the average value of EMD ensembles that filters out the IMFs for the given signal. Moreover, this method also depends on the added noise amplitude to the input signal and the number of trials [6, 9].

6. Conclusion

In this Chapter, Electroencephalograph Signals and their generation process have been discussed; the EEG signal has been compared with fMRI and PET signals. The classification of the EEG signals on the amplitude, frequency, and shape have been elaborated in wave analysis of EEG, and applications of these components are presented.

The artifacts of EEG have been explained in detail. There are two main types of artifacts to be considered; namely, physiological and non-physiological artifacts. Non-physiological contain artifacts such as movement artifacts, electrode pop artifacts, sweat artifacts, and 50/60 Hz noise. Typically, these artifacts are not explicitly monitored, and as such, they need to be filtered out by their characteristics alone. For example, sweat artifacts tend to be of really low frequency, 50/60 Hz noise is contained within a narrow frequency band, and electrode pop artifacts are not necessarily time-aligned in two corresponding electrodes on the two sides of the scalp. Physiological artifacts take the form of ocular artifacts, cardiac artifacts, muscle artifacts, glossokinetic artifacts, and respiratory artifacts. Most of these artifacts can be monitored with another channel, which in turn can be used during the EEG artifact removal.

Subsequently, artifact removal methods have been classified in the form of artifact correction and artifact rejection. The artifact rejection comprises Regression and filtering as the main method. Whereas, artifact correction method comprises Principal Component Analysis (PCA), Independent Component Analysis (ICA), Canonical Correlation Analysis (CCA), Wavelet Transform (WT), and Empirical Mode Analysis (EMD). These all single-stage artifact removal methods and their implementation with results are discussed in the subsequent chapter.

Conflict of interest

The authors declare no conflict of interest.

Author details

Vandana Roy
DoEC, GGITS, Jabalpur, India

*Address all correspondence to: Vandana.roy20@gmail.com

References

[1] McMenamin BW, Shackman AJ, Greischar LL, Davidson RJ. Electromyogenic artifacts and electroencephalographic inferences revisited. Neuroimage. 1 Jan 2011;**54**(1): 4-9. DOI: 10.1016/j.neuroimage.2010. 07.057. Epub 2010 Aug 2. PMID: 20981275; PMCID: PMC2962711

[2] Sweeney KT, McLoone SF, Ward TE. The use of ensemble empirical mode decomposition with canonical correlation analysis as a novel artifact removal technique. IEEE Transactions Biomedical Engineering. 2013;**60**(1):97-105. DOI: 10.1109/TBME.2012.2225427. Epub 2012 Oct 18. PMID: 23086501

[3] Zeng H, Song A, Yan R, Quin H. EOG artifact correction from EEG recording using stationary subspace analysis and empirical mode decomposition. Sensors. 2013;**13**:14839-14859

[4] Soomro MH, Badruddin N, Yusoff MZ. Comparison of blind source separation methods for removal of eye blink artifacts from EEG. 2014 5th International Conference on Intelligent and Advanced Systems (ICIAS). 2014; **2014**:1-6. DOI: 10.1109/ ICIAS.2014.6869470

[5] Liu Q, Liu A, Zhang X, Chen X, Qian R & Chen X. Removal of EMG artifacts from multichannel EEG signals using combined singular spectrum analysis and canonical correlation analysis. Journal of Healthcare Engineering. 2019: 4159676. DOI: 10.1155/2019/4159676

[6] Anastasiadou M, Hadjipapas A, Christodoulakis M, Papathanasiou ES, Papacostas SS, Mitsis GD, Detection and removal of muscle artifacts from scalp EEG recordings in patients with epilepsy, In: IEEE (14th) international conference on bioinformatics and bioengineering (BIBE). US: Boca Raton; 2014. pp. 291–296

[7] Sweeney KT, McLoone SF, Ward TE. The use of ensemble empirical mode decomposition with canonical correlation analysis as a novel artifact removal technique. IEEE Transactions Biomedical Engineering. 2013;**60**:97-105. DOI: 10.1109/TBME.2012.2225427. Epub 2012 Oct 18. PMID: 23086501

[8] Soomro MH, Badruddin N, Yusoff MZ, Jatoi MA, Automatic eye-blink artifact removal method based on EMD-CCA, In: International Conference on Complex Medical Engineering (ICME). 2013. pp. 186–190. DOI: 10.1109/ICCME.2013.6548236

[9] Roy V, Shukla S. Designing efficient blind source separation methods for EEG motion artifact removal based on statistical evaluation. Wireless Personal Communication. 2019;**108**:1311–1327. DOI: 10.1007/s11277-019-06470-3

[10] Xun C, Chen H, Hu P. Removal of muscle artifacts from single-channel EEG based on ensemble empirical mode decomposition and multiset canonical correlation analysis. Journal of Applied Mathematics. 2014;**2014**:10. Article ID: 261347. DOI: 10.1155/2014/261347

[11] Roy V, Shukla S. A methodical health-care model to eliminate motion artifacts from big EEG data. Journal of Organizational and End User Computing. 2017;**29**(4):84-102. DOI: 10.4018/JOEUC.2017100105

Section 3

Biosignal Sensors

Chapter 11

Developmental Studies on Practical Enzymatic Phosphate Ion Biosensors and Microbial BOD Biosensors, and New Insights into the Future Perspectives of These Biosensor Fields

Hideaki Nakamura

Abstract

This chapter summarizes the developmental studies on environmental biosensors of enzymatic phosphate ion (Pi) biosensors for eutrophication and microbial biochemical oxygen demand (BOD) biosensors for organic pollution. In particular, an author focuses on the developmental studies that the author principally conducted, and describe the history and the insights into the future of these fields of environmental biosensors. In our developmental studies on the enzymatic Pi biosensors, we fabricated automatic instruments of a desktop-type and a submersible buoy-type, which was fabricated for remote biosensing of dam water. These instruments employed a luminol-chemiluminescence flow injection analysis (CL-FIA) system and enabled to have practical performances in precise Pi determination, operational stability, and accurate bioavailable Pi measurements. In the microbial BOD biosensor development, the author considered to apply the FIA concept enabling highly repeatable measurements to absorptiometric BOD measurements. Both precise temperature control and accurate time control to incubate measurement mixture of budding yeast cell suspension containing redox color indicator and sample enabled to obtain the highly repeatable results that led to highly sensitive BOD measurements. Looking back on our developmental studies, what the author was thinking at the time and the results obtained are described. Finally, the author discusses the developmental trends of these biosensor fields and new insights into the future perspectives.

Keywords: biosensor instruments, eutrophication, organic pollution, phosphate ion, enzymatic biosensor, BOD, microbial biosensor, budding yeast, CL-FIA, accuracy, precision, automation, remote biosensing, submersible buoy

1. Introduction

Human beings in the global ecosystem are no longer consumers, but wasters. To achieve "Transforming our World: the 2030 Agenda for Sustainable Development (2030 Agenda)" and set the Sustainable Development Goals (SDGs) consisting of 17 global goals in 2015 [1], human beings need to become former consumers and stay within the energy and matter cycles of the global ecosystems. One of the examples is the sixth goal of "Clean Water and Sanitation" in the 17 SDGs. The cause of anthropogenic eutrophication and subsequent organic pollution is the imbalance in the ecological matter cycle that occurs in human social life.

In Japan, the anthropogenic eutrophication and the organic pollution in 1960' had simultaneously been caused by the direct influx of wastewaters from industries and households (**Figure 1a**) [2]. On the other hand, most of such eutrophication in recent years is induced by the anthropogenic influx of nutrient salts, such as phosphate and nitrate salts, which are the essential nutrients of living organisms (**Figure 1b**) [3]. It is known that orthophosphate ion, that is, phosphate ion (Pi) is the most causative nutrient. These nutrient salts are contained in the effluent of sewage treatment plants or industrial wastewater treatment plants, or in leaching water from farms or live stocks [3, 4]. In the cases of these plants, only an ecological decomposer is employed for the biodegradation of organic matters contained in the wastewater (**Figure 1b**). This is the root cause of current eutrophication and subsequent organic pollution. Therefore, such anthropogenic influx of nutrient salts causes the water bloom by phytoplankton as an ecological producer, and the remains of phytoplankton cause organic pollution. To investigate the ecological phenomenon of such anthropogenic eutrophication and subsequent organic pollution, we observed the water ecosystem and water qualities of a eutrophied pond as a model water body [5]. The results led to a study on hydroponics [6] and water chemical remediation (WCR) that was developed for simultaneous removal of Pi and phytoplankton from the anthropogenically eutrophied pond [7]. A series of the studies will be described elsewhere.

In our studies, we have also developed measurement methods for these water pollutions. As one of the ways to measure the degrees of water pollution, several biosensors have been developed. The biosensor consists of a molecular recognition

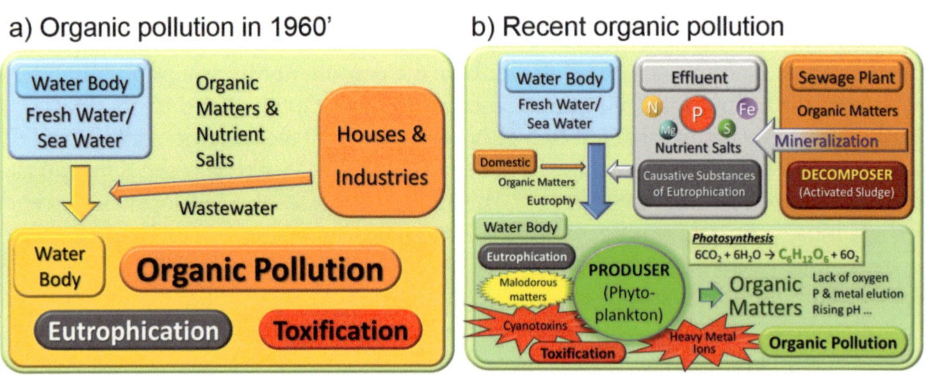

Figure 1.
(a) Schematic diagram in comparison on the causes of organic pollution in the 1960s and the recent past [2]. The schematic diagram of (b) was permitted from Springer Nature [2] and slightly modified for this chapter.

DOI: http://dx.doi.org/10.5772/intechopen.104377

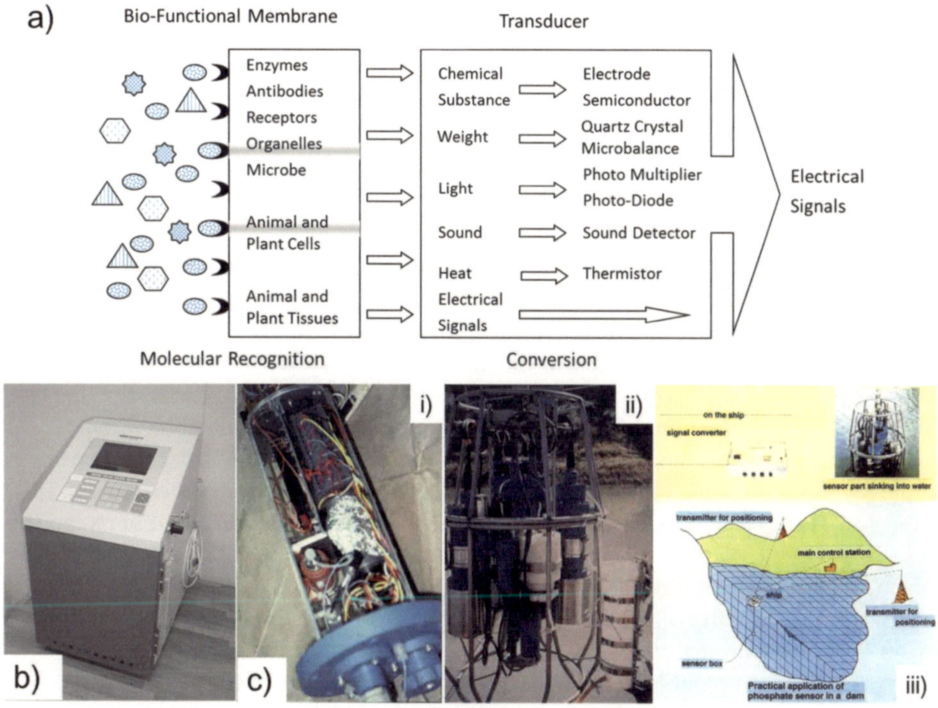

Figure 2.
Biosensor. (a) Principles and (b) automatic Pi biosensor instruments of a desktop-type [8] and (c) a submersible buoy-type [9], (i) a column compactly integrating a Pi biosensor system, (ii) a continuous-remote sensing system for total water-quality monitoring, and (iii) the continuous-remote sensing system is shipped by a boat and sunk vertically (a) and (c) were permitted from Springer Nature [10] and (b) was permitted from Taylor and Francis [11]).

element and a transducer and has the features of a simple and rapid measurement device (**Figure 2a**). The first biosensor was studied for medical use by Updike and Hicks in 1967 and developed to determine glucose concentration employing an enzyme-catalyzed reaction (enzymatic reaction) by glucose oxidase (GOD) [12]. This enzymatic glucose biosensor used a Clark-type electrode [13] and measured dissolved oxygen (DO) consumption caused by the GOD reaction. Since then, biosensors as measurement devices have been developed not only for medical uses [14] but also for food or environmental uses [10]. Thus, many biosensors and their associated techniques have been studied and developed [10]. In particular, the biosensor for environmental use requires highly sensitive and wide-determination range (dynamic range) measurement of the analyte. In addition, depending on what is being analyzed, the environmental biosensors require the feature to perform either specific or nonspecific measurements. Furthermore, for practical use, it is also required the application style of the biosensor, such as on-site use, continuous use, or laboratory use.

To satisfy these requirements, many kinds of biosensors for environmental water pollution have been developed worldwide [3, 10, 15]. In the second section of this chapter, the development of enzymatic Pi biosensors for eutrophication and in the third section, the development of microbial biochemical oxygen demand (BOD) biosensors for eutrophication are described. In the final fourth section, the contents of this chapter are concluded.

2. Development of enzymatic Pi biosensors for eutrophication

In the early times of biosensor development for environmental use, there were many technological problems for practical use. To solve the problems, a wide variety of challenges have been carried out. In this section, the main breakthrough technics for the practical application in the field of biosensor development for eutrophication are described based on the previous literature [3, 10, 14, 15].

2.1 Standard method and consideration to practical estimation performances

As mentioned above, the most causative nutrients of the eutrophication are phosphates, which are classified into Pi, condensed phosphates (pyro-, *meta*-, and other polyphosphates), and organic phosphates. Among the phosphates, the one with the greatest effect of eutrophication is Pi, which is an inorganic phosphate ion.

In Japan, a spectrophotometric molybdenum blue method for Pi determination is employed as the standard method [16], which is based on the method by Lowry and Lopez in 1946 [17]. By this method, Pi concentration can be determined between 0.1 and 3.0 mg/L Pi (3.2–96 μM) at a relative standard deviation (RSD) of 2–10%. The detection limit in this method is 0.03 mg/L Pi (0.32 μM Pi).

These values obtained by the standard method are barely applicable as an indication of the eutrophication (0.64 μM Pi), however, they are insufficient for the estimation of the eutrophication, which is classified into the five categories in lakes (between around 0.032–3.2 μM Pi). In addition, the maximal permissible concentration in Japanese lakes is 0.32 μM Pi for drinking and 3.2 μM Pi for environmental protection [18]. Thus, the influences of Pi on eutrophication are caused at extremely low concentrations. Therefore, it was found that the estimation of the eutrophication requires highly sensitive and wide-range Pi determination techniques.

For ideal estimation of the eutrophication, the standard method has difficulties in both accurate and high-precision measurements. In accurate measurement, dilution of sample solution needs due to that the dynamic range is narrow and causes error. In high-precision measurement, the minimum limit of determination (3.2 μM Pi) is insufficient to estimate the water quality in all categories of eutrophication.

To make ideal estimations for all categories of the eutrophication, a measurement method that was more sensitive and had a wider dynamic range (if it is possible; 0.032–3.2 μM Pi) than the standard methods was needed. However, considering the biosensor performance at that time, such high sensitivity was not realistic. Even if such highly sensitive Pi measurements cannot be made, we should be able to determine 0.32 μM Pi with a biosensor at a concentration that can confirm signs of eutrophication and monitor the quality of the lake water for drinking. In addition, we considered that the maximum limit of Pi determination obtained by the biosensor should be kept at least 3.2 μM or more as the practical dynamic range.

Like the other problems, the standard method is complicated and time-consuming to operate. Further, it requires the use of strong acid and heavy metal ions. The use of such chemicals is subject to limitations when applied to on-site monitoring and continuous monitoring because leakage of the chemicals into the environment has to be prevented. In addition, the standard method affects the influences of co-existing matters in a sample, such as Ca^{2+}, Fe^{3+}, NH_4^+, NO_2^-, NO_3^-, and AsO_4^{3-}.

As is clear here, the standard method is not sufficient to evaluate eutrophication. For this reason, the development of practical Pi biosensors has been performed.

2.2 Development of enzymatic Pi biosensors

It turns out that there were many issues that need to be resolved to actually estimate the eutrophication. Thus, we have set five requirements for the practical application of the Pi biosensors [19].

For practical use, our Pi biosensors are able to;

1. Have a practical Pi determination range (0.32–3.2 μM, no sample dilution required) required for environmental water control,

2. Maintain a practical minimum limit of Pi determination (0.32 μM Pi or less in the calibration curve) required for environmental water control for at least 2 weeks,

Instrument type	**Submersible buoy**[1]	**Desktop**			
Enzymatic system	PO_{psp}	PO_{Av}	MP	MP[2]	IP (PPi)
Ref. No.	[9]	[8]	[20]	[11]	[21]
Requirement					
(1) Calibration:	Satisfied	Satisfied	Satisfied	Satisfied	Satisfied at PPi
Range (at least 0.32–3.2 μM)	0.16–32 μM	96 nM–32 μM	10 nM–32 μM	0.1–30 μM	0.1–100 μM (PPi)
Coefficient	r = 0.998	r = 0.999	r = 0.998	r = 0.998	r^2 = 0.9997
(2) Sability test:	Satisfied	Satisfied	Not performed	Satisfied?	Not performed
as the term to maintain the practical lower limit of Pi determination in the calibration curve (0_32 μM Pi or less	Calibration curves of 0.32–32 μM for 48 days	Calibration curves of 0.16–32 μM for at least 2 weeks	1.0 μM for at least 2 weeks	0.1 μM for at least 2 months	(30 μM PPi for at least 2 weeks)
(3) Sample pretreatment:					
as countermeasures against interfering matters	Not performed	Performed	Performed	Performed and established the method	Not performed
(4) Real sample application:	Performed	Performed	Performed	Performed	Not performed
(5) Automation:	Semi-automated	Automated	Not automated	Not automated	Automated

[1]*Tests with the Pi biosensor on a submersible buoy have not been conducted.*
[2]*Pre-treatment method was investigated in detail for real sample application.*

Table 1.
Looking back on the five requirements that were set for the practical use of our automated CL-FIA systems as Pi biosensors (performed by Nakamura et al.).

3. Establish a pretreatment method for removing interfering matters,

4. Measure a real sample of environmental water, and

5. Automate a biosensor system that meets the above conditions.

We tried to develop practical Pi biosensors that meet these requirements (**Table 1**). As a reference, the history of the studies on the Pi biosensor development has been reviewed in several articles [3, 10, 15].

2.2.1 Development of early time Pi biosensors

A biosensor has characteristics that it can measure analyte using biological reactions by applying the molecular recognizing function in living organisms (**Figure 2a**). A Pi biosensor can measure directly the concentration of the bioavailable Pi existing in the environmental water. This means that the Pi biosensors have the possibility to be able to monitor the status of the water ecosystem. This section briefly explains the history of the development of Pi biosensors with such potential, which is above described [3].

The first Pi biosensor was studied by Guilbalt and Nanjo in 1975. Using the Clark-type DO electrode, they studied an enzymatic Pi biosensor that was based on the inhibition of alkaline phosphatase activity by Pi [22]. By employing the inhibitory reaction, this biosensor lacked sensitivity with the detection limit of 0.1 mM Pi. In addition, the inhibitory reaction is low selectivity in general. In 1990, d'Urso and Coulet studied a two-enzyme Pi biosensor using nucleoside phosphatase and xanthine oxidase [23]. Enzymatically generated hydrogen peroxide (H_2O_2) by the existence of Pi was electrochemically measured. In this study, the Pi biosensor could have a dynamic range between 0.1 and 10 μM Pi. In 1992, Wollenberger et al. improved the two-enzyme system to a multiple-enzyme system for Pi recycling [24]. The Pi biosensor was fabricated by incorporating a Clark-type DO electrode into a flow injection analysis (FIA) system. As the result, this Pi biosensor realized an excellent detection limit at 25 nM Pi. However, this biosensor was not suitable for practical use due to its short lifetimes by using an unstable enzyme. As another reason, it was reported that inosine used as another substrate was also unstable [25].

2.2.2 Development of our practical Pi biosensors

Karube et al. have studied several kinds of enzymatic Pi biosensors using pyruvate oxidase (PO) from *Pediococcus* sp. (PO_{Psp}) [9, 26–28] and genetically engineered PO from *Lactobacillus plantarum* (PO_{Lp}) [29], *Aerococcus viridans* (PO_{Av}) [8], and maltose phosphorylase (MP) [11, 20]. These studies were performed for the practical use of an automatic FIA system (desktop-type; **Figure 2b**) [8] and a remote-controlled automatic continuous Pi monitoring system (submersible buoy-type; **Figure 2c**) [9].

The Pi biosensor using PO is superior to other Pi biosensors because it requires only one step of a catalytic reaction for selective Pi detection. Using PO_{Psp}, the first Pi biosensor was studied by Kubo et al. in 1991 [26]. The Pi biosensor was batch type and used a DO electrode to measure the consumption of DO by the PO_{Psp} catalytic reaction under the existence of Pi, two cofactors (thiamin pyrophosphate; TPP and flavin adenine dinucleotide; FAD) and an enzyme activator (Mg^{2+}). However, the detection limit of 12 μM Pi was insufficient for environmental water control.

In 1996, Ikebukuro et al. examined the combination of a luminol chemiluminescence (CL) reaction and a FIA system for enzymatic Pi biosensor (CL-FIA system) [27]. At that time, the CL reaction was known as a highly sensitive reaction, and the FIA system was also known as a highly repeatable measurement system [30, 31]. The reason why the latter repeatability contributes to high-precision analysis was that the closer the multiple measurement results obtained from the same standard solution were to their average values, the smaller the standard deviation value. Along with this, by increasing the significant difference between the standard measurement value and the blank value, the standard measurement value closer to the blank value could be set as the detection limit. As a result, by combining CL and FIA technics, it was possible to realize a high-precision analytical method due to the synergistic effect of both. This meant that the CL-FIA system can turn the enzymatic Pi biosensors into highly sensitive analytical instruments. Thus, the CL-FIA biosensor systems have been widely studied [32].

In the PO_{Psp} catalytic reaction, hydrogen peroxide was produced and subsequently consumed by a luminol-peroxidase reaction (peroxidase from horseradish, HRP). The CL light resulting from the presence of Pi was detected at a photomultiplier tube (PMT). By the purification of TPP to remove residual phosphates, a detection limit of 74 nM Pi was obtained, although the TPP purification was unsuitable for practical use [28].

In 1997, Nakamura et al. used highly sensitive luminol catalyzing peroxidase from *Arthromyces ramosus* (ARP) [9]. This CL-FIA system was improved to the remote-controlled automatic continuous Pi monitoring system and compactly integrated into a submersible buoy to monitor dam water for drinking (**Figure 2c**) [9, 10]. Then, PO_{Psp} was immobilized onto chitin-chitosan beads filled in a stainless-steel column. In this study, 160 nM Pi was detected without purification of TPP, and by keeping PO_{Psp} activity in the stainless-steel column, 0.32 μM Pi was detected for 48 days. This result was sufficient for practical use of the CL-FIA biosensor system for Pi monitoring. Unfortunately, the manufacturing of PO_{Psp} was stopped.

In 1999, Nakamura et al. reexamined the development of the CL-FIA system for an enzymatic Pi biosensor using a new enzyme, PO_{Av}, which was purified from recombinant *Escherichia coli* [8]. Then, PO_{Av} was densely immobilized onto *N*-hydroxysuccinicacidimido (NHS)-gel beads. Here, the velocity of the enzymatic reaction strongly depends on the temperature. This means that the temperature must be kept constant by precise control to obtain repeatable signals based on the enzymatic reaction. On the other hand, accurate (i.e., absolute) temperature control dose is not essentially needed due to that the enzymatic activity immobilized in the biosensor changes. Thus, in this study, a desktop-type automatic CL-FIA system involving a precise temperature control system was fabricated as a trial enzymatic Pi biosensor instrument (**Figure 2b**). Then, the detection limit was 96 nM Pi. In addition, with sufficient performance at a short measurement time of 2 minutes, a wide linear range of calibration (96 nM and 32 μM Pi) was obtained with an average relative standard deviation (RSD_{av}) of 2.3% (eight points, n = 5) at 25.0 C. In addition, this system kept making calibration curves from 0.16 to 32 μM Pi (five points, n = 3; averaged correlation, r = 1.00) for at least 2 weeks. Thus, the practical utility of the Pi biosensor system was demonstrated.

On the other hand, in 1995, Conrath et al. studied a new electrochemical Pi biosensor using an analyte recycling system consisting of four enzymes, maltose phosphorylase (MP), acid phosphatase (AcP), mutarotase (MUT), and GOD [33]. The four enzymatic system enabled the successful detection of 10 nM Pi. However, the system was too complicated, and we thought it would be difficult to reproduce in manufacturing as well as other multiple-enzyme systems [24]. In 1999, Nakamura et al. modified the MP system and applied it to our CL-FIA biosensor system using a tri-enzymatic reaction of MP-MUT-GOD without the analyte recycling by AcP [20]. Then, we could obtain the same results with Conrath et al. at a detection limit of 10 nM Pi. In addition, an excellent calibration between 10 nM and 30 μM Pi was obtained and stability to detect 1.0 μM Pi was observed for at least 2 weeks.

In 2003, Nakamura et al. improved the MP-MUT-GOD system for freshwater measurements [11]. Our previous studies revealed that the Pi biosensors employing the CL-FIA system were affected by the cations contained in the real sample solutions. Then, we have tried to examine several pretreatment methods to remove the cations from the sample [8, 11, 20]. As the result, we could find and establish a pretreatment method using a cation-exchanging resin. A total of 31 samples of freshwaters were taken from the river and pond. These real samples were pretreated by our method and measured for Pi determination by both this Pi biosensor and the conventional molybdenum-blue method. The results showed that the value from the conventional method was 2.78 times higher than that from the Pi biosensor. One reason for this outcome was considered that there were large differences in the reacting conditions between the Pi biosensor (natural pH) and the conventional method (under strong acid conditions). Therefore, an enzymatic Pi biosensor may determine the more accurate and realistic Pi concentration as free and bioavailable Pi, which is needed to understand the water ecosystem.

Furthermore, Nakamura et al. studied a pyrophosphate ion (PPi) biosensor in 2004 [21]. As well as the Pi concentration, the PPi concentration is also an indicator of the eutrophication and the organic pollution. For the enzymatic PPi biosensor, inorganic pyrophosphatase (IP) was added to the PO_{Av} reaction, and the possibility of this PPi biosensor to environmental water was also shown. In another study, Nakamura et al. also examined the development of a disposable electrochemical Pi biosensor chip for on-site monitoring [34]. Then, a commercially available self-monitoring blood glucose (SMBG) chip was applied to the Pi measurements. Pi was measured with a PO_{Av} or several MP systems coupled with ferricyanide ion (Fe^{3+}) as an electrochemical mediator.

Here, an author looks back on the five requirements that were set for the practical use of our Pi biosensors [8, 9, 11, 20, 21]. In the first requirement, the CL-FIA systems were successfully applied to the Pi biosensors and made it possible to highly sensitive and practical Pi measurements [8, 9, 11, 20, 21]. In the second requirement, our Pi biosensor was able to continue to make practical calibration curves as the stability tests and demonstrate the practicability [8, 9]. In the third requirement, the sample pretreatment method was finally established by the countermeasures against interfering matters [11]. In the fourth requirement, the establishment of the sample pretreatment method was enabled to perform real sample applications [11]. In the fifth requirement, the automation of the Pi and PPi biosensor systems was realized by employing the CL-FIA systems [8, 9, 21].

As described above, we studied several types of Pi biosensors for the estimation of eutrophication, and finally, two trial Pi biosensor instruments of the desktop and the submersible buoy were developed. Although thorough examinations using the real samples were necessarily employing the automatic Pi biosensor instrument for practical use and commercialization, various factors made it impossible to conduct the study (laboratory relocation, running costs, stop production of enzymes, etc.). In conclusion of our study for practical use of the enzymatic Pi biosensors, the highest risk was the stop production of the enzymes. As the general concerns, the development and subsequent practical use of the enzymatic biosensor tend to be expensive running costs for the enzyme. In particular, the FIA system consumes a lot of reagents and our CL-FIA system needs to contain the enzyme (HRP or ARP) in the CL reagent.

2.3 Subsequent development of Pi biosensors and a new insight into the future perspectives of the Pi biosensor fields

Subsequent development of the Pi biosensors by other groups was introduced here. In 2005, Kwan et al. studied a screen-printed electrochemical Pi biosensor using PO. The enzymatic Pi biosensor had a linear calibration range from 75 to 625 μM Pi [35]. The PO reaction needs TPP, which releases Pi. For practical use, an investigation of the storage condition of TPP would be needed. In 2001, Mousty et al. studied an electrochemical tri-enzymatic Pi biosensor employing an MP-MUT-GOD reaction system [36]. This system had a linear calibration range from 1 to 50 μM and was stable for at least 2 weeks. In 1998, Fernandez et al. studied another type of electrochemical tri-enzymatic Pi biosensor [37]. The three enzymes, a substrate, a cofactor, and a mediator, were incorporated into hydrogels. The enzymatic Pi biosensor had a detection limit of 2 mM Pi. Quite complicated principles and unstable enzymes would be a problem for practical use. These enzymatic Pi biosensors had insufficient sensitivity for actual eutrophication. For practical use, the influences of reducing matters in a sample solution on the biosensor response cannot be ignored. In 2013, Lawal and Adeloju studied measures against reducing matters in electrochemical Pi biosensors [38]. For this aim, they used conductive polymer of polypyrrole to the electrochemical bi-enzymatic Pi biosensors and could not observe the obvious influences of uric and ascorbic acids on both amperometry and potentiometric methods. However, the sensitivity of the Pi biosensor was insufficient for natural waters, therefore, the effects of the polypyrrole on the Pi measurement might be unclear. In 2020, Korkut et al. also used the polypyrrole to a PO-Pi biosensor and successfully performed accurate Pi determination of eutrophied water at 91% [39].

The enzymatic Pi biosensors have been developed not only for environmental use but also for medical use (urine Pi) [40, 41] and food use [42]. In the case of food use, in 2020, He and Liu successfully developed a highly sensitive PO-Pi biosensor employing "Nano-Enabled Biosensing" techniques that combined with gold nanorods (AuNRs) as nanomaterials and conductive materials. The PO-Pi biosensor was able to detect 0.4 nM Pi, which is sufficient to estimate eutrophication. On the other hand, these conductive materials have the potential to perform well in both food and medical applications, where samples are high in reducing matters [38, 39, 42].

On the other hand, studies using molecular recognition elements other than enzymes have also been carried out. The molecular recognition elements can be categorized into two types. One is bacterial phosphate-binding proteins (PBPs) and another is an ionophore that is made of lipid or polymer. The PBP is a component of a phosphate transport system and a highly selective recognition element of Pi (K_d = 1 μM) [43]. In bacteria, PBP has the function of transporting Pi into cells and organelles and does not bind other inorganic or organic ions except Pi and arsenate.

In 2002, Kubo et al. studied an electrochemical PBP Pi biosensor. They extracted the PBP from *E. coli* of wild type and detected Pi potentiometrically at a range from 0.1 to 1.5 mM [44]. In 2004, Lyndon et al. applied a mutant PBP for fluorometric Pi biosensor. Then, fluorophore was site-specifically labeled to the mutant PBP. This Pi biosensor showed excellent selectivity and was detected around sub-μM Pi [45], although the stability of PBP should be addressed. In 2019, Sarwar et al. successfully applied a fluorometric PBP-Pi biosensor (mutant PBP-labeled fluorophore), which was purchased from Thermo Fisher Scientific Co., to the estimation for actual eutrophication employing a smartphone camera detection system [46]. They prepared a cassette system for the smartphone using a 3D printer and the paper-based disposal

PBP-Pi biosensor chip using a Xerox printer. This PBP-Pi biosensor had high sensitivity of 1.1 ppb (12 nM) Pi and a response time of only 4 seconds, considering the effect of fluorescence photo-bleaching. One of the notable results in this study is the high reproducibility of the results obtained from the paper-based disposal PBP-Pi biosensor chips using Xerox printing. In general, reproducibility of the results obtained by the disposable type single-use biosensor was one of the problems in practical development. The author has been also energetically studying this problem in the practical study of the SMBG biosensor chips, therefore the author understand the difficulty [47]. In 2020, Franz et al. developed a PBP-Pi biosensor using a mutant PBP-labeled fluorophore and established a new principle of thermophoresis [48]. For Pi detection, they combined the advantages of a biological Pi-receptor based on the PBP with the principle of thermophoresis. The PBP-Pi biosensor enabled the sub-nanomolar Pi determination in sample volumes $\leq$10 μL.

In the cases applying the ionophores to the Pi biosensors, Carey and Riggan in 1994 applied cyclic polyamine to an ion-selective electrode (ISE) for Pi [49]. This Pi sensor specifically detected dibasic phosphate (HPO_4^{2-}) and obtained a linear response between 1.0 μM and 0.1 M Pi. For the real sample application, the influences of sample pH have to be concerned. The ionophores from microbes were used for the Pi biosensors [50, 51]. As an example, the Pi biosensor studied by Wygladacz et al. obtained a linear calibration range from 1.0 μM to 2.5 mM Pi. However, the lifetime was the order of days [51].

Other principles for the Pi biosensors were also studied. In 2001, Schreiter et al. studied a Pi bioavailability assay employing a luminescent cyanobacterial reporter strain for the replacement of the conventional AGP test. The method enabled the highly sensitive detection of Pi from 0.3 to 8 μM, although it took 8 hours of incubation [52]. In 2003, Dollard and Billard studied a *pho A*::*lux*-based bacterial biosensor using a Pi-sensing plasmid and demonstrated the possibility for the assessment of Pi bioavailability [53]. However, the use of genetically engineered Pi biosensor elements is unsuitable in the cases of these leakages into the environment.

In this section, the author explained the representative studies on the development of Pi biosensors and Pi bioavailability assays for eutrophication. The biomaterials, such as enzymes, PBPs, and ionophores, were used for the Pi biosensors. These biomaterials need purification from living organisms. Therefore, the issue of cost and risk of production outage will be a challenge to the practical application of the Pi biosensors in this field. Further, in 2021, Becker et al. calculated the complete environmental factor (E-factor) of the enzyme [54]. The complete E-factor, including required waste and water, was calculated as 37,835 g-waste/g-enzyme. Therefore, the use of such biomaterials will require environmental consideration and not be neglected for the sustainability assessment of bioprocesses in the future. Furthermore, new technologies will be introduced one after another in this field, such as smartphones, 3D printers, nanomaterials, miniaturization, and automation.

3. Development of microbial BOD biosensors for organic pollution

3.1 Standard method and consideration to practical estimation performances

To estimate the degree of organic pollution, several indicators of total organic carbon (TOC), COD, BOD, and DO have been employed. In general, COD is employed for closed water bodies of both natural water and seawater, and BOD is employed for flowing water, such as rivers. The differences in the usage of COD and BOD estimation methods are simply determined by the presence or absence of the flux, which depends on the decomposition rate of organic matters dissolved in the water body by aerobes, although they are often employed as the references in each field.

In the estimation methods for organic pollution, only BOD involves the results obtained by a biological reaction. The conventional standard method of the BOD estimation is referred to as the 5-day BOD (BOD_5) method [55, 56]. It requires 5 days of incubation to obtain the results. The BOD value (mg O_2/L) is calculated from the amount of DO consumed by the aerobic decomposition of organic matters during incubation (primary fermentation). From this principle, BOD is also called biochemical oxygen consumption.

At the peak of organic pollution in advanced countries in the 1960s, the standard method of BOD was limited to the BOD_5 method [55, 56]. The BOD_5 method has several problems that prevent it from satisfying the needs for practical use in wastewater control, that is, this method is time-consuming and requires tedious operations. Therefore, a method that can be used to monitor the BOD value in real-time or continuous was urgently needed.

3.2 Development of microbial BOD biosensors

In 1960', there were many issues that need to be resolved to actually estimate the BOD. To solve these problems, many kinds of BOD biosensors have been studied and developed for practical use [57].

3.2.1 Development of early time BOD biosensors and accomplishment by Dr. Isao Karube in this field

As described above, the BOD_5 method is time-consuming and requires tedious operations. For example, it is not possible to detect the abnormality of wastewater before and after the treatment because it takes 5 days to obtain the measurement result. In other words, even if abnormal wastewater flows into the treatment facility or is not sufficiently treated at the treatment facility, it can be detected only after the wastewater has flowed out to the environmental water. In addition, the tedious operations of the BOD_5 method also make it difficult to make accurate and accurate measurements.

In 1977, Dr. Karube studied a practical microbial biosensor for BOD [58]. The key technique was the immobilization of microbes to a thin collagen membrane. The microbial membrane was put onto the surface of a DO electrode. By the addition of a sample solution into a batch system, microbial respiration was activated by the decomposition of organic matters, and the degree of DO consumption by the microbes was determined by the DO electrode. The microbial BOD biosensor indicating DO consumption (BOD_{DO}) could successfully determine the BOD value at drastically shortened incubation and measurement times (ca. 30 minutes). By the study, the possibilities for solving the problems of wastewater control were enhanced.

In 1979, Hikuma and Karube et al. developed a flow system of the BOD_{DO} biosensor [59]. In the study, omnivorous yeast *Tricbosporon cutaneum* (*Tc*), as a practical microbe, was used in this $BOD_{DO\text{-}Tc}$ biosensor. The microbes were immobilized onto a microporous membrane and attached to the surface of the DO electrode. Based on the study, a flow-type $BOD_{DO\text{-}Tc}$ biosensor was available for practical applications.

Both the desktop-type for rapid measurements and the installation-type for continuous monitoring were sold from the Central Kagaku Co. in 1983. These $BOD_{DO\text{-}Tc}$ biosensor instruments enabled wastewater control by both real-time measurement and continuous monitoring at sewage plants and factories. The $BOD_{DO\text{-}Tc}$ biosensor was established as one of the JIS methods (JIS K 3602) in 1990 [60]. Since then, the $BOD_{DO\text{-}Tc}$ biosensor instrument has also been used in educational settings as a science teaching material [61].

Since the first microbial biosensor was reported, many kinds of microbial biosensors have been studied for not only environmental applications but also food applications, including fermentation. These studies on both environments and foods by microbial biosensing methods were reviewed [3, 10, 15, 62].

Dr. I. Karube was widely studied all-fields of biosensor development as one of the leading scientists in the world. His notable study on biosensor development was summarized in the review [10] and the detailed history of his study on microbial biosensor development was described in one chapter of Encyclopedia [57].

The notable studies on the microbial BOD biosensor development performed by Karube et al. are briefly described as follows. As the study on the BOD biosensors, a microbial fuel cell (MFC) type biosensor has also been developed. However, the MFC biosensor at that time used expensive materials, easily deteriorated electrodes, anaerobes, etc., and had low cathode reaction efficiency due to low electron transfer from the anaerobes to the cathode. In addition, a flow-type cathode chamber of the MFC biosensor has a low exchange efficiency of sample solution, making it difficult to repeat and rapid BOD_{MFC} measurements.

After two types of $BOD_{DO\text{-}Tc}$ biosensor instruments were practically used, the other types of BOD biosensors have been widely studied and developed. One of the practical studies was the development of a bioluminescence BOD biosensor using a luminous bacterium *Photobacterium phosphoreum* (*Pph*) [63]. In 1993, Hyun et al. studied a $BOD_{BL\text{-}Pph}$ biosensor; however, the emission intensity of BL released by *P. phosphoreum* decreased with each measurement. Thus, a reagent-type $BOD_{BL\text{-}Pph}$ biosensor instrument was practically used by Tamiya et al.

Another practical study was the development of portable type instruments for on-site monitoring. To realize the on-site monitoring, it was required to stop using air-supply equipment, to reduce the size of measurement devices, to miniaturize and single-use biosensors, to employ omnivore and vital microbes, etc. Dr. Hiroaki Suzuki has been studying the miniaturization of the biosensors to be used as disposable sensor chips [64]. In 1996, Suzuki and Yang et al. studied $BOD_{DO\text{-}Tc}$ biosensors for on-site monitoring and developed a low-cost paper-based DO electrode [65] and a disposable $BOD_{DO\text{-}Tc}$ biosensor chip [66]. However, in general, the $BOD_{DO\text{-}Tc}$ biosensors were difficult to accurately measure the high BOD value of a sample solution, because the solubility of oxygen into water is limited (8.11 mg O_2/L at 25°C and 1 atm).

To solve the problem, in 2000, Yoshida et al. studied two types of BOD biosensor principles for on-site monitoring. One was a single mediator (SM) type of an electrochemical BOD biosensor [67]. In the study, omnivorous bacteria *Pseudomonas fluorescens* (*Pf*) was isolated from a sewage plant. By using potassium ferricyanide as a highly soluble mediator in water (460 g/L), a $BOD_{SM\text{-}Pf}$ biosensor that does not require air-supply equipment was developed. The principle was applied to a portable type instrument and a disposable $BOD_{SM\text{-}Pf}$ biosensor chip for on-site monitoring [68]. As a result, a wide linear range of calibration (15 and 260 mg O_2/L) was obtained. Another type was an optical BOD biosensor using the redox electron acceptor 2,6-dichlorophenolindophenol (DCIP) sodium salt as a redox color indicator

(RCI). Before the development of a portable type optical instrument, an absorptiometric high-throughput $BOD_{RCI\text{-}Pf}$ measurement method was studied using a microplate reader, which is able to measure 96 samples simultaneously [69]. Based on the principle, the portable type optical $BOD_{RCI\text{-}Pf}$ biosensor instrument was constructed using three pairs of light-emitting diodes (LEDs; 600 nm) and silicon photodiodes (Si-PDs), and a transparent disposable chip containing three biosensing spots [70]. As a result, a linear relationship was observed below 176 mg O_2/L, and the detection limit was 14 mg O_2/L (n = 6, RSD = 10.3%). An excellent correlation coefficient (r^2 = 0.989) was obtained after 600 seconds incubation time. By the study of Yoshida et al., two portable types of the practical BOD_{Pf} biosensor instruments were developed using two types of redox electron acceptors.

On the other hand, in 1999, Chee et al. studied highly sensitive BOD_{DO} biosensors for low BOD measurements [71]. The background of this study was that the spread of sewage treatment facilities improved the water quality of rivers at that time, and it became necessary to measure low BOD including persistent organic matters in the sample solution. To properly measure the river water quality at that time, isolation of the microbe that biodegrades persistent organic matters was needed, and they isolated *Pseudomonas putida* (*Ppu*) from a sewage plant. To enhance the biodegradability of the persistent organic matters by *P. putida*, they examined pretreatment methods of the sample solution and finally established the photocatalytic UV-TiO_2 method [72]. As the result, a practical linear range of calibration (0.5 and 8 mg O_2/L) was obtained using artificial wastewater containing persistent organic matters.

The studies on the practical BOD biosensor were successfully performed by Dr. Karube et al. and the practical instruments including the potable instruments for on-site monitoring were developed.

3.2.2 Development of BOD biosensors that the author principally conducted

After these excellent studies on the practical BOD biosensors by Dr. Karube et al., the author explored other possibilities of BOD biosensors with better functionality, for example, improvements of (1) detection limit, (2) signal repeatability of the microbial biosensor, and (3) suitability of microbe used.

1. The detection limit can be improved to enhance the reaction efficiency of microbial degradation of organic matters. However, most of the microbial biosensors developed to date immobilized the microbes. To enhance the reaction efficiency of microbial degradation of organic matters, microbes should be dispersed to uniform the suspension.

2. The signal repeatability of the microbial biosensor can be enhanced by a fully unified operation of repeating measurements under the same conditions. It is important to keep constant at least both temperature and reaction time. This enhancement also leads to highly sensitive measurements. This is because by increasing the significant difference between the standard measurement value and the blank value, the standard measurement value closer to the blank value can be set as the detection limit (it is known that the reproducibility of the signals obtained by the microbial biosensor is around 10% (as RSD value) [70]).

3. On the other hand, the improvement of microbial suitability can also be achieved by employing easily available, omnivorous, and vital microbe.

Then, the author tried to satisfy these requirements by employing the absorptiometric BOD_{RCI} measurement method and a temperature-controlled three-cuvette-stir system [73, 74]. As the usable (easily available, omnivorous, and vital) microbe, Baker's dry yeast *Saccharomyces cerevisiae* (*Sc*) was used after liquid culturing. *S. cerevisiae* is budding yeast; therefore, it was suitable for forming uniform suspension in the cuvette. On the other hand, *T. cutaneum*, which is conventionally used for the BOD biosensors and makes flocks by sticking together, was not suitable for this study because it was filamentous fungi. In this method, DCIP was used as RCI of a high absorption coefficient (*epsilon* = 1.45×10^5 cm^{-1} M^{-1}) to enhance the sensitivity of the absorptiometry. Then, the absorbance of DCIP decreased due to degradation of organic matters by *S. cerevisiae* in the measurement suspensions, and the absorbance change between before and after incubation was measured as the time difference method (**Figure 3**).

In general, the suspension is not suitable for absorptiometry due to the occurrence of light scattering. However, by a combination of the cuvette-stir system and the time difference method, the influences of the light scattering were efficiently canceled and only absorbance change of DCIP was accurately determined. Further, by repeating the exact same measurement operation three times, the fluctuation of the measured value became small, and the reproducibility was improved, so that highly precise measurement became possible. As a result, the significant difference from the blank value became large, and highly sensitive measurement became possible.

$BOD_{RCI\text{-}Sc}$ measurement method: As a result, a calibration curve between 1.1 and 22 mg O_2/L (r = 0.988, six points, n = 3, RSD = 1.77%) was obtained by this highly sensitive $BOD_{RCI\text{-}Sc}$ measurement method when the incubation mixture was incubated for exact 10 minutes at 30°C. Employing salt-tolerant yeast *S. cerevisiae*

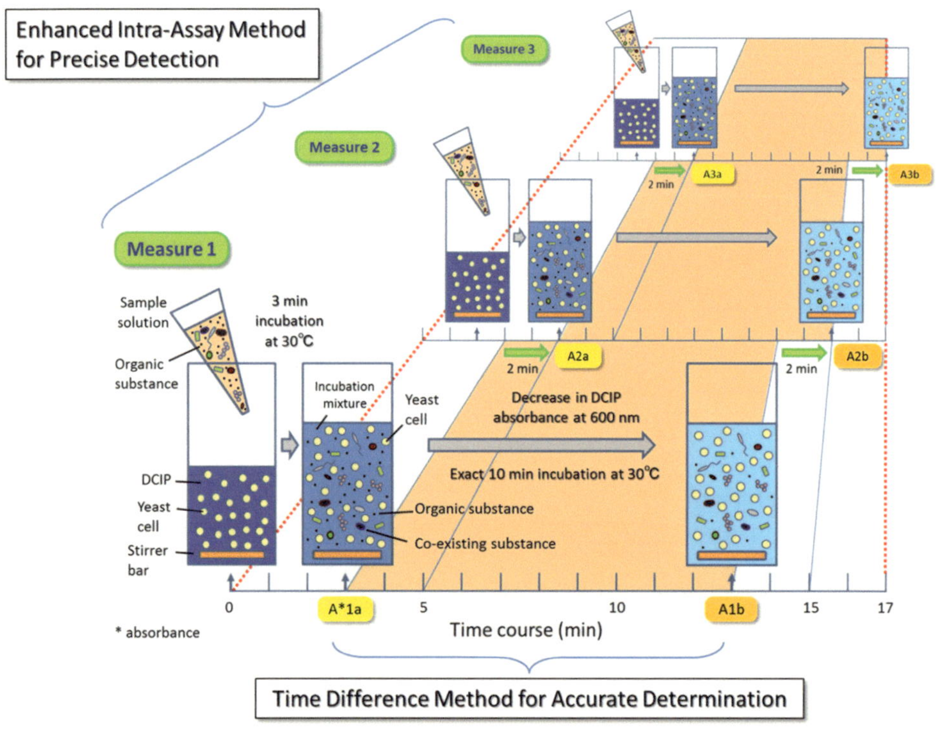

Figure 3.
A key principle for the simple absorptiometric measurement method using redox color indicator [73].

ARIF KD-003 (*Sc*II), a $BOD_{RCI\text{-}ScII}$ measurement method was also studied for seawater [75]. In these studies, the highly sensitive $BOD_{RCI\text{-}Sc}$ measurement method was developed by enhancing the repeatability of the measurements and by employing the usable yeast. From the future perspective of this study, the $BOD_{RCI\text{-}Sc}$ measurement method might be improved by applying it to an absorptiometric-FIA system.

$BOD_{DM\text{-}Sc}$ biosensor: As the other application of *S. cerevisiae* to a BOD biosensor, the author also studied a mediator type BOD biosensor. By applying a double mediator (DM) system coupled with ferricyanide and a lipophilic mediator, menadione, electrochemical signals were obtained from the eukaryote *S. cerevisiae* cells [76]. For practical use, the author designed a package-free disposable microbial biosensor chip containing living microbial cells [77] and the biosensor chip was applied to a DM-type $BOD_{DM\text{-}Sc}$ biosensor [78]. Under the optimal conditions, a calibration curve was obtained with a practical range of 6.6–220 mg O_2/L (five points, n = 3, RSD = 6.6%). Thus, the $BOD_{DM\text{-}Sc}$ biosensor was developed as the third generation of the BOD biosensor [3, 10].

$BOD_{CL\text{-}Sc}$ measurement method: By applying the principle of the BOD_{DM} biosensor, the author next studied a chemiluminescence BOD ($BOD_{CL\text{-}Sc}$) measurement method. Because Yamashoji et al. in 2004 already established luminol CL assay for the viable microbial detection method using ferricyanide and menadione [79]. Their principle was based on hydrogen peroxide (H_2O_2) determination produced by the reaction of the viable microbes and menadione. After optimization of the measurement conditions, a practical correlation between $BOD_{CL\text{-}Sc}$ value and amount of organic matters assimilated by *S. cerevisiae* was observed with a range of 11–220 mg O_2/L (six points, n = 3, RSD = 3.71%) at the incubation time of only 5 minutes [80, 81]. Then, the detection limit was 5.5 mg O_2/L.

$BOD_{DM:Trinder\text{-}Sc}$ measurement method: As one of the reagents for H_2O_2 measurement, there is a modified Trinder's reagent. It is an absorptiometric H_2O_2 measurement method using peroxidase (POD), 4-aminoantipyrine (4-AA), and *N*-ethyl-*N*-(2-hydroxy-3-sulfopropyl)-3,5-dimethylaniline sodium salt (MAOS). Applying this reagent, we already developed a surface plasmon resonance (SPR) biosensor for H_2O_2 measurement using a modified Trinder's reagent as a color indicator [82]. This reagent had high selectivity, however, POD was unsuitable for applying to the microbial biosensor due to take cost. On the other hand, H_2O_2 reacted as the reactant in $BOD_{CL\text{-}Sc}$ method. This meant that H_2O_2 or active oxygen species might also react as the reactant in $BOD_{DM\text{-}Sc}$ method. To verify the possibility, MAOS and 4-AA, which were used in the modified Trinder's reagent, were added to the principle of the $BOD_{DM\text{-}Sc}$ method. As the result obtained without the use of POD as the biocatalyst, correlations between $BOD_{DM:Trinder\text{-}Sc}$ value and amount of organic matters assimilated by *S. cerevisiae* were observed in several measurement conditions, although further practical examinations are required [83].

In the studies that the author principally conducted, excellent functions in the BOD biosensor were achieved in (1) the practical detection limit, (2) the signal reproducibility, and (3) the suitability of the microbe used. In addition, some principles of both microbial BOD biosensors and measurement methods have been studied for practical use, but none of the studies the author have principally conducted has reached practical use. The most practical BOD measurement method in the studies might be the $BOD_{RCI\text{-}Sc}$ measurement method. The reasons are as follows:

1. Practically suitable microbe (easily available, omnivorous, and vital yeast)

2. Very simple operation (just added three solutions into a cuvette; a *S. cerevisiae* cell suspension, a DCIP solution, and a sample solution)

3. Rapid measurement time (only 10 minutes incubation)

4. Highly sensitive measurements (highly repeatable results were obtained by employing a temperature-controlled three-cuvette-stir system and provided highly precise results, enabling highly sensitive measurements; and it was also important to use RCI of high absorption coefficient)

5. Practical dynamic range (same as available BOD biosensor instrument)

6. The patent registered for practical use (the patent right did not continue [74])

For future study, automatic instrumentation of the BOD biosensor would be required having the features that we obtained. Then, further suitability of the microbe might be needed to be considered, for example, use of thermally killed microbes [84] or cell crushed microbes, or direct use of available dry yeast [85].

3.3 Subsequent development of BOD biosensors and a new insight into the future perspectives of the BOD biosensor fields

Even after our studies on the BOD biosensors have been reported, the studies on next-generation BOD biosensors are ongoing. In this section, the progress of our studies on the BOD biosensors performed by other groups is introduced.

In our studies that the author principally conducted, the most practical BOD biosensor or measurement method was the $BOD_{RCI\text{-}Sc}$ measurement method. Unfortunately, we did not achieve the instrumentation. However, in 2021, Azevedo et al. developed an automated *S. cerevisiae*-based spectrophotometric instrument using methylene blue (MB) dye as a RCI, although this instrument was not for BOD measurement, but also possible to measure BOD [86]. The instrument consists of a sequential injection analysis (SIA) flow system, which enables high throughput measurements with small quantities of reagent consumption. On the other hand, DCIP has been used not only as a RCI but also as a redox mediator for electrochemical BOD_{SM} biosensors. For example, Reshetilov et al. developed several types of electrochemical microbial biosensors using DCIP as the redox mediator [87]. In 2017, Niyomdecha et al. fabricated a practical electrochemical FIA type microbial biosensor system for highly precise BOD measurements [88]. They used MB dye as a redox mediator and successfully obtained highly sensitive results of the detection limit at 0.1 mg O_2/L. This study demonstrated that highly reproducible results provided highly precise results, enabling highly sensitive measurements.

As recent progress of the DM-type microbial biosensors, several groups were reported. For example, in 2017, Gao et al. reported a DM-type *S. cerevisiae* biosensor for toxicity of wastewater and co-immobilized *S. cerevisiae*, menadione, and ferricyanide onto a glassy carbon electrode by electrodeposition of a chitosan hydrogel and nanocrystalline diamond particles [89]. In this study, it seems that *S. cerevisiae* and two mediators were successfully immobilized into the matrix without leakage and made it possible to distribute toxic matters into the matrix. However, this biosensor has a complication of the fabrication, therefore reproducible fabrication of the biosensor electrodes might be difficult. In 2017, Zaitseva et al. developed a batch-type BOD_{DM} biosensor employing yeast *Debaryomyces hansenii* (*Dh*) and ferrocene-MB mediator system [90]. The $BOD_{DM\text{-}Dh}$ biosensor had practical characteristics of a short measurement time of 10 min, a minimum limit of determination of 2.5 mg O_2/L, and long-time stability of 43 days. Then, they assumed as a new insight that lipophilic mediators, such as MB and DCIP, are capable of penetrating inside the microbial cell through the lipid membrane, taking electrons, and passing them on to the electrode immobilized ferrocene. If their assumption is true, new future perspectives in microbial electron transfer techniques can be opened.

As recent progress of the $BOD_{CL\text{-}Sc}$ biosensor, in 2018, Costa et al. developed a practical SIA microfluidic system of a $BOD_{CL\text{-}Sc}$ biosensor [91]. The SIA system was programmed to precisely control the flow of multiple channels in an accurate time, making it easier to obtain highly reproducible results. In addition, the incubation time under constant temperature for *S. cerevisiae* to assimilate the organic matters in the sample solution was also precisely controlled by setting the stopped period. If hydrogen peroxide is not used, highly sensitive measurements might be obtained by reduction of the background signal, and if the mixed solution could be agitated during incubation, both reaction efficiency and reproducibility might simultaneously be improved.

As the other progress, MFC biosensors have many potentials not only as BOD biosensors but also as self-powered devices for biosensors [92]. As a new insight into the future perspectives of the BOD biosensor fields, the author have one idea that is our past application study on a damped glycolytic oscillation induced in living yeast cells for toxicity assays (**Figure 4**) [93, 94]. We extracted six indexes from the wave shape and observed that these indexes were changed depending on both toxicity and the concentration of each toxic matter. By applying this principle, wave changes depending on both bioavailability and the concentration of the organic matters dissolved in a sample solution might be determined. In fact, excellent correlation was obtained between one of the indexes and the concentration of glucose (r = 0.9989, 2.5 μM–0.25 M, 12 points).

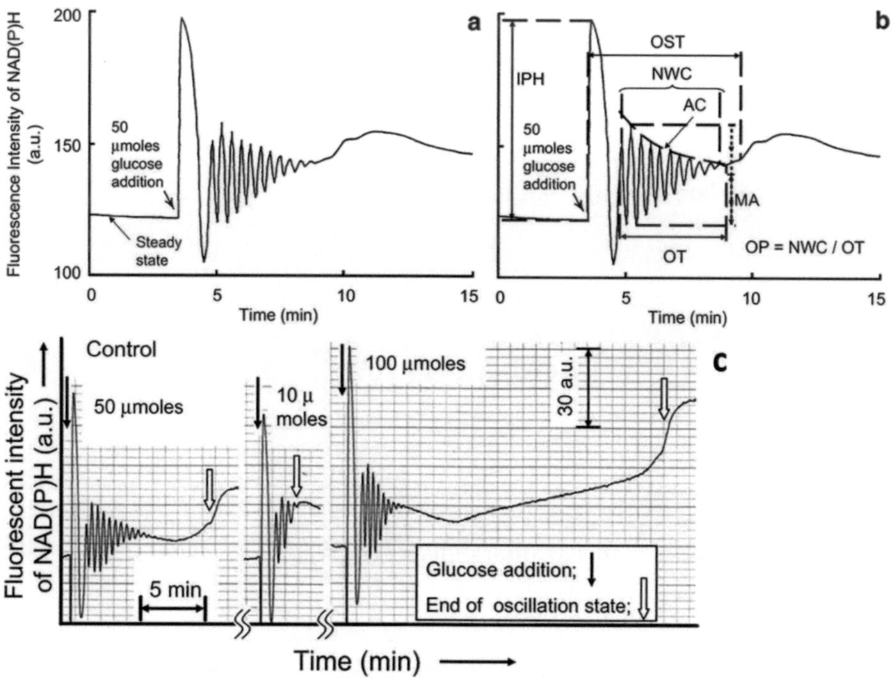

Figure 4.
(a) Typical damped glycolytic oscillation induced in living yeast cells. (b) Six indexes in an oscillation wave shape. (c) Response to glucose. These were permitted from Springer Nature [93].

Glycolysis is an important system that plays a central role in metabolism [14]. If this metabolic oscillation is applied to environmental monitoring, it may be possible to continuously sense the state of the aquatic environment perceived by organisms living in aquatic ecosystems in real-time. By doing so, for example, not only the index of BOD concentration but also the nutritional status of water quality and the substantial effect of heavy metals and antibiotics can be understood through the metabolic status of microbes employed for biosensing.

4. Conclusion

In this chapter, the author described the study on biosensor development for both eutrophication and organic pollution as one of my studying fields. By focusing on the two keywords of eutrophication and organic pollution, the author was able to summarize for the first time a series of our developmental flows and their aims. In conclusion, our biosensors introduced here could not be put into practical use. Nonetheless, the author hope that the practical use of both Pi and BOD biosensors as a replacement of the conventional standard methods will be realized based on the knowledge obtained by our developmental study.

Acknowledgements

In the relevant studies of the present chapter, the author acknowledges Professor Dr. Isao Karube (February 2020 passed away), his laboratory members, the relevant parties, for their mentoring, collaborations, and supports, and also acknowledge my laboratory members for the contributions to their experiments.

Conflict of interest

The authors declare no conflict of interest.

Author details

Hideaki Nakamura
Department of Liberal Arts, Tokyo University of Technology, Tokyo, Japan

Address all correspondence to: nakamurahd@stf.teu.ac.jp

References

[1] United Nations. The Sustainable Development Goals. 2015. Available from: https://www.un.org/sustainabledevelopment/ [Accessed: February 23, 2022]

[2] Nakamura H. Current status of water environment and their microbial biosensor techniques—Part I: Current data of water environment and recent studies on water quality investigations in Japan, and new possibility of microbial biosensor techniques. Analytical and Bioanalytical Chemistry. 2018;**410**(17):3953-3965. DOI: 10.1007/s00216-018-0923-z

[3] Nakamura H. Recent organic pollution and its biosensing methods. Analytical Methods. 2010;**2**(5):430-444. DOI: 10.1039/b9ay00315k

[4] Breida M, Younssi SA, Ouammou M, Bouhria M, Hafsi M. Pollution of water sources from agricultural and industrial effluents: Special attention to $NO3^-$, Cr(VI), and Cu(II). In: Eyvaz M, Yüksel E, editors. Water Chemistry. London: IntechOpen; 2019. pp. 39-68. DOI: 10.5772/intechopen.86921

[5] Nakamura H. Water chemical remediation for simultaneous removal of phosphate ion and blue-green algae from anthropogenically eutrophied pond. In: Eyvaz M, Yüksel E, editors. Water Chemistry. London: IntechOpen; 2019. pp. 21-38. DOI: 10.5772/intechopen.88490

[6] Nakamura H, Suka N, Kita Y, Yasue N, Sakamaki T, Ito M, et al. Investigations of eco-balance and water quality in a holding pond—Organic pollution caused by eutrophication and its effects on water quality (in Japanese). Bulletin of Tokyo University of Technology. 2010;**5**:69-77

[7] Nakamura H, Taguchi M, Yokoyama H, Hirabayashi K, Abiko S, Gotoh M, et al. Study on highly-effective purification of eutrophied freshwater applying hydroponic culture (in Japanese). Bulletin of Tokyo University of Technology. 2010;**5**:43-52

[8] Nakamura H, Tanaka H, Hasegawa M, Masuda Y, Arikawa Y, Ikebukuro K, et al. An automatic flow-injection analysis system for determining phosphate ion in river water using pyruvate oxidase G (from *Aerococcus viridans*). Talanta. 1999;**50**(4):799-807. DOI: 10.1016/S0039-9140(99)00137-X

[9] Nakamura H, Yamamoto H, Kubo I, Suzuki M, Hayashi K, McNiven SJ, et al. A chemiluminescent FIA biosensor for phosphate ion monitoring using pyruvate oxidase. Biosensors and Bioelectronics. 1997;**12**(9-10):959-966. DOI: 10.1016/S0956-5663(97)00032-8

[10] Nakamura H, Karube I. Current research activities in biosensors. Analytical and Bioanalytical Chemistry. 2003;**377**(3):446-468. DOI: 10.1007/s00216-003-1947-5

[11] Nakamura H, Hasegawa M, Arikawa Y, Nomura Y, Ikebukuro K, Karube I. Improvement of a CL-FIA system using maltose phosphorylase for the determination of phosphate ion in freshwater. Analytical Letters. 2003;**36**:1805-1817. DOI: 10.1081/AL-120023615

[12] Updike SJ, Hicks GP. The enzyme electrode. Nature. 1967;**214**(5092):986-988. DOI: 10.1038/214986a0

[13] Clark LC Jr, Wolf R, Granger D, Taylor Z. Continuous recording of blood oxygen tensions by polarography. Journal

of Applied Physiology. 1953;**6**(3):189-193. DOI: 10.1152/jappl.1953.6.3.189

[14] Nakamura H. Biosensors: Monitoring human health for the SDGs sustainable development goals. Biomedical Journal of Scientific and Technical Research. 2018;**9**(2):1-4. DOI: 10.26717/BJSTR.2018.09.001761

[15] Nakamura H. Current status of water environment and their microbial biosensor techniques—Part II: Recent trends in microbial biosensor development. Analytical and Bioanalytical Chemistry. 2018;**410**(17):3967-3989. DOI: 10.1007/s00216-018-1080-0

[16] Japanese Industrial Standard (JIS) Committee. Testing Methods for Industrial Wastewater (JIS K 0102; in Japanese). 2008 ed. JIS Committee; 1964

[17] Lowry OH, Lopez JA. The determination of inorganic phosphate in the presence of labile phosphate esters. Journal of Biological Chemistry. 1946;**162**:421-428

[18] Testing Methods for Drinking Waters (Tutorial Edition). Tokyo: Japan Water Works Association (JWWA); 1993

[19] Nakamura H. Phosphate ion determination in water for drinking using biosensors [digest of doctoral dissertation]. Bunseki Kagaku. 2001;**50**(8):581-582. DOI: 10.2116/bunsekikagaku.50.581

[20] Nakamura H, Hasegawa M, Nomura Y, Arikawa Y, Matsukawa R, Ikebukuro K, et al. Development of a highly sensitive chemiluminescence flow-injection analysis sensor for phosphate-ion detection using maltose phosphorylase. Journal of Biotechnology. 1999;**75**(2-3):127-133. DOI: 10.1016/S0168-1656(99)00150-9

[21] Nakamura H, Yamazaki R, Shirai T, Sano H, Nakami Y, Ikebukuro K, et al. Development of an enzymatic flow injection chemiluminescence system for determining inorganic pyrophosphate ion. Analytica Chimica Acta. 2004;**518**(1-2):45-49. DOI: 10.1016/j.aca.2004.05.057

[22] Guilbault GG, Nanjo M. A phosphate-selective electrode based on immobilized alkaline phosphatase and glucose oxidase. Analytica Chimica Acta. 1975;**78**(1):69-80. DOI: 10.1016/S0003-2670(01)84753-X

[23] d'Urso EM, Coulet PR. Phosphate-sensitive enzyme electrode: A potential sensor for environment control. Analytica Chimica Acta. 1990;**239C**:1-5. DOI: 10.1016/S0003-2670(00)83827-1

[24] Wollenberger U, Schubert F, Scheller FW. Biosensor for sensitive phosphate detection. Sensors and Actuators B. 1992;**7**(1-3):412-415. DOI: 10.1016/0925-4005(92)80335-U

[25] Male KB, Luong JHT. An FIA biosensor system for the determination of phosphate. Biosensors and Bioelectronics. 1991;**6**(7):581-587. DOI: 10.1016/0956-5663(91)80023-Q

[26] Kubo I, Inagawa I, Sugawara T, Arikawa Y, Karube I. Phosphate sensor composed from immobilized pyruvate oxidase and an oxygen electrode. Analytical Letters. 1992;**24**:1711-1717. DOI: 10.1080/00032719108053007

[27] Ikebukuro K, Kubo I, Inagawa M, Sugawara T, Nakamura H, Arikawa Y, et al. Phosphate sensing system using pyruvate oxidase and chemiluminescence detection. Biosensors and Bioelectronics. 1996;**11**(10):959-965. DOI: 10.1016/0956-5663(96)87655-X

[28] Ikebukuro K, Nishida R, Yamamoto H, Arikawa Y, Nakamura H, Suzuki M, et al. A novel biosensor system for the

determination of phosphate. Journal of Biotechnology. 1996;**48**(1-2):67-72. DOI: 10.1016/0168-1656(96)01398-3

[29] Suzuki M, Kurata H, Inoue Y, Shin H, Kubo I, Nakamura H, et al. Reagentless phosphate ion sensor system for environmental monitoring. Denki Kagaku. 1998;**66**(6):579-583. DOI: 10.5796/kogyobutsurikagaku.66.579

[30] Ruzicka J, Hansen EH. Flow injection analyses: Part I. A new concept of fast continuous flow analysis. Analytica Chimica Acta. 1975;**78**(1):145-157. DOI: 10.1016/S0003-2670(01)84761-9

[31] Estela JM, Cerda V. Flow analysis techniques for phosphorus: An overview. Talanta. 2006;**66**(2):307-331. DOI: 10.1016/j.talanta.2004.12.029

[32] Miro M, Estela JM, Cerd' V. Potentials of multisyringe flow injection analysis for chemiluminescence detection. Analytica Chimica Acta. 2005;**541**(1-2):57-68. DOI: 10.1016/j.aca.2004.06.075

[33] Conrath N, Grundig B, Huwel K, Cammann K. A novel enzyme sensor for the determination of inorganic phosphate. Analytica Chimica Acta. 1995;**309**(1-3):47-52. DOI: 10.1016/0003-2670(95)00065-8

[34] Nakamura H, Gotoh M, Karube I. Japanese Patent Application Raid-Open Disclosure P2005/073399A. Tokyo: Japan Patent Office (JPO); 2005

[35] Kwan RCH, Leung HF, Hon PYT, Barford JP, Renneberg R. A screen-printed biosensor using pyruvate oxidase for rapid determination of phosphate in synthetic wastewater. Applied Microbiology and Biotechnology. 2005;**66**:377-383. DOI: 10.1007/s00253-004-1701-8

[36] Mousty C, Cosnier S, Shan D, Mu S. Trienzymatic biosensor for the determination of inorganic phosphate. Analytica Chimica Acta. 2001;**443**:1-8. DOI: 10.1016/S0003-2670(01)01188-6

[37] Fernandez JJ, Lopez JR, Correig X, Katakis I. Reagentless carbon paste phosphate biosensors: Preliminary studies. Sensors and Actuators, B. 1998;**47**:13-20. DOI: 10.1016/S0925-4005(98)00003-3

[38] Lawal AT, Adeloju SB. Polypyrrole based amperometric and potentiometric phosphate biosensors: A comparative study B. Biosensors and Bioelectronics. 2013;**40**(1):377-384. DOI: 10.1016/j.bios.2012.08.012

[39] Korkut S, Göl S, Kilic MS. Poly(pyrrole-co-pyrrole-2-carboxylic acid)/pyruvate oxidase based biosensor for phosphate: Determination of the potential, and application in streams. Electroanalysis. 2020;**32**(2):271-280. DOI: 10.1002/elan.201900517

[40] Kulkarni SJ, Karve MS. Fabrication of enzyme-based optical biosensor for estimation of inorganic phosphate in a urine sample. SN Applied Sciences. 2020;**2**:1118. DOI: 10.1007/s42452-020-2748-6

[41] Kilic MS. A novel flow-injection rhodium nanoparticles modified phosphate biosensor and its operation in artificial urine. Electroanalysis. 2021;**33**(8):1963-1977. DOI: 10.1002/elan.202100154

[42] He B, Liu H. Electrochemical biosensor based on pyruvate oxidase immobilized AuNRs@ Cu_2O-NDs as electroactive probes loaded poly (diallyldimethylammonium chloride) functionalized graphene for the detection of phosphate. Sensors and Actuators B: Chemical. 2020;**304**:127303. DOI: 10.1016/j.snb.2019.127303

[43] Leucke H, Quiocho FA. High specificity of a phosphate transport protein determined by hydrogen

bonds. Nature. 1990;**347**:402-406. DOI: 10.1038/347402a0

[44] Kubo I. Potentiometric phosphate-sensing system utilizing phosphate-binding protein. Analytical and Bioanalytical Chemistry. 2002;**372**:273-275. DOI: 10.1007/s00216-001-1138-1

[45] Salins LLE, Deo SK, Daunert S. Phosphate binding protein as the biorecognition element in a biosensor for phosphate. Sensors and Actuators B: Chemical. 2004;**97**(1):81-89. DOI: 10.1016/j.snb.2003.07.019

[46] Sarwar M, Leichner J, Naja GM, Li CZ. Smart-phone, paper-based fluorescent sensor for ultra-low inorganic phosphate detection in environmental samples. Microsystems & Nanoengineering. 2019;**5**:56. DOI: 10.1038/s41378-019-0096-8

[47] Nakamura H. Microstructured electrochemical SMBG biosensor chip design development for sustainable mass production based on the strategic platform patent map. In: Rai M, Reshetilov A, Plekhanova Y, Ingle AP, editors. Macro, Micro, and Nano-Biosensors. Cham: Springer; 2021. pp. 285-323

[48] Franz P, Gassl V, Topf A, Eckelmann L, Iorga B, Tsiavaliaris G. A thermophoresis-based biosensor for real-time detection of inorganic phosphate during enzymatic reactions. Biosensors and Bioelectronics. 2020;**169**:112616. DOI: 10.1016/j.bios.2020.112616

[49] Carey CM, Riggan WB. Cyclic polyamine ionophore for use in a dibasic phosphate-selective electrode. Analytical Chemistry. 1994;**66**(21):3587-3591. DOI: 10.1021/ac00093a009

[50] Wróblewski W, Wojciechowski K, Dybko A, Brzózka Z, Egberink RJM, Snellink-Ruël BHM, et al. Uranyl salophenes as ionophores for phosphate-selective electrodes. Sensors and Actuators B: Chemical. 2000;**68**(1-3):313-318. DOI: 10.1016/S0925-4005(00)00450-0

[51] Wygladacz K, Qin Y, Wroblewski W, Bakker E. Phosphate selective fluorescent sensing microspheres based on uranyl salophene ionophores. Analytica Chimca Acta. 2008;**614**:77-84. DOI: 10.1016/j.aca.2008.02.069

[52] Schreiter PPY, Gillor O, Post A, Belkin S, Schmid RD, Bachmann TT. Monitoring of phosphorus bioavailability in water by an immobilized luminescent cyanobacterial reporter strain. Biosensors and Bioelectronics. 2001;**16**:811-818. DOI: 10.1016/S0956-5663(01)00224-X

[53] Dollard MA, Billard P. Whole-cell bacterial sensors for the monitoring of phosphate bioavailability. Journal of Microbiological Methods. 2003;**55**:221-229. DOI: 10.1016/S0167-7012(03)00164-7

[54] Becker M, Lütz S, Rosenthal K. Environmental assessment of enzyme production and purification. Molecules. 2021;**26**(3):573. DOI: 10.3390/molecules26030573

[55] American Public Health Association (APHA). Standard Methods for the Examination of Waters and Wastewater. 16th ed. Washington, DC: APHA; 1986. pp. 525-531

[56] JIS Committee. Testing Methods for Industrial Wastewater (JIS K 0102). Tokyo: JIS Committee; 1964

[57] Nakamura H, Karube I. Microbial biosensors. In: Grimes CA, Dickey EC, Pishko MV, editors. Encyclopedia of Sensors. 1st ed. Vol. 6. California: American Scientific Publishers; 2005. pp. 87-126

[58] Karube I, Matsunaga T, Mitsuda S, Suzuki S. Microbial electrode BOD sensors. Biotechnology and Bioengineering. 1977;**19**:1535-1547. DOI: 10.1002/bit.260191010

[59] Hikuma M, Suzuki H, Yasuda T, Karube I, Suzuki S. Amperometric estimation of BOD by using living immobilized yeasts. European Journal of Applied Microbiology and Biotechnology. 1979;**8**:289-297. DOI: 10.1007/BF00508793

[60] JIS Committee. Apparatus for the Estimation of Biochemical Oxygen Consumption (BODs) with Microbial Sensor (JIS K 3602). Tokyo: JIS Committee; 1990

[61] Central Kagaku Co. Biosensor Type Quick BOD Measuring Instrument Quick BOD α5000 Type. Available from: https://aqua-ckc.jp/products/bod5000.html [Accessed: February 23, 2022]

[62] Nakamura H, Shimomura-Shimizu M, Karube I. Development of microbial sensors and their application. In: Renneberg R, Lisdat F, editors. Biosensing for the 21st Century. Advances in Biochemical Engineering/Biotechnology. Vol. 109. Berlin: Springer; 2008. pp. 351-394. DOI: 10.1007/10_2007_085

[63] Hyun CK, Inoue N, Tamiya E, Takeuchi T, Karube I. A novel BOD sensor based on bacterial luminescence. Biotechnology and Bioengineering. 1993;**41**(11):1107-1111. DOI: 10.1002/bit.260411114

[64] Suzuki H. Microfabrication of chemical sensors and biosensors for environmental monitoring. Materials Science and Engineering: C. 2000;**12**(1-2):55-61. DOI: 10.1016/S0928-4931(00)00158-2

[65] Yang Z, Suzuki H, Sasaki S, Karube I. Design and validation of a low-cost paper-based oxygen electrode. Analytical Letters. 1997;**30**:1797-1807. DOI: 10.1080/00032719708001698

[66] Yang Z, Suzuki H, Sasaki S, Karube I. Disposable sensor for biochemical oxygen demand. Applied Microbiology and Biotechnology. 1996;**46**:10-14. DOI: 10.1007/s002530050776

[67] Yoshida N, Yano K, Morita T, McNiven SJ, Nakamura H, Karube I. A mediator-type biosensor as a new approach to biochemical oxygen demand estimation. The Analyst. 2000;**125**(12):2280-2284. DOI: 10.1039/b005995l

[68] Yoshida N, Hoashi J, Morita T, McNiven SJ, Nakamura H, Karube I. Improvement of a mediator-type biochemical oxygen demand sensor for on-site measurement. Journal of Biotechnology. 2001;**88**(3):269-275. DOI: 10.1016/S0168-1656(01)00282-6

[69] Yoshida N, McNiven SJ, Morita T, Nakamura H, Karube I. A simple, multiple simultaneous spectrophotometric method for biochemical oxygen demand determination using DCIP as the electron acceptor. Analytical Letters. 2002;**35**(9):1541-1549. DOI: 10.1081/AL-120006729

[70] Yoshida N, McNiven SJ, Yoshida A, Morita T, Nakamura H, Karube I. A compact optical system for multi-determination of biochemical oxygen demand using disposable strips. Field Analytical Chemistry and Technology. 2001;**5**(5):222-227. DOI: 10.1002/fact.10001

[71] Chee GJ, Nomura Y, Karube I. Biosensor for the estimation of low biochemical oxygen demand. Analytica

Chimica Acta. 1999;**379**:185-191. DOI: 10.1016/S0003-2670(98)00680-1

[72] Chee GJ, Nomura Y, Ikebukuro K, Karube I. Biosensor for the evaluation of biochemical oxygen demand using photocatalytic pretreatment. Sensors and Actuators B: Chemical. 2001;**80**:15-20. DOI: 10.1016/S0925-4005(01)00883-8

[73] Nakamura H, Kobayashi S, Hirata Y, Suzuki K, Mogi Y, Karube I. A spectrophotometric biochemical oxygen demand determination method using DCIP as the redox color indicator and eukaryote *Saccharomyces cerevisiae*. Analytical Biochemistry. 2007;**369**(2): 168-174. DOI: 10.1016/j.ab.2007.06.040

[74] Nakamura H, Karube I. Method for Measuring Activity of Microorganism. Registration No. JP4868405. Tokyo: Japan Patent Office (JPO); 2011

[75] Nakamura H, Mogi Y, Hattori H, Kita Y, Hattori D, Yoshimura A, et al. Absorption-based highly sensitive and reproducible biochemical oxygen demand measurement method for seawater using salt-tolerant yeast *Saccharomyces cerevisiae* ARIF KD-003. Analytica Chimica Acta. 2008;**620**(1-2):127-133. DOI: 10.1016/j.aca.2008.05.008

[76] Baronian K, Downard AJ, Lowen RK, Pasco N. Detection of two distinct substrate-dependent catabolic responses in yeast cells using a mediated electrochemical method. Applied Microbiology and Biotechnology. 2002;**60**:108-113. DOI: 10.1007/s00253-002-1108-3

[77] Nakamura H, Gotoh M, Karube I. Method of Measuring BOD. Registration No. JP4798502. Tokyo: JPO; 2011

[78] Nakamura H, Suzuki K, Ishikuro H, Kinoshita S, Koizumi R, Okuma S, et al. A new BOD estimation method employing a double mediator system by ferricyanide and menadione using the eukaryote *Saccharomyces cerevisiae*. Talanta. 2007;**72**(1):210-216. DOI: 10.1016/j.talanta.2006.10.019

[79] Yamashoji S, Asakawa A, Kawasaki S, Kawamoto S. Chemiluminescent assay for detection of viable microorganisms. Analytical Biochemistry. 2003;**333**(2): 303-308. DOI: 10.1016/j.ab.2004.05.043

[80] Nakamura H, Karube I. Method for Measuring Activity of Eukaryotic Microorganism. Registration No. JP4899156. Tokyo: JPO; 2012

[81] Nakamura H, Abe Y, Koizumi R, Suzuki K, Mogi Y, Hirayama T, et al. A chemiluminescence biochemical oxygen demand measuring method. Analytica Chimica Acta. 2007;**602**(1):94-100. DOI: 10.1016/j.aca.2007.08.050

[82] Nakamura H, Mogi Y, Akimoto T, Naemura K, Kato T, Yano K, et al. An enzyme-chromogenic surface plasmon resonance biosensor probe for hydrogen peroxide determination using a modified Trinder's reagent. Biosensors and Bioelectronics. 2008;**24**(3):455-460. DOI: 10.1016/j.bios.2008.04.022

[83] Nakamura H. New possibility for an absorptiometric microbial biosensor principle involving a modified Trinder's reaction and a lipophilic mediator's reaction. Current Topics in Analytical Chemistry;**2020**(11):59-66

[84] Tan TC, Qian Z. Dead *Bacillus subtilis* cells for sensing biochemical oxygen demand of waters and wastewaters. Sensors and Actuators B: Chemical. 1997;**40**:65-70. DOI: 10.1016/S0925-4005(97)00013-0

[85] Jarque S, Bittner M, Hilscherová K. Freeze-drying as suitable method to

achieve ready-to-use yeast biosensors for androgenic and estrogenic compounds. Chemosphere. 2016;**148**:204-210. DOI: 10.1016/j.chemosphere.2016.01.038

[86] Azevedo AMO, Vilaranda AG, Neves AFDC, Sousa MJ, Santos JLM, Saraiva MLMFS. Development of an automated yeast-based spectrophotometric method for toxicity screening: Application to ionic liquids, GUMBOS, and deep eutectic solvents. Chemosphere. 2021;**277**:130227. DOI: 10.1016/j.chemosphere.2021.130227

[87] Kharkova AS, Arlyapov VA, Turovskaya AD, Avtukh AN, Starodumova IP, Reshetilov AN. Mediator BOD biosensor based on cells of microorganisms isolated from activated sludge. Applied Biochemistry and Microbiology. 2019;**55**:189-197. DOI: 10.1134/S0003683819010083

[88] Niyomdecha S, Limbut W, Numnuam A, Asawatreratanakul P, Kanatharana P, Thavarungkul P. A novel BOD biosensor based on entrapped activated sludge in a porous chitosan-albumin cryogel incorporated with graphene and methylene blue. Sensors and Actuators B: Chemical. 2017;**241**:473-481. DOI: 10.1016/j.snb.2016.10.102

[89] Gao G, Fang D, Yu Y, Wu L, Wang Y, Zhi J. A double-mediator based whole cell electrochemical biosensor for acute biotoxicity assessment of wastewater. Talanta. 2017;**167**:208-216. DOI: 10.1016/j.talanta.2017.01.081

[90] Zaitseva AS, Arlyapov VA, Yudina NY, Alferov SV, Reshetilov AN. Use of one-and two-mediator systems for developing a BOD biosensor based on the yeast *Debaryomyces hansenii*. Enzyme and Microbial Technology. 2017;**98**:43-51. DOI: 10.1016/j.enzmictec.2016.12.005

[91] Costa SPF, Cunha E, Azevedo AMO, Pereira SAP, Neves AFDC, Vilaranda AG, et al. Microfluidic chemiluminescence system with yeast *Saccharomyces cerevisiae* for rapid biochemical oxygen demand measurement. ACS Sustainable Chemistry & Engineering. 2018;**6**(5):6094-6101. DOI: 10.1021/acssuschemeng.7b04736

[92] Cui Y, Lai B, Tang X. Microbial fuel cell-based biosensors. Biosensors. 2019;**9**:92. DOI: 10.3390/bios9030092

[93] Nakamura H, Suzuki M. New concept for a toxicity assay based on multiple indexes from the wave shape of damped metabolic oscillation induced in living yeast cells—Part I: Characterization of the phenomenon. Analytical and Bioanalytical Chemistry. 2007;**389**(4):1225-1232. DOI: 10.1007/s00216-007-1517-3

[94] Nakamura H, Suzuki M. New concept for a toxicity assay based on multiple indexes from the wave shape of damped metabolic oscillation induced in living yeast cells—Part II: Application to analytical toxicology. Analytical and Bioanalytical Chemistry. 2007;**389**(4):1233-1241. DOI: 10.1007/s00216-007-1513-7

Chapter 12

Nanostructures in Biosensors: Development and Applications

Gizem Karabulut, Nuray Beköz Üllen and Selcan Karakuş

Abstract

In recent years, there has been significant interest in advanced nanobiosensor technologies with their exceptional properties for real-time monitoring, ultra-sensing, and rapid detection. With relevant experimental data, highly selective and hypersensitive detection of various analytes is possible using biosensors based on nanostructures. In particular, biosensors focus on vital issues such as disease early diagnosis and treatment, risk assessment of quality biomarkers, food-water quality control, and food safety. In the literature, there has been great attention to the preparation and sensing behavior of several nanomaterials-based sensors, such as polymer frameworks, metal-organic frameworks, one-dimensional (1D) nanomaterials, two-dimensional (2D) nanomaterials, and MXenes-based sensors. This chapter gives points to all aspects of fabrication, characterization, mechanisms, and applications of nanostructures-based biosensors. Finally, some smart advanced sensing systems for ultra-sensing nanoplatforms, as well as a comprehensive understanding of the sensor performances, current limitations, and future outlook of next-generation sensing materials, are highlighted.

Keywords: biosensor, nanostructures, sensing nanoplatform

1. Introduction

Today, as a result of rapid industrialization, global problems bring about pollution, diseases, and many other problems. Early detection, prevention, and elimination of these problems have become very important for the continuity of the ecological system. Due to increasing technological developments, the rapid, precise, high-sensitivity, and reusable detection of these situations is made possible with biosensors. Biosensors are innovative, effective, and independent analytical devices that respond selectively and reversibly depending on the concentration or activity of the analyte to be determined in the sample [1–3]. With a brief historical overview of biosensors from past to present, in 1962, the first electrochemical enzymatic biosensor was invented by Clark et al. to detect glucose in biological samples due to the oxygenation of blood samples by reducing oxygen on the surface of the platinum electrode [1]. With this discovery, Leland C. Clark is referred to as the "father of the biosensor." In 1962, Clark determined the concentration of glucose by immobilization of the glucose oxidase on the surface of the amperometric enzyme electrode. In 1962, Montalvo and Guilbault reported the first potentiometric urease enzyme sensor for the detection of the ammonium ion activity due to the enzyme-catalyzed hydrolysis [4]. Another fascinating work was presented by Opitz and Lubbers with the development of the optical biosensor for the detection of alcohol in 1975, which made the field of sensors very remarkable and rapid developments in this area continued [5]. One year later, Clemens et al. developed an electrochemical glucose biosensor for a bedside type of artificial bedside pancreas as a prominent work in the field of biotechnology [6]. At the beginning of the twentieth century, researchers at the University of Cambridge found a pen-sized detector for monitoring blood sugar levels [5]. In the light of ongoing research, different biosensors have been developed by integrating nanostructures for the selective detection of specific analytes. When biosensors were applied to pesticide determination, Ivanov et al. [7] emphasized that an enzymatic layer makes it difficult to operate the biosensor in real samples, especially in field conditions, and reduces the sensitivity and reproducibility of the results obtained. With this approach, they experimentally demonstrated the importance of producing new low-cost disposable pesticide biosensors in which the ultrathin film of the enzyme is directly immobilized to the surface. As a result of rapidly developing technologies in the last 20 years, Chinnappan et al. [8] proposed as an alternative to existing allergen detection methods. It was shown that graphene oxide (GO)-based biosensors for the detection of major shrimp allergens (tropomyosin) with affinity (30 nM) and LOD (2 nM) values in the low nanomolar range were highly sensitive when compared with traditional sensors. For an example of work on the detection of bacterial pathogens originating from water, Yaghoobi et al. [9] demonstrated the successful usage of the green selective, sensitive, stable, repeatable, and reproducible electrochemical biosensor in *Streptococcus Pneumoniae bacteria* with a low limit of detection (0.0022 ng/ml ~ 622 bacteria) and a high sensitivity (3432.9 Ω $(\text{ng/ml})^{-1}$). A glassy carbon electrode (GCE) was modified with DNA-lead nanoparticles (Pb NPs) for sensitive and selective detection of the bacteria. In a study on biosensors for early detection of cancer, Alves et al. (2022) developed a novel electrochemical biosensor for monitoring of breast cancer by immobilizing the biotin-C3 and biotin-H_2 peptides in the screen-printed electrodes/poly 3-(3-aminophenyl) propionic acid/avidin system [10]. As we advanced deeper into the pandemic, we saw the need for advanced sensor technologies as a solution in the public health response to COVID-19. As it is known, since December 2019, humanity has been going through a historical process related to the coronavirus [COVID-19]. The urgency of developing a fast, easily accessible, and highly sensitive biosensor to monitor COVID-19 in all countries has emerged. In particular, the importance of developing and researching biosensors that do not give false-negative results for viruses that are at risk of rapid transmission and have lethal effects, which is another problem for humanity, has been understood. Dai et al. reported the development of a novel COVID-19 biosensor highly-sensitive and rapid enzymatic detection of the COVID-19 spike antigen without sample labeling for the accurate and rapid diagnosis of SARS-CoV-2 infection [11]. In this study, the anti-SARS-CoV-2 spike monoclonal antibodies were immobilized onto the surface of biosensor for the specific recognition of the SARS-CoV-2 spike antigen. Thus, it has been proven by rapid development and successful experimental results that biosensors have a wide range of applications such as environmental applications, drug delivery, diagnostics, biomedicine, food quality and safety [12].

In particular, biosensors have a wide range of applications, such as environmental applications, drug delivery, diagnostics, biomedicine, food quality and safety, etc. [12]. The global biosensor market was valued at $15.5 billion in 2015, but it was expected to grow to $24.9 billion by 2021 [13]. In other words, it has shown an increase of 60.6% in 6 years, an indication that it has a widespread usage network day by day. A biosensor is a compact device containing a biological or biomimetic sensing element. It consists of bioreceptor, electronic system, and transducer component [14]. The target analytes are the structures to be detected in the sample. Bioreceptors are structures that produce a measurable signal as a result of physicochemical changes that occur through interaction with the analyte as a result of physical or chemical bonding. These can be enzymes, nucleic acids (DNA or RNA), antibodies, tissues, aptamers, organelles, etc. [2, 12, 15]. After analyte and bioreceptor interaction, a number of physicochemical changes may occur, such as pH change, mass change, electron transfer, heat transfer, etc. [16]. When a physicochemical signal such as specific temperature, sound, light, weight or pressure is produced by the interaction of the bioreceptor with the analyte, the transducer converts it into a readable or measurable electrical signal [17]. Generally, biosensors can be classified according to the type of biorecognition element and transducer [18, 19]. Based on the biorecognition element, biosensors can be classified as antibody, enzyme, antigen, or oligonucleotide-based biosensors. Based on the transducer, biosensors can be classified as optical, electrochemical, magnetic, amperometric, potentiometric, piezoelectric, acoustic, or thermometric-based biosensors. In **Figure 1**, the schematic diagram of the classification and application areas of biosensors was presented. With the unique sensing performance of nanostructure-based biosensors, a variety of chemical and biosensing nanoplatforms have been reported.

In sensor applications needing continuous monitoring of many analytes, e.g., pesticides, drugs, heavy metals, and bacteria residues detection in real samples, volatile organic compounds (VCOs), biomarkers, specific allergens detection in blood, glucose have been investigated [16]. As known, biosensors are under the influence of more than one scientific area and require a multidisciplinary study. Therefore, it is a very suitable area for development. Recently, developments in nanotechnology and, accordingly, nanotechnological applications of biosensors have attracted attention in the scientific world. In general, the impact of nanotechnology and nanomaterials on the development of biosensors, recent innovations in this area, and future expectations are reviewed in this chapter.

2. Biosensors with a nanotechnological approach

Nanotechnological developments have played an important role in the development of biosensors along with many other scientific research areas [15]. Nano-sized materials can exhibit unique properties compared with their bulk structures. This has also been advantageous in biosensor applications and has revolutionized them. It enables rapid analysis of multiple analytes at any time and place [20]. The selectivity, detection, non-toxicity, biocompatibility, reversibility, fast response, and sensitivity required for transducer materials can be met by nanomaterials [15, 21]. The fact that nanomaterials can be synthesized in different sizes, shapes, distributions, and compositions makes them unique for biosensor applications [14]. The nanotechnological approach is indispensable for biosensor design, as it ensures superior optoelectronic, electrical conductivity, catalytic activity, and biocompatibility properties as a result of a high surface-to-volume ratio [14, 17]. Due to these unique multi-functional properties, many researchers have recently focused on the use of various nanomaterials in biosensors. There are several reported techniques to fabricate electrodes to develop highly sensitive, selective, and rapid nanosensors for biosensing applications. Various

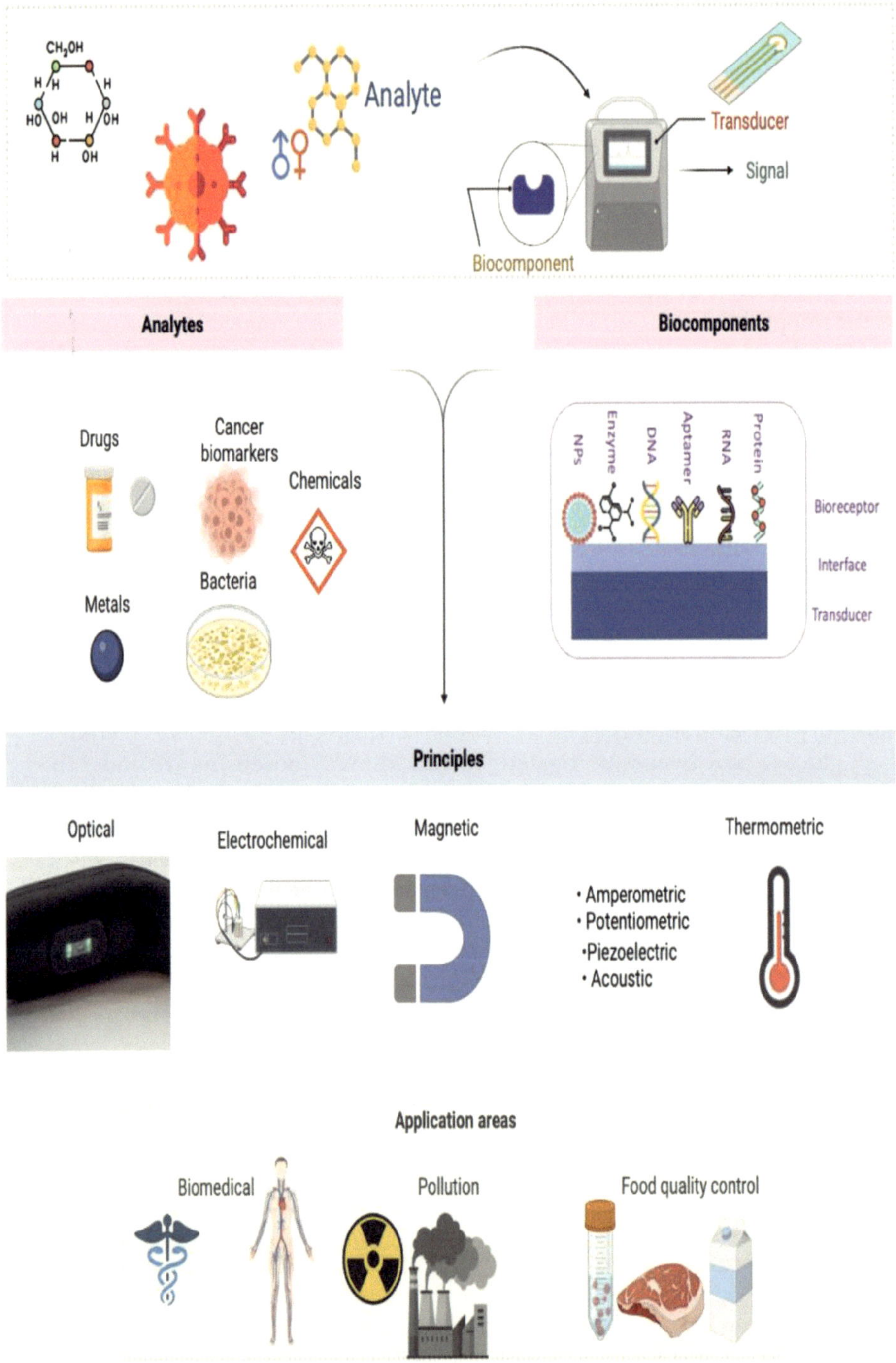

Figure 1.
The schematic diagram of the classification and application areas of biosensors.

strategies, such as using nanocomposite structures, indium tin oxide (ITO)-polymer, conductive polymer nanoparticles, screen-printing water-based carbon ink method, surface molecular imprinting method, inkjet printing method, recrystallization method, injection molding method, and charge transfer method, have been used for the fabrication of high-performance biosensors [22]. It is known that nanomaterials have good detection sensitivity with a high specific surface area and homogeneous particle distribution. In particular, graphene, GO, and reduced graphene oxide (rGO) metal oxide nanocomposites are the preferred nanomaterials for the production of electrochemical sensors. In the last decade, graphene and graphene-based nanocomposites have been investigated to design biosensors with improved performance. In 2016, Eftekhari-Sis et al. developed a novel GO/5-carboxy fluorescein-labeled DNA-based nano-biosensor for monitoring of the mutation in exon 19 of the EGFR gene in lung cancer [23]. Bao et al. (2019) proposed an effective 3D graphene/copper oxide nano-flowers-based acetylcholinesterase electrochemical biosensor for the detection of malathion [24]. The experimental results showed that the proposed biosensor had a low detection limit of 0.31 ppt in concentration, ranging from 1 ppt to 15.555 ppb due to the excellent conductivity and adsorption property of the CuO NFs nanocomposite electrode. In 2021, a novel non-enzymatic PAN: β-rhombohedral borophene-based non-enzymatic electrochemical biosensor has been prepared for the detection of glucose by Taşaltın [25]. The two-dimensional (2D) PAN: β-rhombohedral borophene combined non-enzymatic glucose biosensor was developed, and the proposed biosensor detected glucose with a low LOD of 0.099 mM in a concentration range from 1.5 to 12 mM and a rapid response time (30 s) due to the electrochemical oxidation of glucose. Up to date, 0D–2D nanomaterials-based nanobiosensors have been reported with high sensing performance in the form of polymer-based, metal-based, carbon-based, and composite-based nanosystems.

2.1 Polymer-based nanobiosensors

Polymer-based nanostructures are used for purposes such as to improve cell permeability, to increase therapeutic application, to control dosage frequency and amounts due to their adjustable nanoscale properties in order to improve efficiency in the use of biosensors. Although there are stand-alone applications, polymer-based nanostructures are generally used in composite-based biosensor systems and are preferred in areas such as drug delivery systems, nanomedicines, catalysts, wastewater treatment, etc. Polymer-based nanostructures used in biosensors can be in forms such as polymeric dendrimers, micelles, nanogels, polymersomes, and polymer nanoparticles [26]. In literature, Vais et al. [27] developed a novel DNA biosensor for the detection of *Trichomonas vaginalis* via an electropolymerized poly(ortho-aminophenol) (POAP) thin-film-based transducer. The POAP film was developed as an electrochemical nanotransducer and acted as a redox active indicator. In this pursuit, the POAP nanotranducer exhibited long-time stability, good reproducibility, high selectivity for *Trichomonas vaginalis*, and reusability. It has also been reported that POAP film has significant potential in the development of biosensors for DNA immobilization in biomedical applications. In another study, Singh et al. [28] studied a novel L-asparaginase (L-ASP) immobilization by obtaining a polymer-based carrier of gelatin alginate nanoparticles (GANp) synthesized by the ionic gelation method. The produced nanoparticles in the study were tested as a polymer nanoparticle-based fiber optic asparagine biosensor. The tested biosensor works on the basis of detecting the fluorescence intensity of Rhodamine 6G with L-ASP as a bioreceptor when there is an ammonia release occurring in the presence of asparagine. The authors stated that the polymer-based nanostructure of GANp was successful in L-ASP immobilization and offered a selective, sensitive, reusable, and reproducible solution for the asparagine biosensor and that it could also be used in leukemia patients. In 2020, Zahed et al. [29] successfully developed a flexible poly (3, 4-ethylene dioxythiophene)-poly (styrene sulfonate) (PEDOT:PSS) anchored 3-dimensional (3D) porous laser-induced graphene-based electrochemical glucose and pH biosensor with a highly sensitivity by modifying the surface electrode with PEDOT:PSS/graphene. In this report, various advantages of conductive PEDOT:PSS, such as high electrical conductivity, solution workability, chemical stability, and biocompatibility, have been brought to the fore in biosensor applications. Tran et al. [30] highlighted the development of conducting polymer-based electrochemical biosensors for the detection of proteins and nucleic acids as biomarkers for COVID-19. Different methods of SARS-CoV-2 by biosensor have been highlighted, such as detection of virus and antigen, viral RNA, and antibody in next-generation diagnostic technologies. In this study, different detecting mechanisms such as gene interaction, protein-protein interaction, protein-aptamer interaction, protein-antibody interaction, antigen-specific antibody response, receptor binding domain interaction, and SARS-CoV-2-angiotensin-converting enzyme 2 (ACE2) interaction for electrochemical virus biosensors were presented. However, the desired success in COVID-19 sensors has not been achieved due to some disadvantages such as weak interaction forces, uncontrollable reactions, large diffusional barriers, poor water solubility, and poor stability.

2.2 Metal-based nanobiosensors

Metal-based structures at the nanoscale are used in many fields due to their functionability, catalytic and electrical properties, surface plasmon resonance behavior, charge conduction, and sensing properties, and these properties provide unique advantages, especially for biosensor applications. Core@shell nanomaterials have been successfully synthesized by different methods, such as the hydrothermal method [31], sonochemical method [32], microwave irradiation [33], laser ablation [34] etc. In 2022, Mallick et al. highlighted the requirement of metal@metal oxide (M@MO) core@shell nanoparticles (NPs) with chemical, physical properties, and unique morphologies at the nanoscale in high-performance biosensor applications [35]. Various characterization methods such as photoluminescence (PL), UV-visible spectrophotometer, dynamic light scattering (DLS), scanning electron microscopy (SEM), wet-scanning electron microscopy (wet-SEM), field-emission scanning electron microscopy (FESEM), energy-dispersive X-ray spectroscopy (EDX), transmission electron microscopy (TEM), Fourier-transform infrared spectroscopy (FTIR), Raman spectrometer, X-ray photoelectron spectroscopy (XPS), and X-ray diffraction (XRD) are used to characterize nanostructures. However, thanks to new studies demonstrating advancements in nanotechnology, it is proven that the sensing performance of chemosensors and biosensors improves depending on the size and shape of nanostructures, including TiO_2, SnO_2, CuO, ZnO, WO_3, and Fe_2O_3 nanoparticles with different morphologies.

Metals (Au, Ag, Pt, etc.) and metal oxides (ZnO, ZrO_2, CuO, Fe_2O_3, TiO_2, etc.) were investigated in metal-based biosensor studies. Among metal nanoparticles, noble metal nanoparticles (such as silver (Ag) and gold (Au) NPs) have been widely studied for use in biosensor applications [21, 36]. In particular, Ag NPs and Au NPs have been used for the detection of heavy metals such as cadmium, arsenic, mercury, etc. [21]. Santhosh et al. [37] synthesized novel plant-derived Ag NPs and tested them for the detection of heavy metals. In this study, waste *Allium cepa L* peels were prepared as a plant extract and then Ag NPs were synthesized in a greener way by chemical precipitation via using the plant extract.

The synthesized Ag NPs were tested in the solution of various heavy metal salts and a significant color change was observed in the $HgCl_2$ solution. This result paves the way for the detection of mercury in the liquid phase by observation, which is easy and does not require any tools. The authors stated that green-produced Ag NPs can be used as a simple and inexpensive sensing partner in biosensor applications. In light of the metal-based nanosystems with sensing performances, Hasan et al. [38] worked on developing a gold nanoparticle-based biosensor that provides observation in a colorimetric way for the early diagnosis of ovarian cancer, which is one of the most common cancer types in women. In their study, a novel aptamer-based fluorescence sensor was develpoed for the detection of platelet-derived growth factor (PDGF). It aimed to develop a biosensor based on the fact that Au NPs show significant color change after aggregation. The authors stated that after aptamers and platelets were added to the Au NPs solution, aggregations occurred and changed the particle size of the NPs. In this case, the color of the solution changed from a pinkish color to a purplish color. Also, they said that the aptamers and Au NPs-based structure have potential for such applications by providing the observability of such an important disease in a simple, fast, inexpensive, and effective way for early diagnosis. Another metal-based nanostructure widely used in biosensor applications is metal-oxide nanoparticles (MO NPs). Many different forms of synthesized nano-sized metal oxides have many uses as transducers in biosensors, and many studies are being conducted on them [17]. Karakuş et al. [39] synthesized novel green polyphenol matrix CuO nanoparticles with the help of matcha tea powder extract by a low-cost, easy, green, and fast sonochemical method and then studied the development of the biosensor for the smartphone-based digital colorimetric detection of ammonia. In the study, the prepared CuO NPs solution was coated onto the gold electrochemical transducer by drop-casting and then dried at 40°C, and CuO NPs-based electrochemical biosensors were prepared. It was clear that the prepared biosensor carried out with the detection of color changes by performing red-green-blue (RGB) analysis in the examinations with the help of a smartphone provides an easy and highly selective detection of ammonia at nano levels.

2.3 Carbon-based nanobiosensors

Carbon is one of the most special elements in the material science world. It can be used in many areas thanks to its different atomic array versions, such as graphene, graphite, fullerenes, and nanotubes. Two general approaches, such as top-down (laser ablation, chemical ablation, electrochemical, and sonication) and bottom-up (ultrasonication, solvothermal, electrochemical, hydrothermal, and microwave methods), have been used for synthesizing carbon dots, carbon nanotubes, carbon nanorods, and carbon fibers. Due to its ability to improve electrical, mechanical, physical, and chemical properties, it was used in various fields. In recent years, various studies have been carried out on carbon-based nanobiosensors in biosensor applications [40]. Sreekanth et al. [41] studied the detection of cadmium metal in water with multi-walled carbon nanotube enhanced nanobiosensors. Heavy metals, especially cadmium, are harmful to both nature and humans and pose a serious threat to human health. In this study, a nanobiosensor was developed to detect cadmium (Cd) metal with a DNA-assisted electrochemical technique. In the study, the glassy carbon electrode (GCE) was decorated with a multi-walled carbon nanotube, and dsDNA was immobilized on the carbon nanotube decorated GCE. Furthermore, heavy metal detection was examined by using differential pulse voltammetry (DPV) analysis. In the presence of Cd (II) ions, dsDNA interacts with Cd to form ssDNA. ssDNA binds with ethyl green (EG), and this provides a noticeable change in reduction peak current. Higher reduction peak currents are observed at increasing Cd concentrations. The developed nanobiosensor has demonstrated the potential of multi-walled carbon nanotubes in nanobiosensor applications with its ability to detect Cd at a limit of detection (2 nM) and sensitivity (5 nA nM^{-1}). In addition, Ballen et al. focused on the development of cantiveler biosensors to detect the presence of cadmium. In their studies, they developed urease, (GO), and urease/GO-based nanobiosensors and investigated the properties of nanobiosensors for the detection of Cd. The urease nanobiosensor has a detection limit of 0.03776 ppb, while the GO/urease nanobiosensor has a more advanced detection limit of 0.01831 ppb [42]. In another study, Taşaltın et al. studied a nanobiosensor enhanced with rGO synthesized by an ultrasonic microwave assisted method for propamocarb pesticide detection. It has been reported that the developed biosensor in the study has superior properties such as high selectivity (101.1 $\mu A \mu M^{-1}$ cm^{-2}), rapid response (1 min), a wide linear range (1–5 μM), and a low detection limit (0.6 μM) of pesticide [43]. In another study, Elugoke et al. [44] fabricated a novel electrochemical biosensor based on a modified electrode with carbon quantum dots and CuO nanocomposite for the detection of dopamine using square wave voltammetry (SWV). The electrochemical results showed that the carbon quantum dots-CuO nanocomposite-based biosensor exhibited a low LOD of 25.4 μM in a wide linear range from 1 to180 μM. Furthermore, it was proposed that the sensing mechanism was based on the negative charge of the oxygen-containing functionalities on the modified electrode, which attracted the positively charged analyte. With a similar approach, Gaidukevic et al. [45] prepared a sensitive electrochemical rGO-based biosensor for the determination of dopamine in the presence of malonic acid and P_2O_5 additives. Experimental results showed that the proposed biosensor exhibited high sensitivity of 28.64 μA μM^{-1} cm^{-2} and a low LOD value of 0.11 μM for the detection of dopamine. Additionally, it was reported that the sensing mechanism of the redox reaction of analyte was changed due to the change from reversible to irreversible transition. The biosensing mechanism of the redox reaction of analyte was changed due to the change from a reversible to an irreversible transition. In addition, the electrochemical process was a phenomenon occurring in the surface adsorption-controlled reaction.

2.4 Composite nanobiosensors

Another most commonly used material type is composite materials, in nanobiosensor applications. These materials have been developed with the combination of the desired properties of two or more materials in their structure, and these materials have also come to the fore in applications thanks to their superior properties [46]. So far, sensor studies have been reported on many nanomaterials-based biosensors that focused on flexible, stretchable, and wearable sensors to determine target analytes such as heart rate, blood pressure, breathing rate, serum electrolyte, temperature, creatinine, albumin, urea, DNA, RNA, and glucose. Based on the use of composite nanomaterials, Ebrahimi et al. developed a microRNA-199a-5p targeted electrochemical nanobiosensor for Triple-Negative Breast Cancer. The composite nanobiosensor was prepared using gold nanorods, GO, and graphene electrode glass. Fetal bovine serum and human serum samples were studied for detection of microRNA-199a-5p in this study. It was stated that high selectivity and sensitivity were observed in both sample environments. It has been reported that the prepared composite nanobiosensor offers an important potential due to its detection even at low concentrations [47]. In another study, Karakuş et al. studied glucose detection by developing an electrochemical nanobiosensor prepared with polyacrylonitrile (PAN) and rGO. It has been stated that due to the redox mechanism provided by rGO, it allows glucose detection with high stability and sensitivity. It has been stated that compared with the PAN-based sensor, the nanobiosensor supplemented with rGO provides glucose detection with higher sensitivity [48]. This shows the importance of developing composite structures for nanobiosensor applications. In another study, Baytemir et al. studied the detection of glucose with an electrochemical nanobiosensor and developed a nickel phthalocyanine-borophene composite based nanobiosensor. It has been reported that the borophene-doped nanobiosensor exhibits high electrical conductivity and sensitivity compared with the NiPc nanobiosensor. It was also stated that the composite nanobiosensor exhibited a lower limit of detection value [49]. In another study, Samak et al. developed a novel nanobiosensor for H_2S detection that is coupled with a DNA/sulfide fluorophore (SF) and a hybrid composite (alumina nanorods and GO nanosheet). In the study, it was stated that composite structures that can be produced in a controllable way are important in nanobiosensor applications and that the prepared composite nanobiosensor for sensitive and selective H_2S detection in wastewater can be developed [50]. As seen from the literature, composite structures have an important potential for nanobiosensor applications and can be used in many different areas. In **Table 1**, comparison of developed nanobiosensor for the detection of specific analytes was presented.

2.5 MXene nanobiosensors

Discovered in 2011 and attracting great attention in recent years, especially in advanced nanosensor technologies, MXene is a 2D transition metal carbide and nitride material with different functional groups (-O, -OH, and -F). MXene sensors have been great attention with their excellent electrical, biological, chemical, surface, and mechanical properties in various applications such as water treatment systems, energy storage materials, photothermal systems, and sensor applications.

Recently, various types of 2D nanomaterials have been produced in small quantities for other applications outside the sensor field, whereas scale of production for healthcare applications poses a major challenge. In addition, it has been proven that most of the 2D materials produced have properties such as hydrophobic and instability in the air environment. Therefore, 2D MXene materials have a strong influence in the field of modern science, with the development of issues with superior metallic conductivity, ease of processing, hydrophilic character, chemical stability, and layered morphology. Soomro et al. developed a novel photo-electrochemical $NiWO_4$-MXene sensor for the detection of the prostate-specific antigen [63]. According to the experimental results, it was found that the sensor had a wide detection range from 1.2 $fg.mL^{-1}$ to 0.18 $mg.mL^{-1}$ and a low detection limit of 0.15 $fg.mL^{-1}$ for the prostate-specific antigen. In another study, Qin et al. reported that MXene/V_2O_5/$CuWO_4$-based sensor had a highly selective against ammonia at room temperature in few seconds [64]. Ranjbar et al. studied the sensing performance of the novel wearable conductive polymer/MXene-based pressure sensor for the human detection and information transmission using cotton fabric [65]. In another study, Zhu et al. developed a novel acetone sensor using ZnO/$Ti_3C_2T_x$-MXene composite nanomaterials [66]. The few-layered ZnO/Ti3C2Tx-MXene composite nanomaterial was prepared by a hydrothermal method Furthermore, the proposed nanosensor exhibited a

Biosensor	Bioreceptor	Detection	Results		Ref.
Polymer-based nanobiosensor	Polypyrole	H_2O_2 and glucose	Detection range for H_2O_2	10 mM–10 mM	[51]
			Linear range	1–5 mM	
	Polypyrole	Prostate cancer	LOD	2.0 pg. mL^{-1}	[52]
			Linear range	0.01–4.0 ng mL^{-1}	
Metal-based nanobiosensor	DNA-CuO nanoparticles	Single nucleotide polymorphism anemia	LOD	0.64 nM	[53]
			Linear range	2 nM to 12 nM	
	Gold nanoparticles	Thyroid disease diagnosis	LOD	0.001 µIU/mL	[54]
			Linear variation	100 µIU/mL	
	Cu Nanocluster	Detection of $VEGF_{165}$ biomarker	LOD	12 pM	[55]
			Linear range	10–800 pM	
	Gold nanoparticles	Prolactin hormone	Linear range	1–40 ng ml^{-1}	[56]
			LOD	0.8 ng ml^{-1}	
			Sensitivity	10 pg. ml^{-1}	
Carbon-based nanobiosensor	GO/urease	Cadmium	LOD	0.01831 ppb to 0.03776 ppb	[42]
	Multi-walled carbon nanotube	Cadmium	LOD	2 nM in a linear range of 2 nM–10.0 nM.	[41]
	Graphene	IgE detection	LOD	47 pM in a linear range 50 pM to 250 nM	[57]

DOI: http://dx.doi.org/10.5772/intechopen.108508

Biosensor	Bioreceptor	Detection	Results		Ref.
Composite nanobiosensor	Molecularly imprinted polymers/ carbon quantum dots	Hemoglobin (Hb)	Linear range	0.77–7.7 nM	[58]
			LOD	0.77 nM	
			Recovery in serum sample	86.8% to 93.9%	
	l-Glutathione modified Poly(3,4-ethylenedioxythiophene): polystyrene sulfonate/ carboxylated multiwall carbon nanotubes	Cadmium (II) ions	Sensitivity	10.69 μA/ppm	[59]
			LOD	1 ppb	
	rGO/gold nanocomposite	miRNA-122 biomarker	LOD	1.73 pM in a range from 10 μM to 10 pM	[60]
MXene nanobiosensor	$NiO/Ti_3C_2T_x$ MXene	H_2O_2	LOD	0.34 μM in a range from 0.01–4.5 mM	[61]
MXene composite biosensor	MXene@Ag nanoclusters and amino-functionalized multi-walled carbon nanotubes	Carbendazim	LOD	0.1 nM in a range from 0.3 nM–10 μM	[62]

Table 1.
Comparison of developed nanobiosensor for the detection of specific analytes.

high-sensing response nearly six times higher than that of the ZnO in a concentration range of 14.4–100 ppm of acetone at 320°C due to the large specific surface area and layered structure. Finally, the sensing mechanism was proposed based on the large specific surface area, sufficient adsorption and reaction sites, a large number of oxygen functional groups (-O, -OH) of MXene nanostructures, and the surface of the modified electrode for sensing gas molecules.

3. Future trends of sensing nanomaterials

With these developed nanomaterial-based sensors, various sensors with excellent sensing performance values have been fabricated, and their sensing performances have been observed to detect the target analyte in a short time. Accordingly, previous results show that advanced biosensors are low-cost, easier to use, selective, rapid, and sensitive. In addition, the synthesis methods of large-scale nanostructure-based sensors are still a hot topic. Considering the nanostructures outlined in this review, it is clear that many nanosensors, each with their own unique superior properties and advantages, are suitable for incorporation into biosensing nanoplatforms. In particular, MXene and its composites appear to be a promising choice for use in forensic biosensors due to their ultra-sensitivity and superior electrochemical properties that provide a broad absorption spectrum. The use of MXene and MXene composites with various detection systems such as antibodies, genes, viruses, biomarkers, and enzymes allows the fabrication of rapid and ultra-sensitive biosensors with very low LOD values. As research in the field continues to expand, there is no doubt that portable and flexible biosensors for real-time mobile detection of illicit drugs, early detection of disease, environmental pollutants, and biological traces will become universal in sensor applications and facilitate quality of life. However, it has also been shown that nanosensors can rapidly detect the target molecule among mixed components at very low concentrations, and detection research in the health field is gaining momentum. It is seen that successful experimental data have been obtained in the field of development and sensing mechanisms of 2D materials-based nanobiosensors, which is an interesting subject for biomedical and environmental applications. As a result, there are not enough reports on the research of sensitive, selective, and effective nanostructure-based sensors with different morphologies. For this reason, nanostructure-based sensors with high sensing potential are being investigated and will guide future studies in a wide spectrum of science.

DOI: http://dx.doi.org/10.5772/intechopen.108508

Author details

Gizem Karabulut[1], Nuray Beköz Üllen[1] and Selcan Karakuş[2]*

1 Department of Metallurgical and Materials Engineering, Istanbul University-Cerrahpasa, Istanbul, Turkey

2 Faculty of Engineering, Department of Chemistry, Istanbul University-Cerrahpasa, Istanbul, Turkey

*Address all correspondence to: selcan@iuc.edu.tr

References

[1] Vigneshvar S, Sudhakumari CC, Senthilkumaran B, Prakash H. Recent advances in biosensor technology for potential applications - An overview. Frontiers in Bioengineering and Biotechnology. 2016;**4**:11. DOI: 10.3389/FBIOE.2016.00011/BIBTEX

[2] Tetyana P, Shumbula PM, Njengele-Tetyana Z. Biosensors: Design, Development and Applications. In: Ameen S, Akhtar MS, Shin H, editors. Nanopores. London: IntechOpen; 2021. DOI: 10.5772/intechopen.97576

[3] Malhotra S, Verma A, Tyagi N, Kumar V. Biosensors: Principle, types and applications. International Journal of Advance Research and Innovative Ideas in Education. 2017;**3**:3639-3644

[4] Dhawan G, Sumana G, Malhotra BD. Recent developments in urea biosensors. Biochemical Engineering Journal. 2009;**44**:42-52. DOI: 10.1016/J.BEJ.2008.07.004

[5] Kulkarni MB, Ayachit NH, Aminabhavi TM. Biosensors and microfluidic biosensors: From fabrication to application. Biosensors. 2022;**12**:543. DOI: 10.3390/BIOS12070543

[6] Naresh V, Lee N. A review on biosensors and recent development of nanostructured materials-enabled biosensors. Sensors. 2021;**21**:1109. DOI: 10.3390/S21041109

[7] Ivanov AN, Evtugyn GA, Gyurcsányi RE, Tóth K, Budnikov HC. Comparative investigation of electrochemical cholinesterase biosensors for pesticide determination. Analytica Chimica Acta. 2000;**404**:55-65. DOI: 10.1016/S0003-2670(99)00683-2

[8] Chinnappan R, Rahamn AA, AlZabn R, Kamath S, Lopata AL, Abu-Salah KM, et al. Aptameric biosensor for the sensitive detection of major shrimp allergen, tropomyosin. Food Chemistry. 2020;**314**:126133. DOI: 10.1016/J.FOODCHEM.2019.126133

[9] Yaghoobi A, Abiri R, Alvandi A, Arkan E, Mohammadi G, Farshadnia T, et al. An efficiently engineered electrochemical biosensor as a novel and user-friendly electronic device for biosensing of Streptococcus Pneumoniae bacteria. Sensing and Bio-Sensing Research. 2022;**36**:100494. DOI: 10.1016/J.SBSR.2022.100494

[10] da Fonseca Alves R, Martins IC, Franco DL, Silva AdG, de Souza Santos P, Goulart LR, et al. A novel peptide-based electrochemical biosensor for breast cancer characterization over a poly 3-(3-aminophenyl) propionic acid matrix. Biosensors & Bioelectronics. 2022;**205**:114081. DOI: 10.1016/J.BIOS.2022.114081

[11] Dai Z, Xu X, Wang Y, Li M, Zhou K, Zhang L, et al. Surface plasmon resonance biosensor with laser heterodyne feedback for highly-sensitive and rapid detection of COVID-19 spike antigen. Biosensors & Bioelectronics. 2022;**206**:114163. DOI: 10.1016/J.BIOS.2022.114163

[12] Fatima T, Bansal S, Husain S, Khanuja M. Biosensors. In: Maruccio G, Narang J, editors. Electrochemical Sensors: From Working Electrodes to Functionalization and Miniaturized Devices. United Kingdom: Elsevier. 2022:1-30. DOI: 10.1016/B978-0-12-823148-7.00001-5

[13] Sadana A, Sadana N. Market size and economics for biosensors. In: Sadana A,

Sadana N, editors. Fractal Analysis of the Binding and Dissociation Kinetics for Different Analytes on Biosensor Surfaces. Elsevier; 2008:317-334. DOI: 10.1016/B978-044453010-3.50014-1

[14] Purohit B, Vernekar PR, Shetti NP, Chandra P. Biosensor nanoengineering: Design, operation, and implementation for biomolecular analysis. Sensors International. 2020;**1**:100040. DOI: 10.1016/J.SINTL.2020.100040

[15] Thomas S, Saji KJ, Jayaraj MK. An introduction to biosensors. Nanomaterials for Sensing and Optoelectronic Applications. 2022:91-107. DOI: 10.1016/B978-0-12-824008-3.00013-8

[16] Velasco-Garcia MN, Mottram T. Biosensor technology addressing agricultural problems. Biosystems Engineering. 2003;**84**:1-12. DOI: 10.1016/S1537-5110(02)00236-2

[17] Kumar R, Chauhan G, Martinez-Chapa SO. Metal oxides and their composites as flow-through biosensors for biomonitoring. In: Mondal K, editor. Metal Oxides for Biomedical and Biosensor Applications. Elsevier; 2022:291-319. DOI: 10.1016/B978-0-12-823033-6.00010-7

[18] Huang X, Zhu Y, Kianfar E. Nano Biosensors: Properties, applications and electrochemical techniques. Journal of Materials Research and Technology. 2021;**12**:1649-1672. DOI: 10.1016/J.JMRT.2021.03.048

[19] Freeman MH, Hall JR, Leopold MC. Monolayer-protected nanoparticle doped xerogels as functional components of amperometric glucose biosensors. Analytical Chemistry. 2013;**85**:4057-4065. DOI: 10.1021/AC3037188/SUPPL_FILE/AC3037188_SI_001.PDF

[20] Dede S, Altay F. Biosensors from the first generation to nano-biosensors. International Advanced Researches and Engineering Journal. 2018;**02**:200-207

[21] Bose S, Maity S, Sarkar A. Nanomaterials as biosensor for heavy metal detection. Food, Medical, and Environmental Applications of Nanomaterials. 2022:493-526. DOI: 10.1016/B978-0-12-822858-6.00018-2

[22] Sadana A, Sadana N. Fabrication of Biosensors. Handbook of Biosensors and Biosensor Kinetics. 2011:35-60. DOI: 10.1016/B978-0-444-53262-6.00003-6

[23] Eftekhari-Sis B, Aliabad MA, Karimi F. Graphene oxide based nanobiosensor for the detection of deletion mutation in exon 19 of EGFR gene, leading to lung cancer. Materials Letters. 2016;**183**:441-443. DOI: 10.1016/J.MATLET.2016.07.031

[24] Bao J, Huang T, Wang Z, Yang H, Geng X, Xu G, et al. 3D graphene/copper oxide nano-flowers based acetylcholinesterase biosensor for sensitive detection of organophosphate pesticides. Sensors and Actuators B: Chemical. 2019;**279**:95-101. DOI: 10.1016/J.SNB.2018.09.118

[25] Taşaltın C. Glucose sensing performance of PAN: β-rhombohedral borophene based non-enzymatic electrochemical biosensor. Inorganic Chemistry Communications. 2021;**133**:108973. DOI: 10.1016/J.INOCHE.2021.108973

[26] Fatima S, Quadri SN, Parveen S, Beg S, Rahman M, Ahmad FJ, et al., Polymeric nanoparticles for potential drug delivery applications in cancer. In: Beg S, Choudhry H, Ahmad FJ, Rahman M,

Souto EB, editors. Nanoformulation Strategies for Cancer Treatment. Elsevier: 2021:65-88. DOI: 10.1016/B978-0-12-821095-6.00009-4

[27] Dehdari Vais R, Heli H, Sattarahmady N, Barazesh A. A novel and ultrasensitive label-free electrochemical DNA biosensor for Trichomonas vaginalis detection based on a nanostructured film of poly(ortho-aminophenol). Synthetic Metals. 2022;**287**. DOI: 10.1016/J.SYNTHMET.2022.117082

[28] Singh A, Verma N, Kumar K. Fabrication and characterization of L-asparaginase entrapped polymeric nanoparticles for asparagine biosensor construction. Materials Today: Proceedings. 2022;**67**:591-597. DOI: 10.1016/J.MATPR.2022.05.227

[29] Zahed MA, Barman SC, Das PS, Sharifuzzaman M, Yoon HS, Yoon SH, et al. Highly flexible and conductive poly (3, 4-ethylene dioxythiophene)-poly (styrene sulfonate) anchored 3-dimensional porous graphene network-based electrochemical biosensor for glucose and pH detection in human perspiration. Biosensors & Bioelectronics. 2020;**160**:112220. DOI: 10.1016/J.BIOS.2020.112220

[30] van Tran V, Tran NHT, Hwang HS, Chang M. Development strategies of conducting polymer-based electrochemical biosensors for virus biomarkers: Potential for rapid COVID-19 detection. Biosensors & Bioelectronics. 2021;**182**:113192. DOI: 10.1016/J.BIOS.2021.113192

[31] Vlazan P, Ursu D, Sfirloaga P, Rusu EV, Ursu DH, Irina-Moisescu C, et al. Structural and electrical properties of TiO2/ZnO core-shell nanoparticles synthesized by hydrothermal method. Materials Characterization. 2015:153-158. DOI: 10.1016/j.matchar.2015.01.017

[32] Ghows N, Entezari MH. Sono-synthesis of core–shell nanocrystal (CdS/TiO2) without surfactant. Ultrasonics Sonochemistry. 2012;**19**:1070-1078. DOI: 10.1016/J.ULTSONCH.2012.01.009

[33] Womiloju AA, Höppener C, Schubert US, Hoeppener S, Womiloju AA, Schubert US, et al. Microwave-assisted synthesis of core–shell nanoparticles-insights into the growth of different geometries. Particle and Particle Systems Characterization. 2020;**37**:2000019. DOI: 10.1002/PPSC.202000019

[34] Kazakevich PV, Simakin AV, Voronov VV, Shafeev GA, Starikov D, Bensaoula A. Formation of core-shell nanoparticles by laser ablation of copper and brass in liquids. Solid State Phenomena. 2005;**106**:23-26. DOI: 10.4028/WWW.SCIENTIFIC.NET/SSP.106.23

[35] Mallick S, Singh KR, Nayak V, Singh J, Singh RP. Potentialities of core@shell nanomaterials for biosensor technologies. Materials Letters. 2022;**306**:130912. DOI: 10.1016/J.MATLET.2021.130912

[36] Ghosh G. Early detection of cancer: Focus on antibody coated metal and magnetic nanoparticle-based biosensors. Sensors International. 2020;**1**:100050. DOI: 10.1016/J.SINTL.2020.100050

[37] Santhosh A, Theertha V, Prakash P, Smitha Chandran S. From waste to a value added product: Green synthesis of silver nanoparticles from onion peels together with its diverse applications. Materials Today: Proceedings. 2021;**46**:4460-4463. DOI: 10.1016/J.MATPR.2020.09.680

[38] Hasan MR, Sharma P, Pilloton R, Khanuja M, Narang J. Colorimetric biosensor for the naked-eye detection of ovarian cancer biomarker PDGF using citrate modified gold nanoparticles. Biosensors and Bioelectronics X. 2022;**11**. DOI: 10.1016/J.BIOSX.2022.100142

[39] Karakuş S, Baytemir G, Taşaltın N. Digital colorimetric and non-enzymatic biosensor with nanoarchitectonics of Lepidium meyenii-silver nanoparticles and cotton fabric: real-time monitoring of milk freshness. Applied Physics A: Materials Science & Processing. 2022;**128**:1-11. DOI: 10.1007/S00339-022-05529-6/FIGURES/10

[40] Eivazzadeh-Keihan R, Bahojb Noruzi E, Chidar E, Jafari M, Davoodi F, Kashtiaray A, et al. Applications of carbon-based conductive nanomaterials in biosensors. Chemical Engineering Journal. 2022;**442**:136183. DOI: 10.1016/J.CEJ.2022.136183

[41] Sreekanth SP, Alodhayb A, Assaifan AK, Alzahrani KE, Muthuramamoorthy M, Alkhammash HI, et al. Multi-walled carbon nanotube-based nanobiosensor for the detection of cadmium in water. Environmental Research. 2021;**197**:111148. DOI: 10.1016/J.ENVRES.2021.111148

[42] Ballen SC, Steffens J, Steffens C. Stability characteristics of cantilever nanobiosensors with simple and complex molecules for determination of cadmium. Sensors and Actuators A: Physical. 2021;**324**:112686. DOI: 10.1016/J.SNA.2021.112686

[43] Taşaltın N, Karakuş S, Taşaltın C, Baytemir G. Highly sensitive and selective rGO based Non-Enzymatic electrochemical sensor for propamocarb fungicide pesticide detection. Food Chemistry. 2022;**372**:131267. DOI: 10.1016/J.FOODCHEM.2021.131267

[44] Elugoke SE, Fayemi OE, Adekunle AS, Mamba BB, Nkambule TTI, Ebenso EE. Electrochemical sensor for the detection of dopamine using carbon quantum dots/copper oxide nanocomposite modified electrode. FlatChem. 2022;**33**:100372. DOI: 10.1016/J.FLATC.2022.100372

[45] Gaidukevic J, Aukstakojyte R, Barkauskas J, Niaura G, Murauskas T, Pauliukaite R. A novel electrochemical sensor based on thermally reduced graphene oxide for the sensitive determination of dopamine. Applied Surface Science. 2022;**592**:153257. DOI: 10.1016/J.APSUSC.2022.153257

[46] Das S, Das S. Properties for polymer, metal and ceramic based composite materials. Encyclopedia of Materials: Composites. 2021:815-821. DOI: 10.1016/B978-0-12-803581-8.11897-1

[47] Ebrahimi A, Nikokar I, Zokaei M, Bozorgzadeh E. Design, development and evaluation of microRNA-199a-5p detecting electrochemical nanobiosensor with diagnostic application in Triple Negative Breast Cancer. Talanta. 2018;**189**:592-598. DOI: 10.1016/J.TALANTA.2018.07.016

[48] Karakus S, Tasaltin C, Gürol I, Baytemir G, Tasaltin N. Design of the polyacrylonitrile-reduced graphene oxide nanocomposite-based non-enzymatic electrochemical biosensor for glucose detection. Journal of Materials Science: Materials in Electronics. 2022;**33**(23):18400-18409. DOI: 10.1007/S10854-022-08694-9

[49] Baytemir G, Gürol İ, Karakuş S, Taşaltın C, Taşaltın N. Nickel phthalocyanine-borophene nanocomposite-based electrodes

for non-enzymatic electrochemical detection of glucose. Journal of Materials Science: Materials in Electronics. 2022;**33**:16586-16596. DOI: 10.1007/S10854-022-08551-9/TABLES/2

[50] Samak NA, Selim MS, Hao Z, Xing J. Controlled-synthesis of alumina-graphene oxide nanocomposite coupled with DNA/sulfide fluorophore for eco-friendly "Turn off/on" H2S nanobiosensor. Talanta. 2020;**211**:120655. DOI: 10.1016/J.TALANTA.2019.120655

[51] Weng B, Morrin A, Shepherd R, Crowley K, Killard AJ, Innis PC, et al. Wholly printed polypyrrole nanoparticle-based biosensors on flexible substrate. Journal of Materials Chemistry B. 2014;**2**:793-799. DOI: 10.1039/C3TB21378A

[52] Yazdani Z, Yadegari H, Heli H. A molecularly imprinted electrochemical nanobiosensor for prostate specific antigen determination. Analytical Biochemistry. 2019;**566**:116-125. DOI: 10.1016/J.AB.2018.11.020

[53] Kasiri M, Rahaie M. A visible and colorimetric nanobiosensor based on DNA-CuO nanoparticle for detection of single nucleotide polymorphism involved in sickle cell anemia disease. Materials Today Communications. 2021;**27**:102423. DOI: 10.1016/J.MTCOMM.2021.102423

[54] Saxena R, Srivastava S. A sensitive and one-step quantification of thyroid stimulating hormone using nanobiosensor. Materials Today: Proceedings. 2019;**18**:1351-1357. DOI: 10.1016/J.MATPR.2019.06.600

[55] Moghadam FM, Rahaie M. A signal-on nanobiosensor for VEGF165 detection based on supraparticle copper nanoclusters formed on bivalent aptamer. Biosensors & Bioelectronics. 2019;**132**:186-195. DOI: 10.1016/J.BIOS.2019.02.046

[56] Faridli Z, Mahani M, Torkzadeh-Mahani M, Fasihi J. Development of a localized surface plasmon resonance-based gold nanobiosensor for the determination of prolactin hormone in human serum. Analytical Biochemistry. 2016;**495**:32-36. DOI: 10.1016/J.AB.2015.11.016

[57] Wang X, Zhu Y, Olsen TR, Sun N, Zhang W, Pei R, et al. A graphene aptasensor for biomarker detection in human serum. Electrochimica Acta. 2018;**290**:356-363. DOI: 10.1016/J.ELECTACTA.2018.08.062

[58] Zhou T, Ashley J, Feng X, Sun Y. Detection of hemoglobin using hybrid molecularly imprinted polymers/carbon quantum dots-based nanobiosensor prepared from surfactant-free Pickering emulsion. Talanta. 2018;**190**:443-449. DOI: 10.1016/J.TALANTA.2018.08.030

[59] Sayyad PW, Sontakke KS, Farooqui AA, Shirsat SM, Tsai M-L, Shirsat MD. A novel three-dimensional electrochemical Cd(II) biosensor based on l-glutathione capped poly(3,4-ethylenedioxythiophene):polystyrene sulfonate/carboxylated multiwall CNT network. Journal of Science: Advanced Materials and Devices. 2022;**7**:100504. DOI: 10.1016/J.JSAMD.2022.100504

[60] Kasturi S, Eom Y, Torati SR, Kim CG. Highly sensitive electrochemical biosensor based on naturally reduced rGO/Au nanocomposite for the detection of miRNA-122 biomarker. Journal of Industrial and Engineering Chemistry. 2021;**93**:186-195. DOI: 10.1016/J.JIEC.2020.09.022

[61] Ramachandran R, Zhao C, Rajkumar M, Rajavel K, Zhu P, Xuan W, et al. Porous nickel oxide microsphere

and Ti3C2Tx hybrid derived from metal-organic framework for battery-type supercapacitor electrode and non-enzymatic H_2O_2 sensor. Electrochimica Acta. 2019;**322**:134771. DOI: 10.1016/J.ELECTACTA.2019.134771

[62] Zhong W, Gao F, Zou J, Liu S, Li M, Gao Y, et al. MXene@Ag-based ratiometric electrochemical sensing strategy for effective detection of carbendazim in vegetable samples. Food Chemistry. 2021;**360**:130006. DOI: 10.1016/J.FOODCHEM.2021.130006

[63] Soomro RA, Jawaid S, Zhang P, Han X, Hallam KR, Karakuş S, et al. NiWO4-induced partial oxidation of MXene for photo-electrochemical detection of prostate-specific antigen. Sensors and Actuators B: Chemical. 2021;**328**:129074. DOI: 10.1016/J.SNB.2020.129074

[64] Ranjbar F, Hajati S, Ghaedi M, Dashtian K, Naderi H, Toth J. Highly selective MXene/V2O5/CuWO4-based ultra-sensitive room temperature ammonia sensor. Journal of Hazardous Materials. 2021;**416**:126196. DOI: 10.1016/J.JHAZMAT.2021.126196

[65] He J, Shi F, Liu Q, Pang Y, He D, Sun W, et al. Wearable superhydrophobic PPy/MXene pressure sensor based on cotton fabric with superior sensitivity for human detection and information transmission. Colloids and Surfaces A: Physicochemical and Engineering Aspects. 2022;**642**:128676. DOI: 10.1016/J.COLSURFA.2022.128676

[66] Zhu Y, Ma Y, Wu D, Jiang G. Preparation and gas sensing properties of ZnO/MXene composite nanomaterials. Sensors Actuators A Physics. 2022;**344**:113740. DOI: 10.1016/J.SNA.2022.113740

Chapter 13

Biological Sensing Using Infrared SPR Devices Based on ZnO

Hiroaki Matsui

Abstract

Biological detection based on surface plasmon resonances (SPRs) on metallic Ga-doped zinc oxide (ZnO: Ga) film surfaces is introduced as one of the interesting functionalities of ZnO. SPRs on ZnO: Ga films (ZnO-SPRs) have attracted much attention as alternative plasmonic materials in the infrared (IR) range. This chapter focuses on the structure and optical properties of ZnO-SPR with different layer structure from experimental and theoretical approaches. First, the plasmonic properties of single ZnO: Ga films excited by Kretschmann-type SPRs were investigated. Second, an insulator–metal–insulator structure with a ZnO: Ga film applied as a metal layer is introduced. Finally, hybrid layer structures with the capping of thin dielectric layers to ZnO-SPR (dielectric-assisted ZnO-SPR) were fabricated to enhance SPR properties in the IR range. The biological sensing on ZnO-SPR is experimentally demonstrated by measuring biological interactions. This work provides new insights for fabricating biological sensing platforms on ZnO materials.

Keywords: oxide semiconductor, surface plasmon, near-infrared, biological detection, zinc oxide, heterointerface

1. Introduction

The impurity dopants in zinc oxide (ZnO) produce interesting optical, electrical and magnetic functionalities. For example, photoluminescence behaviors are observed by doping with rare-earth and transition-metal atoms [1–4]. Ferromagnetic properties are found by the incorporation of transition-metal atoms into the host [5–7]. Above all, the donor dopants, such as Ga and Al ions, lead to the metallic conductivity of ZnO which has been widely used as transparent electrodes [8, 9]. The metallic properties of ZnO are also prospective candidates for alternatively plasmonic materials in the infrared (IR) range [10–13]. Unlike classical plasmonic materials such as Ag and Au metals, plasmonic resonances can be controlled by changing electron density in ZnO. Additionally, the electronic structure of ZnO is composed of 4*s* and 2*p* orbitals, providing no inter-band transition such as those shown by Ag and Au metals [14]. The inter-band transition of ZnO only shows in the ultra-violet range. This band system produces a low optical loss in the IR range. Thus far, different geometries such as dots, wires, and films have been chosen to study surface plasmon resonances (SPRs) [15–17]. These SPR-related studies have shown the unprecedented capabilities of ZnO for use as alternatives to metals in IR applications.

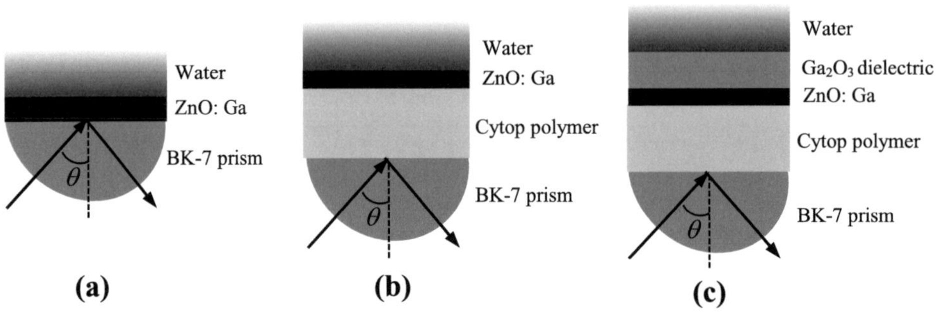

Figure 1.
Schematic figures of SPR sensing platforms of (a) single, (b) IMI and (c) hybrid samples.

It is known that ZnO is one of the interesting materials in biological sensing.

Optical and electrical techniques detect biomolecular interactions on ZnO film surfaces. The piezoelectric responses of ZnO have been applied to biosensors based on surface acoustic waves [18]. Electrochemical impedance is needed to use transparent electrodes based on ZnO [19]. These interesting properties of ZnO as biocompatible materials have generated much attention as solid oxide substrates for highly sensitive biosensing platforms. Our group has investigated layer samples of ZnO to improve the optical technology associated with SPRs. In particular, layer samples could readily be employed in biological sensing based on propagation-type SPRs. The benefits of layer samples with large surface areas render film platforms more attractive for industrial applications. Recently, SP waves, which are excited by traverse magnetic polarization, have been produced in ZnO-based optical fibers as biochemical sensing probes [20, 21]. Surface-enhanced infrared absorptions have also been confirmed on ZnO film surfaces using a prism-based SPR method [22, 23]. These previous studies indicate the potential of ZnO-based SPR (ZnO-SPR) biosensors and have motivated the study of biological sensing.

In this chapter, we discuss the structural and optical properties of ZnO-SPR from experimental and theoretical approaches. We first outline single layers' SPR properties based on ZnO: Ga, which is referred to as a single sample. The single sample is excited by Kretschmann-type SPRs using attenuated total reflection (ATR) optics. Second, the utilization of an insulator–metal–insulator (IMI) structure to a ZnO-SPR (IMI sample) is introduced in relation to the long-range SP mode. Finally, we fabricate hybrid layer structures with the capping of thin dielectric layers to ZnO-SPR (dielectric-assisted ZnO-SPR; hybrid sample) to enhance SPR properties in the IR range. Schematic pictures of single, IMI and hybrid samples are shown in **Figure 1**. Each sample's detection sensitivity is discussed from the viewpoint of electric-field distribution (E-field), propagation and penetration depths of SP waves. Finally, biological sensing on ZnO-SPR is experimentally demonstrated by measuring biological interactions between biotin and streptavidin. This study introduces SPR devices based on ZnO for biological sensing.

2. SPRs properties of single ZnO layer surfaces

This section deals with the correlation between SPR phenomena and evanescent fields on metallic ZnO: Ga film surfaces. The fabrication of ZnO: Ga film is introduced as follows [13]. ZnO: Ga films with 5% Ga content were grown on BK-7 glass substrates at 260°C using the pulsed laser ablation (PLD) method. ArF excimer laser pulses (193 nm, 3 Hz, and 1 J/cm^2) were irradiated on a ZnO: Ga ceramic target in an O_2 atmosphere of 10^{-4} Pa. The film thickness (t) was controlled within 41 to 180 nm range. A BK-7 glass substrate with a refractive index of 1.517 was applied using an ATR system with a BK-7 optical prism. SPR reflectance (R_p/R_s) was measured using a Kretschmann-type ATR system connected to a Fourier-transform NIR spectrometer, where R_p and R_s indicate the p- and s-polarized reflection lights, respectively. The spectral intensity of SPR reflectance was acquired in the wavenumber range of 7000–4000 cm^{-1}. For theoretical calculations, SPR reflectance spectra and their electric-field (E-field) depths were simulated by Fresnel relations of an N-multilayer model to calculate reflection coefficients under s- and p-polarized configurations [13, 24].

Figure 2(a) shows SPR reflectance spectra of a 174 nm-thick film as a function of incident angle (θ) from 62° to 72° in 2° increments. The peak position gradually shifted to higher wavenumbers with increasing incident angle, also confirmed by calculated SPR reflectance spectra (**Figure 2(b)**). The SPR behavior was not observed in the film samples with small thicknesses below 100 nm. The screened bulk plasmon resonances appeared in place of SPRs. **Figure 2(c)** shows a dispersion curve of a 164 nm-thick film sample, revealing consistency between the experimental

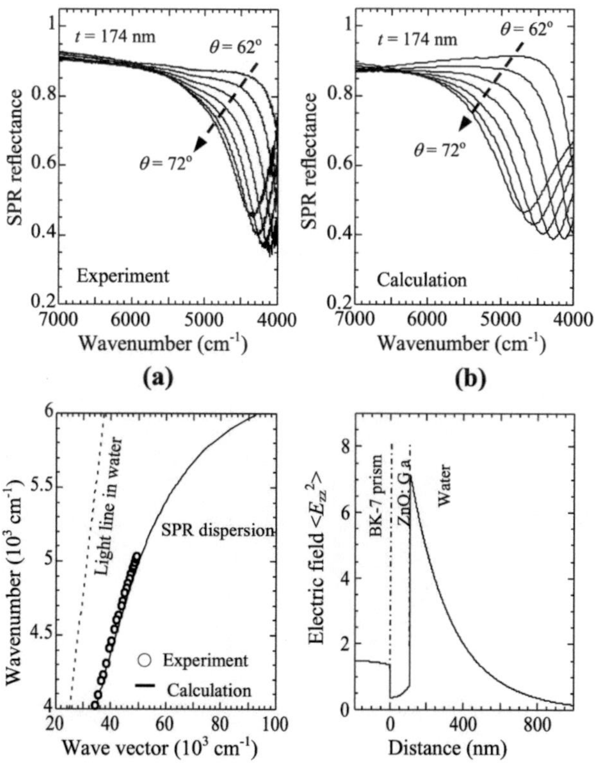

Figure 2.
(a) Experimental and (b) calculated SPR reflectance spectra of a 174 nm-thick ZnO: Ga film. Water was selected as the dielectric medium. The incident angle of light (Θ) was changed from 62° to 72°. (c) Experimental and calculated dispersion curves of SPRs. A dotted line indicates a light line in a water medium. (d) a depth-dependent mean square evanescent field at calculated at an SPR peak position of θ = 72.

(black circles) and calculated (black line) data, which were derived from the single SPR mode at the water-ZnO: Ga film interface. The result of *E*-field depth also evidenced this result. **Figure 2(d)** shows a depth profile of a mean-square evanescent field $<E_{zz}^2>$ at 4500 cm^{-1} of the *p*-polarized component along the z-direction. Here, the *x* and y directions are parallel to the film, while the *z* direction is normal to the film. The film sample had a $< E_{zz}^2 >$ value of 7.3 with a penetration depth (δ_W) of 200 nm into the water medium, where δ_W was determined at the depth at which the field decays by a factor of 1/*e*. The ZnO: Ga film provided a narrow field depth in the IR range, which was essentially different from Au film-based SPRs [25].

The SPR performance was evaluated by examining the bulk sensitivity using a change in the refractive index of glucose-water mixed solution. **Figure 3(a)** shows the SPR reflectance spectra at $\theta = 75°$ for a 107 nm-thick ZnO: Ga film using different glucose contents (0, 1 and 5 g/dL) [24]. The peak position systematically shifted to lower wavenumbers with increasing glucose content in water, showing a peak shift (Δv) of 22 cm^{-1} at 1 g/dL. Furthermore, we experimentally and theoretically evaluated the sensitivity (S_{exp} and S_{cal}) at a wavenumber of 4500 cm^{-1}. The detection sensitivity was expressed by the following expression:

$$S = \Delta v / \Delta n \quad (1)$$

where Δn indicates the per unit change in the refractive index. The experimental S_{exp} was determined to be 8300 cm^{-1}/RIU (RIU: refractive index unit), which was similar to the calculated value (8600 cm^{-1}/RIU) (**Figure 3(b)**).

This section introduced the SPR responses of single ZnO: Ga film surfaces in the IR range. We could clearly observe the SPR spectra and their field distributions. The bulk sensitivity was evaluated using the glucose-water solution to estimate sensing performance. However, the bulk sensitivity requires improvement for real-time monitoring of biological interactions.

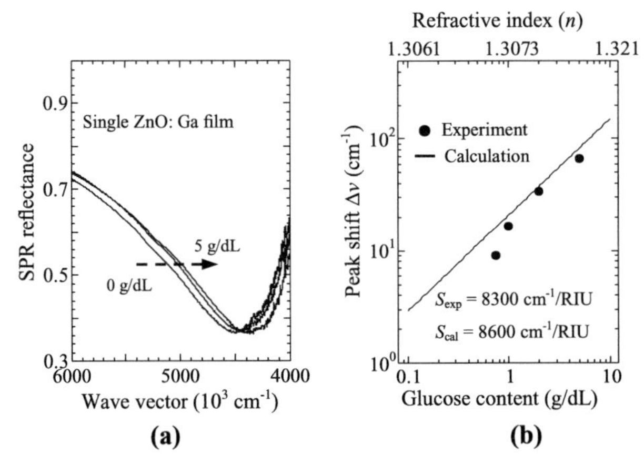

Figure 3.
*(a) SPR reflectance spectra of the single film measured with varying glucose content in water from 0, 1 and 5 g/dL. (b) Correlation between peak shift (Δv) and glucose content in water for the single film. The change in refractive index (n) of a mixed solution consisting of glucose and water is also described in the upper horizontal axis. Black line and dots indicate calculated and experiment data (**Figure 4(b)** and (**c**) of [24]). Copyright by the American Institute of Physics.*

3. IMI structures for sensing performance

The evanescent depth of SPR plays an essential role in determining the sensing performance of plasmonic devices [26]. Above all, an IMI structure can control the evanescent field by changing the thickness of the metal layer [27]. This IMI structure is applied to slightly asymmetric dielectric media [28]. The slightly asymmetric IMI structure can provide benefits for aqueous sensing solutions. To date, no attention has been paid to the SPR property based on a ZnO-related IMI structure. The employment of IMI geometry to SPR excitations on ZnO: Ga films remains unclear. In this section, we introduce asymmetric IMI structures consisting of water, ZnO: Ga, and a cytop polymer. In particular, water-based IMI structures are one of the interesting sensing platforms in SPR applications. The benefits of SPR are confirmed from the bulk sensitivity based on index changes. We discuss the sensing performance of ZnO-SPR based on the proof-of-concept of an IMI structure.

The fabrication of IMI samples was performed as follows. The refractive index of a cytop polymer is kept close to water, which can excite SPRs using IMI structures with ZnO: Ga films. A Cytop polymer (perfluropolymer) film (1.8 mm-thickness) was deposited on BK-7 glass substrates using a polymer content of 9% in fluoride solvent by a spin coating method (2500 rpm for 50s). The coated polymer films were annealed at 220°C for 2 h in the air to evaporate the solvent. ZnO: Ga films were fabricated on polymer/glass substrates using PLD at room temperature. ArF excimer laser pulses (193 nm, 5 Hz, and 1 J/cm^2) were focused on ZnO: Ga targets in an O_2 flow of 10^{-4} Pa [29].

The IMI sample SPR reflectance spectra are shown in **Figure 4(a)**. The peak positions gradually moved within the 4000 to 6000 cm^{-1} range with an increasing incident angle from 60.5° to 64° in 2° increments [29]. The SPR spectra were observed even at a film thickness of 22 nm. The SPR peak dependence on the incident angle of light for the IMI sample was higher than that for the single ZnO film. In addition, the IMI sample showed narrower spectral features than those of the single ZnO films. These behaviors were also confirmed by theoretical SPR spectra (**Figure 4(b)**) [29].

The SP mode of an IMI structure is separated into two types of plasmon branches comprising the short-range and long-range SP modes. The dispersion curves of both SP modes can be described using the Maxwell relations in a planar structure [30]:

$$\left(\frac{\varepsilon_2(v)}{\varepsilon_1(v)}+\frac{\gamma_2(v)}{\gamma_1(v)}\right)\cdot\left(\frac{\varepsilon_0(v)}{\varepsilon_1(v)}+\frac{\gamma_0(v)}{\gamma_1(v)}\right).e^{2\gamma_1(\omega)t}=\left(\frac{\varepsilon_2(v)}{\varepsilon_1(v)}-\frac{\gamma_2(v)}{\gamma_1(v)}\right)\cdot\left(\frac{\varepsilon_0(v)}{\varepsilon_1(v)}+\frac{\gamma_0(v)}{\gamma_1(v)}\right) \quad (2)$$

$$\gamma_i^2=k^2-\grave{o}_i\left(\frac{v}{c}\right)^2 \quad (i = 0, 1, 2) \quad (3)$$

where $\varepsilon_i(v)$ $(i = 0, 1, 2)$ represents the dielectric function in each layer, i.e., water, ZnO: Ga, and cytop polymer layers, respectively. **Figure 4(c)** shows a dispersion curve of the IMI sample, revealing two plasmon branches of short-range and long-range SP modes. The experimental data were similar for the long-range SP mode, which was due to the phase-matching of wave vectors of SPRs at the water–ZnO: Ga–cytop polymer interfaces. An SP wave of the long-range mode is expected to show a longer propagation distance than that of the single-mode. The following equation can

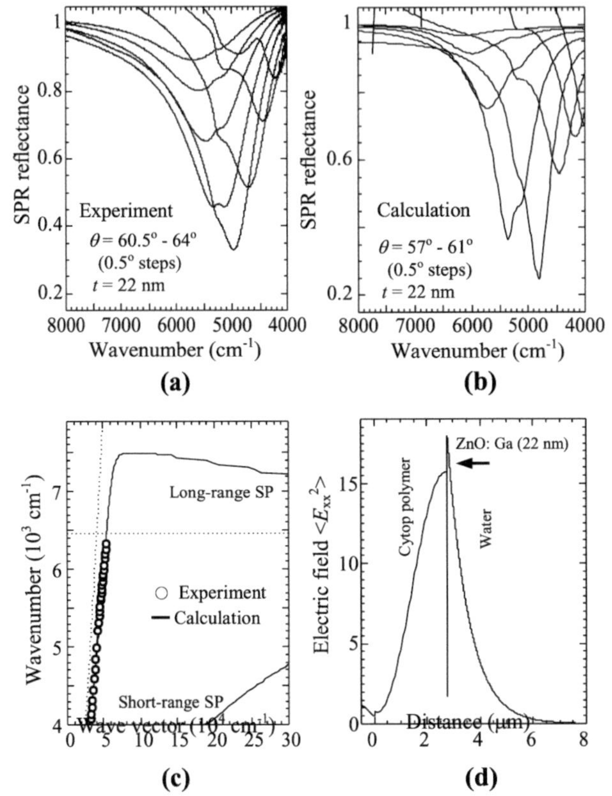

Figure 4.
*(a) Experimental and (b) calculated SPR reflectance spectra of the ZnO IMI sample with a film thickness (t) of 22 nm. Water was selected as the dielectric medium. (c) Experimental and calculated dispersion curves of the ZnO IMI sample (t = 22 nm). A dot line indicates light line in water medium. Long-range and short-range SP modes are represented in the figure. (d) a depth-dependent mean square evanescent field at calculated at 4500 cm^{-1} for the IMI sample (**Figures 4(d)** and **5(c)** of [29]). Copyright by the American Institute of Physics.*

express the propagation distance (L_{prop}): $L_{prop} = 1/2 \times \mathrm{Im}[k_x]$ [31], which represents the length from the launch point where the evanescent field power decays by a factor of $1/e$. The L_{prop} value of the IMI sample was approximately 10 μm, which was longer than that of the single film (L_{prop} = 3 μm). The difference in SPR response between the IMI sample and single films was related to the propagation distance.

Figure 4(d) shows a depth profile of a mean-square evanescent field at 4500 cm^{-1} of the p-polarized component [29]. The value of $<E_{zz}^2>$ was estimated to be 18.0, which was higher than that of the single film. Besides, the δ_w value in the water medium was in the vicinity of 1 μm. The penetration depth clearly expanded when using the IMI sample, relating to the long propagation distance and the high angle dependence of SPR reflectance spectra.

Figure 5(a) shows the SPR reflectance spectra (θ = 58.25°) of the IMI sample, revealing a large Δv of 82 cm^{-1} at 1 g/dL, which was higher than that of the single film [29]. Additionally, the sensitivity was measured at 4500 cm^{-1}, which resulted in a large S_{exp} value of 30,530 cm^{-1}/RIU. This value was close to the theoretical estimation (S_{cal} = 33,000 cm^{-1}/RIU). The enhanced sensitivity was attributed to the evanescent field depth and longer propagation distance of the SPR, which was compared with the single film (**Figure 5(b)**) [29].

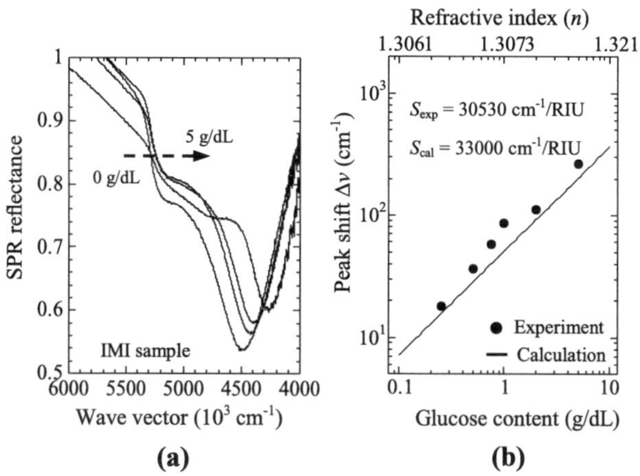

Figure 5.
*(a) SPR reflectance spectra of the IMI sample measured with varying glucose content in water from 0, 1, and 5 g/dL. (b) Correlation between peak shift (Δv) and glucose content in water for the IMI sample. The change in refractive index (n) of a mixed solution consisting of glucose and water is also described in the upper horizontal axis. Black line and dots indicate calculated and experiment data (**Figure 4(b)** and (**c**) of [29]). Copyright by the American Institute of Physics.*

In this section, we investigated the SPR properties and sensing performance of the IMI sample. The SPR spectra of the IMI sample displayed narrower features than those of the single film. This result provided the extended evanescent field depth and the long propagation distance. Consequently, the sensitivity of the IMI sample was markedly enhanced compared to that of the single film.

4. Dielectric-assisted ZnO-SPR

In Sections 2 and 3, we introduced the SPR properties of the single film and IMI sample. The single film showed broad SPR resonances and weak evanescent fields. The use of an IMI structure increased the evanescent field because of the long-range SP mode. However, the IMI sample produced a large sensing volume on the sample surface due to the long penetration depth, where it is not easy to detect small changes in the refractive index near the sample surfaces. Therefore, there is a need to find new strategies for circumventing the structural limitations of ZnO-SPRs in terms of penetration depth and evanescent field. Consequently, we propose a new structural concept based on dielectric-assisted SPRs to overcome some difficulties associated with ZnO-SPRs for real-time monitoring of biological interactions.

When sufficiently thick dielectric layers are placed on Ag and Au-metal layer surfaces, waveguide modes are supported in addition to the conventional SP mode [32, 33]. However, the sensing performance of a waveguide is comparable to that of a classical SPR. However, the Ag and Au-based SPR devices with thin dielectric layers (e.g., Al_2O_3 and SiO_2) show SP waves along the thin dielectric layer surfaces with a thickness insufficient to support a waveguide mode. The SP waves of dielectric-assisted SPRs sufficiently penetrate the analyte region, unlike the waveguide mode. Therefore, the introduction of thin dielectric layers on top of Ag and Au metallic films has been reported to improve the sensing performance in the visible range [34].

In this section, we report on the capping of thin dielectric layers to a ZnO-SPR sensing platform to enhance the detection sensitivity in the IR range. Here, we define dielectric-assisted ZnO-SPR devices as "hybrid samples". The insertion of dielectric layers changes the *E*-field distribution and penetration depth, providing enhanced detection sensitivity. The improvement in sensing performance is discussed from the viewpoint of penetration depth and *E*-field of the SP waves. Finally, we introduce the sensing capabilities of the hybrid samples by measuring the biological interactions between biotin and streptavidin.

The fabrication of hybrid samples was conducted as follows. Cytop polymer films (2.2 μm thickness) were deposited on BK-7 glass substrates. Metallic ZnO: Ga films with a thickness of 22 nm were fabricated on the polymer-coated substrates using a PLD method at room temperature (RT). Fabrication conditions of the polymer and ZnO: Ga films were the same as those of the IMI sample. In this study, we selected Ga_2O_3 as a dielectric layer. 190 m-thick Ga_2O_3 dielectric layers were deposited over ZnO: Ga layers on the polymer/glass substrates at RT in an O_2 flow of 10^{-4} Pa using the PLD method [35].

Figure 6(a) shows a hybrid sample's experimental SPR reflectance spectra with a Ga_2O_3 thickness of 190 nm [35]. The peak positions moved within the 4000–5500 cm^{-1}

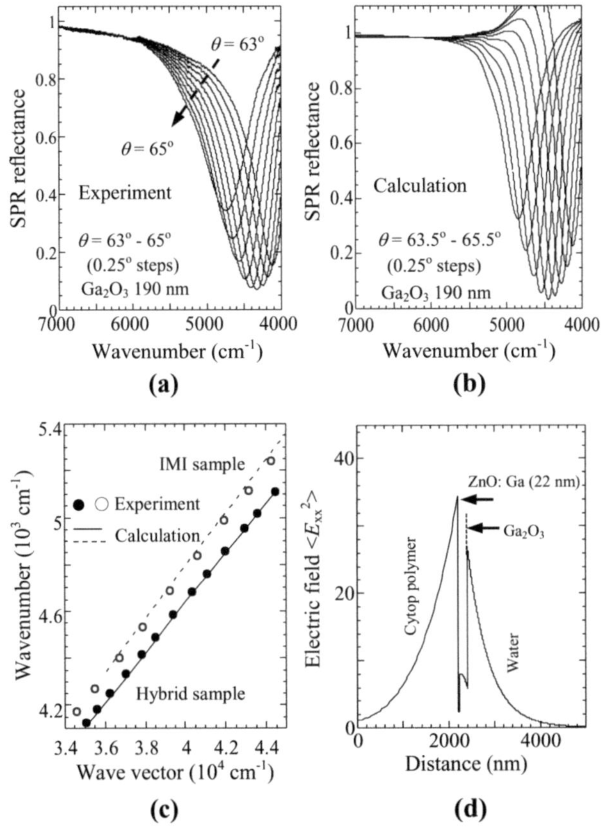

Figure 6.
*(a) Experimental and (b) calculated SPR reflectance spectra of the hybrid sample with a Ga_2O_3 thickness of 190 nm. Water was selected as the dielectric medium. (c) Experimental and calculated dispersion curves of the IMI sample and hybrid sample. Black open and closed circles indicate experimental data. Dotted and straight lines represent calculation data. (d) a depth-dependent mean square evanescent field at calculated at 4500 cm^{-1} for the hybrid sample (***Figures 4(c), 6(d)*** and ***(h)*** of [35]). Copyright by the American Chemical Society.*

range as the incident angle increased in 2.5° increments. The dependence of the SPR peak on the incident angle of light for the hybrid sample was higher than that for the IMI sample. The hybrid sample exhibited narrower spectral features than those of the IMI sample. These SPR behaviors were further reproduced by theoretical SPR spectra (**Figure 6(b)**) [35]. The difference in SPR response between the hybrid and IMI samples is attributed to the propagation length. An experimental L_{prop} of approximately 14 mm was obtained for the hybrid sample, which was greater than that of the IMI sample (L_{prop} = 10 μm). **Figure 6(c)** shows the dispersion curves of the hybrid and IMI samples [35]. The dispersion curve of the IMI sample was close to the light line in free space due to the long-range SP mode. However, the dispersion curve of the hybrid sample shifted to higher SP wave vectors by insertion of a Ga_2O_3 layer on top of a ZnO: Ga layer surface, leading to changes in the optical properties of the SPR reflectance spectra. Besides, the use of Ga_2O_3 dielectric layer was effective in reducing the penetration depth in the water medium. **Figure 6(d)** shows a depth profile of a mean-square evanescent field at 4500 cm^{-1} of the *p*-polarized component [35]. The value of $<E_{zz}^2>$ was increased up to 34.5, which was higher than that of the IMI sample. Additionally, the δ_w value in the water medium was suppressed to 400 nm. The reduced penetration depth was related to an increase in SP wave vector by inserting the dielectric layer to the IMI sample.

Figure 7(a) shows the SPR reflectance spectra of the hybrid sample [35]. The dip peaks shifted to lower wavenumbers with increasing glucose concentration. A wavenumber shift of 19 cm^{-1} at 1 g/dL was observed from the SPR reflectance spectra taken at θ = 63°. The S_{exp} and S_{cal} of the hybrid sample were 18,700 and 19,200 cm^{-1}/RIU, respectively. These values were smaller than those of the IMI sample [35]. (**Figure 7(b)**). This was due to the reduced penetration depth of the hybrid sample. Furthermore, there is a need to evaluate the sensitivity (*S*) and spectral linewidth (FWHM: full-width half-maximum) when considering the performance of a biosensor. The figure-of-merit (FoM) is defined by the following relation:

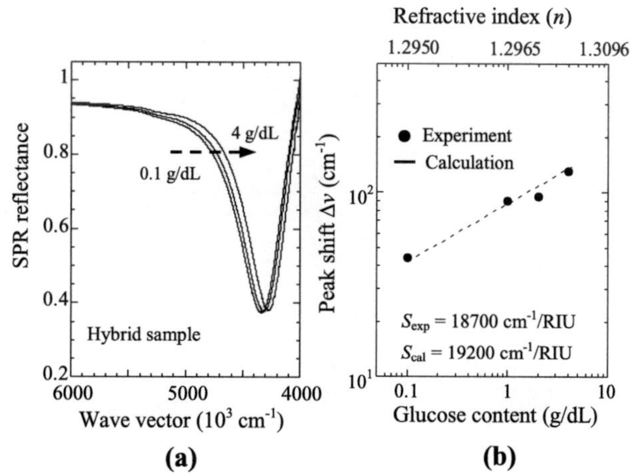

Figure 7.
*(a) SPR reflectance spectra of the hybrid sample measured with varying glucose content in water (0, 1, 1, 2 and 4 g/dL). (b) Correlation between peak shift (Δv) and glucose content in water for the hybrid sample. The change in refractive index (n) of a mixed solution consisting of glucose and water is also described in the upper horizontal axis. Black line and dots indicate calculated and experiment data (**Figure 8** of [35]). Copyright by the American Chemical Society.*

$$FoM = S / \text{FWHM} \quad (4)$$

This relation is used to quantify the general performance of a biosensor [36]. This normalization allows for comparison with other sensing platforms. The hybrid sample provided a higher FoM value (51.0 RIU^{-1}) than did the IMI sample (36.1 RIU^{-1}). The enhanced FoM was attributed to the narrowing of the spectral linewidth resulting from the insertion of the Ga_2O_3 layer.

5. Real-time monitoring of biological interactions

We evaluated the SPR sensing performance of the hybrid sample using the biological interactions between biotin-PEG-DPPE and streptavidin. PEG and DPPE indicate poly(ethylene glycol) and 1, 2 dipalmitoyl-*sn*-glycerol-3-phosphatidylethanolamine, respectively. The high binding affinity and irreversible binding of the molecular pair of biotin-streptavidin is a powerful tool to measure changes in the SPR reflectance, which has medical applications such as antigen–antibody reactions and allergic reactions. We conducted surface modifications before the biological experiments using self-assembled monolayer (SAM) formation.

The Ga_2O_3 layer surface of the hybrid sample was chemically modified using a SAM of *n*-octadecylphosphonic acid [$C_{18}H_{37}PO(OH)_2$:ODPA] to form a CH_3-terminated SAM (CH_3-SAM). This CH_3-SAM is commonly used to obtain hydrophobic surfaces because of the strong hydrogen bonding acid–base character of the $-PO(OH)_2$ group [37]. The hybrid samples were immersed in ODPA (5 mM in ethanol) at RT for 48 h after O_2 plasma irradiation. The surface states and chemical composition of the SAM-coated sample were investigated using X-ray photoemission spectroscopy (XPS). **Figure 8(a)** shows the typical Ga(3d), P(2p), C(1 s), and O(1 s)

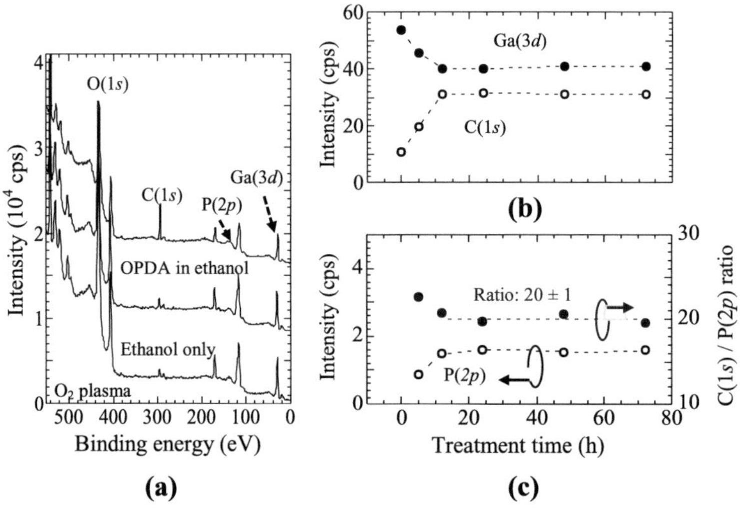

Figure 8.
(a) XPS core-level spectra of Ga(3d), P(2p), C(1 s) and O(1 s)-related peaks following different surface modifications. The XPS spectra were taken after surface treatments of ODPA in ethanol, ethanol only and O_2 plasma. (b) Ga(3d)- and C(1 s)-related peak intensities as a function of OPDA treatment time. (c) P(2p)-related peak and intensity ratio of C(1 s) and P(2p) as a function of OPDA treatment time (Figure 10 of [35]). Copyright by the American Chemical Society.

peaks for different surface treatments [35]. The P(2*p*) peak of the ODPA-coated sample was observed at 136 eV, which was not obtained for the ethanol or O_2 plasma-treated samples. This result clarified the formation of CH_3-SAM on the sample surface. Immersion of the hybrid samples in a toluene solution of ODPA reduced the peak intensities related to Ga(3*d*) and Ga(3*p*) assigned to Ga–O within 20 min owing to the adsorption of ODPA (**Figure 8(b)**) [35]. The ratio of the surface carbon concentration to the phosphorous concentration was 20 ± 1, which was similar to 18, the value expected from the molecular formula of ODPA (**Figure 8(c)**). These XPS results revealed the formation of ODPA on the hybrid samples [35].

Biological interactions were conducted as follows [35]. The hybrid and IMI samples were washed with ethanol several times and then dried using nitrogen gas. Both samples were first exposed to a phosphate-buffered saline (PBS) solution with pH = 7.4 [PBS (1) process], until a stable SPR signal was obtained. Next, both samples were exposed to a solution of biotin-PEG-DPPE (100 μg/mL in PBS) for 35 min, followed by washing with PBS for 5 min [PBS (2) process]. After the sample surfaces were treated with biotin-PEG-DPPE, bovine serum albumin (BSA) was introduced to confirm non-specific protein adsorption to the sample surfaces [BSA process], followed by another PBS wash [PBS (3) process]. PBS solutions with different streptavidin concentrations (0–10 μg/dl in PBS) were then introduced [Streptavidin process].

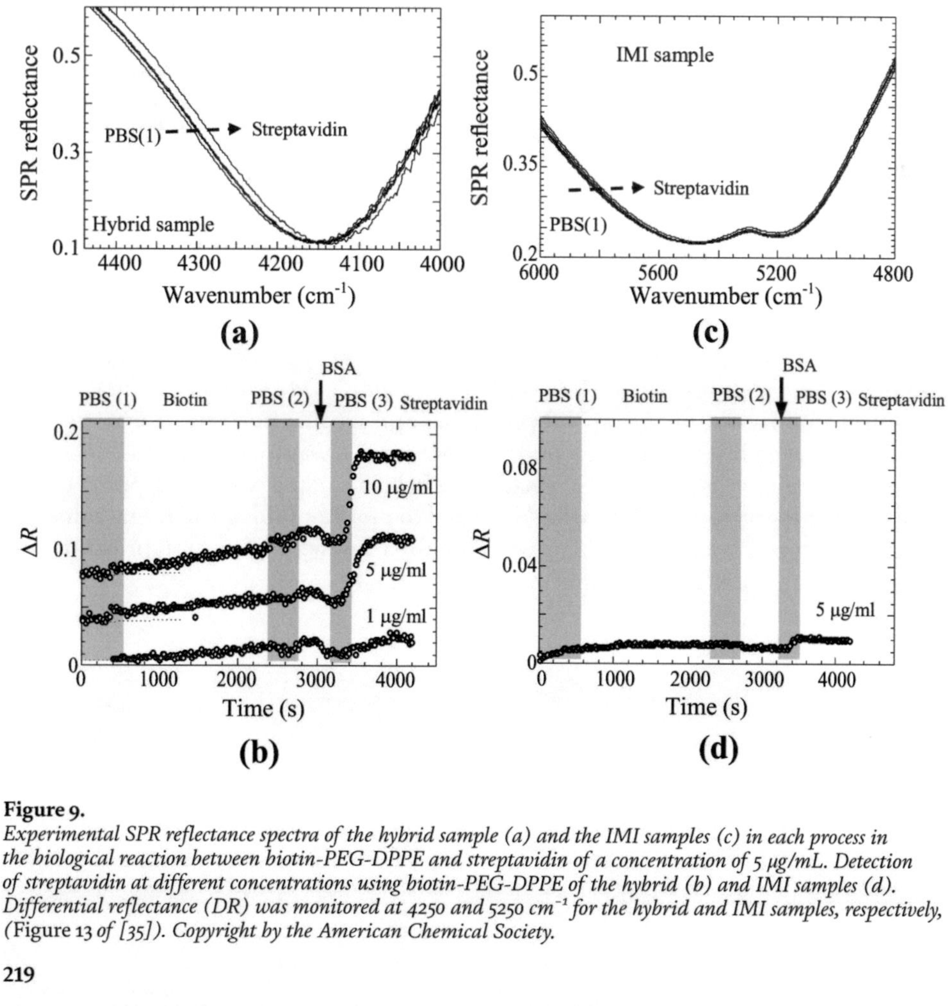

Figure 9.
Experimental SPR reflectance spectra of the hybrid sample (a) and the IMI samples (c) in each process in the biological reaction between biotin-PEG-DPPE and streptavidin of a concentration of 5 μg/mL. Detection of streptavidin at different concentrations using biotin-PEG-DPPE of the hybrid (b) and IMI samples (d). Differential reflectance (DR) was monitored at 4250 and 5250 cm^{-1} for the hybrid and IMI samples, respectively, (Figure 13 *of [35]). Copyright by the American Chemical Society.*

The streptavidin concentrations were used to monitor the specific biological bonding of biotin and avidin [38].

Figure 9(a) shows the SPR reflectance spectra measured after each process [35]. The SPR peak position shifted to small wavenumbers after the surfaces were treated with biotin-PEG-DPPE and streptavidin. The SPR peak shift (Δv) was observed to be 14 cm^{-1}. The SPR peak shift was evaluated by monitoring the reflectance difference (ΔR) at 4250 cm^{-1} induced by biotin-streptavidin binding (**Figure 9(b)**) [35]. The ΔR values were changed slightly through surface treatment with biotin-PEG-DPPE. The streptavidin binding to biotin-PEG-DPPE remarkably depended on the streptavidin concentration. However, the IMI sample did not exhibit a significant change in ΔR during the biotin-streptavidin binding (**Figure 9(c)** and **(d)**) [35]. The time-dependent ΔR of the hybrid and IMI samples was attributed to the biotin-streptavidin binding. The use of the Ga_2O_3 layer on top of the ZnO: Ga layer surface successfully allowed for monitoring of the biological interactions. This resulted from the higher *E*-field and shorter field depth of the hybrid sample compared with those of the IMI sample.

The present detection limit of the hybrid samples was approximately 1 μg/ml (15 nM) due to the background noises. Industrial applications are expected to detect bio-molecule concentration at the ng/dl (~ pM) level. The spectral features of the present ZnO-SPRs were markedly influenced by the interface roughness, relating to the sensing activity for biomolecular detection. Recently, high-sensitive SPR detection at the pM levels of small biomolecules (e.g. biotin) using nanophotonic devices such as cavity structures and metamaterials with layer structures have been reported [39–41]. Recently, biological sensing based on ZnO-related SPR and metamaterials are reported by some papers [42–44]. Therefore, monitoring biological interactions at the pM level could be realized by enhancing the structural and crystalline quality of ZnO-SPR sensors. The detection sensitivity of ZnO-SPR is expected to improve the employment of new nano-plasmonic structures such as cavities and metamaterials.

6. Conclusion

This chapter reported on the structural and optical properties of ZnO-SPR with different layer structures (single, IMI, and hybrid samples) from experimental and theoretical approaches. First, the SPR properties and sensing performance of the single sample were investigated. Second, the IMI sample was introduced in ZnO-SPR devices to enhance sensing activity. Finally, the hybrid sample with the capping of thin dielectric layers to ZnO-SPR was developed to monitor biological interactions between biotin and streptavidin. This work highlights new insights for fabricating biological sensing platforms on ZnO materials.

Author details

Hiroaki Matsui
The University of Tokyo, Bunkyo-ku, Tokyo, Japan

*Address all correspondence to: hiroaki@ee.t.u-tokyo.ac.jp

References

[1] Jadwisienczak WM, Lozykoqski HJ, Xu A, Patel B. Visible emission from ZnO doped with rare-earth ions. Journal of Electronic Materials. 2002;**31**:776-684. DOI: 10.1007/s11664-002-0235-z

[2] Badalawa W, Matsui H, Osone T, Hasuike N, Harima H, Tabata H. Correlation between structural and luminescent properties in Eu^{3+}-doped ZnO epitaxial layers. Journal of Applied Physics. 2011;**109**:053502. DOI: 10.1063/1.3549633

[3] Panda J, Sasmal I, Nath TK. Magnetic and optical properties of Mn-doped ZnO vertically aligned nanorods synthesized by hydrothermal technique. AIP Advances. 2016;**6**:035118. DOI: 10.1063/1.4944837

[4] Babikier M, Wang D, Wang J, Li Q, Sun J, Yan Y, et al. Cu-doped ZnO nanorod arrays: The effects of copper precursor and concentration. Nanoscale Research Letters. 2014;**9**:199. DOI: 10.1186/1556-276X-9-199

[5] Neal JR, Behan AJ, Ibrahim RM, Blythe HJ, Ziese M, Fox AM, et al. Room-temperature magneto-optics of ferromagnetic transition-metal-doped ZnO thin films. Physical Review Letters. 2006;**96**:197208. DOI: 10.1103/PhysRevLett.96.197208

[6] Matsui H, Tabata H. Lattice, band and spin engineering on $Zn_{1-}xCo_xO$. Journal of Applied Physics. 2013;**113**:183525

[7] Ali N, Singh B, Khan ZA, Vijava AR, Tarafder K, Ghosh S. Origin of ferromagnetism in Cu-doped ZnO. Scientific Reports. 2019;**9**:2461. DOI: 10.1038/s41598-019-39660-x

[8] Jin ZC, Hamberg I, Granqvist CG. Optical properties of sputter-deposited ZnO: Al thin films. Journal of Applied Physics. 1988;**64**:5117. DOI: 10.1063/1.342419

[9] Yamamoto N, Makino H, Osone N, Ujihara A, Ito T, Hokari H, et al. Structural, electrical and optical properties of highly transparent conductive ZnO films. Thin Solid Films. 2012;**520**:4131. DOI: 10.3169/itej.66.555

[10] Buonsanti R, Llordes A, Aloni S, Helms BA, Milliron DJ. Tunable infrared absorption and visible transparency of colloidal aluminum-doped zinc oxide nanocrystals. Nano Letters. 2011;**11**:4706. DOI: 10.1021/nl203030f.nnichsen

[11] Sachet E, Losego MD, Guske J, Franzen S, Maria JP. Mid-infrared surface plasmon resonance in znc oxide semiconductor thin films. Applied Physics Letters. 2013;**102**:051111. DOI: 10.1063/1.4791700

[12] Naik GJ, Kim J, Boltasseva A. Oxides and nitrides as alternative plasmonic materials in the optical range. Optical Materials Express. 2011;**1**(6):1090-1099. DOI: 10.1364/OME.1.001090

[13] Badalawa W, Matsui H, Ikehata A, Tabata H. Surface plasmon modes guided by ZnO: Ga layers bounded by different dielectrics. Applied Physics Letters. 2011;**99**:011913. DOI: 10.1063/1.3608313

[14] Sönnichsen C, Franzl F, von Plessen G, Feldmann J. Plasmon resonances in large noble-metal clusters. New Journal of Physics. 2002;**4**:93. DOI: 10.1088/1367-2630/4/1/393

[15] Kalusniak S, Sadofev S, Hennberger F. ZnO as a tunable metal: New types of surface plasmon polaritons.

Physical Review Letters. 2014;**112**:137401. DOI: 10.1103/PhysRevLett.112.137401

[16] Kim J, Dutta A, Memarzadeh B, Kildishev AV, Mosallaei H, Boltasseva A. Mint: Zinc oxide based plasmonic multilayer resonator: Localized and gap surface plasmon in the infrared. ACS Photonics. 2015;**2**:1224. DOI: 10.1021/acsphotonics.5b00318

[17] Nader N, Vangala S, Hendrickson JR, Leedy KD, Look DC, Guo J, et al. Investigation of plasmon resonance tunneling through subwavelength hole arrays conductive ZnO films. Journal of Applied Physics. 2015;**118**:173106. DOI: 10.1063/1.4934875

[18] Cao X, Cao S, Guo H, Li T, Jie Y, Wang N, et al. Piezotronic effect enhanced label-free detection of DNA using a schottky-contacted ZnO nanowire biosensor. ACS Nano. 2016;**10**:8038-8044. DOI: 10.1021/acsnano.6b04121

[19] Wang C, Huang N, Zhuang H, Jiang X. Enhanced performance of nanocrystalline ZnO DNA biosensors via introducing electrochemical covalent biolinkers. ACS Applied Materials & Interfaces. 2015;7:7605-7612. DOI: 10.1021/acsmi.5b00040

[20] Wang Y, Dong J, Luo Y, Tang J, Lu H, Yu J, et al. Indium tin oxide coated two-mode fiber for enhanced SPR sensor on near-infrared region. IEEE Photonics Journal. 2017;**9**:4801309. DOI: 10.1109/JPHOT.2017.2757513

[21] Minn K, Anopchenko A, Yang J, Lee HWH. Excitation of epsilon-near-zero resonance in ultra-thin indium tin oxide shell embedded nanostructured optical fiber. Scientific Reports. 2018;**8**:2342. DOI: 10.1038/s41598-018-19633-2

[22] Martínez J, Ródenas A, Aguiló M, Fernadez T, Solis J, Diaz F. Mid-infrared surface plasmon resonance polariton chemical sensing on fiber-coupled ITO coated glass. Optics Letters. 2016;**41**:2493-2496. DOI: 10.1364/OL.41.002493

[23] Kalusniak S, Sadofev S, Hennberger F. Resonant interaction of molecular vibrations and surface plasmon polaritons: The weak coupling regime. Physical Review B. 2014;**90**:125423. DOI: 10.1103/PhysRevB.90.125423

[24] Matsui H, Ikehata A, Tabata H. Surface plasmon sensors on ZnO: Ga layer surfaces: Electric field distributions and absorption-sensitivity enhancements. Applied Physics Letters. 2015;**106**:011905. DOI: 10.1063/1.4905211

[25] Ikehata A, Itoh T, Ozaki Y. Surface plasmon resonance near-infrared spectroscopy. Analytical Chemistry. 2004;**76**:6461-6469. DOI: 10.1021/ac049003a

[26] Yang F, Sambles JR, Bradberry GW. Long-range surface modes supported by thin films. Physical Review B. 1991;**44**:5855. DOI: 10.1103/PhysRevB.44.5855

[27] Dionne JA, Swealtlock LA, Atwater HA, Polman P. Planar metal plasmon waveguides: Frequency-dependent dispersion, propagation, localization, and loss beyond the free electron model. Physical Review B. 2005;**72**:075405. DOI: 10.1103/PhysRevB.72.075405

[28] Wendier L, Haupt R. Long-range surface plasmon - polariton in asymmetric layer structures. Journal of Applied Physics. 1986;**59**:3289. DOI: 10.1063/1.336884

[29] Matsui H, Ikehata A, Tabata H. Asymmetric plasmon structures on

ZnO: Ga for high sensitivity in the infrared range. Applied Physics Letters. 2016;**109**:191601. DOI: 10.1063/1/4966598

[30] Economou EM. Surface plasmons in thin films. Physical Review B. 1969;**182**:539. DOI: 10.1104/PhysRev.182.539

[31] Dastmalchi B, Tassin P, Koschny T, Soukoulis CN. A new perspective on plasmonics: Confinement and propagaton length of surface plasmons for different materials and geometries. Advanced Optical Materials. 2015;**3**:177. DOI: 10.1002/adom.201500446

[32] Hayashi S, Nesterenko DV, Rahmouni A, Sekkat Z. Observation of Fano line shapes arising from coupling between surface plasmon polariton and waveguide modes. Applied Physics Letters. 2016;**108**:051101. DOI: 10.1063/1.4940984

[33] Abbas A, Linman MJ, Cheng Q. Sensitivity comparison of surface plasmon resonance and plasmon-waveguide resonance biosensors. Sensors and Actuators A. 2011;**156**:169-175. DOI: 10.1016/j.snb.2011.04.008

[34] Lahav A, Shalabaney A, Abdulhalim I. Surface plasmon sensor with enhanced sensitivity using top nano dielectric layer. Journal of Nanophotonics. 2009;**3**:031501. DOI: 10.1117/1.3079803

[35] Kuranaga Y, Matsui H, Ikehata Am Shimoda Y, Noiri M, Ho YL, Delaunay JJ, et al. Enhancing detection sensitivity of ZnO-based infrared plasmonic sensors using capped dielectric Ga_2O_3 layers for real-time monitoring of biological interactions. ACS Applied Bio Materials. 2020;**3**:6331-6342. DOI: 10.1021/acsabm.0c00792

[36] Otte MA, Sepúlveda B, Ni W, Juste JP, Liz-Marzán LM, Lechuga LM. Identification of the optimal spectra region for plasmonic and nanoplasmonic sensing. ACS Nano. 2010;**4**:349-357. DOI: 10.1021/nn901024e

[37] Li F, Shishkin E, Mastro MA, Uite JK, Eddy CR, Edgar JH, et al. Photopolymerization of self-assembled monolayers of Diacetylentic Alkylphophonic acids on group-III nitride substrates. Langmuir. 2010;**26**:10725-10730. DOI: 10.1021/la100273q

[38] Seto H, Yamashita C, Kamba S, Kondo T, Hasegawa M, Matsumoto M, et al. Biotinylation of silicon and nickel surfaces and detection of streptavidin as biosensor. Langmuir. 2013;**29**:9457-9463. DOI: 10.1021/la401068n

[39] Sreekanth KV, Sreejith S, Mishra A, Chen X, Sun H, Lim CT, et al. Biosensing with the singular phase of an ultrathin metal-dielectric nanophotonic cavity. Nature Communications. 2018;**9**:369. DOI: 10.1038/s41467-018-02860-6

[40] Shinohara S, Tanaka D, Okamoto K, Tamada K. Colorimetric plasmon sensors with multilayered metallic nanoparticle sheets. Physical Chemistry Chemical Physics. 2015;**17**:186060-118612. DOI: 10.1039/C5CP02564H

[41] Sreekanth KV, Sreejith S, Alapan Y, Sitti M, Lim CT, Singh R. Microfluidics integrated lithography-free nanophotonic biosensors for the detection of small molecules. Advanced Optical Materials. 2019;**7**:1801313. DOI: 10.1003/adom.201801313

[42] Guo S, Wu X, Li Z, Tong K. High-sensitivity biosensor-based enhanced SPR by ZnO/MoS2 nanowires array layer with graphene oxide nanosheet. International Journal of Optics. 2020;**2020**:7342737. DOI: 10.1155/2020/342737

[43] Xu H, Song Y, Zhu P, Zhao W, Liu T, Wang Q, et al. Alcohol sensor based on surface plasmon resonance of ZnO nanoflowers/Au structure. Materials. 2022;**15**:189. DOI: 10.3390/ma15010189

[44] Mei GS, Menon PS, Hegde G. ZnO for performance enhancement of surface plasmon biosensor: A review. Materials Research Express. 2020;7:012003. DOI: 10.1088/2053-1591/ab66a7

Chapter 14

Development of Simple and Portable Surface Acoustic Wave Biosensors for Applications in Biology and Medicine

Marlon S. Thomas

Abstract

There has been a renewed interest in the development of surface acoustic wave (SAW) biosensors because they hold great promise for opening new frontiers in biology and medicine. The promise of SAW technology is grounded in the advantages SAW devices hold over traditional laboratory techniques used in biological and medical laboratories. These advantages include having smaller sizes to allow greater portability, using smaller sample volumes, requiring lower power requirements, the ability to integrate them into microfluidic platforms, and their compatibility with smart devices such as smartphones. The devices offer high sensitivity and can be designed to allow microfluidic interfacing. Other major advantages of SAW-based technologies include the fact that they can be operated remotely in harsh conditions without the need for an AC power supply. Their compatibility with lab-on-a-chip systems allows the creation of fully integrated devices with the ability to isolate the sample from the operator. In this mini-review, we will discuss SAW devices and their ability to enable a variety of applications in Biology and Medicine. The operating principles of the SAW biosensors will be discussed along with some technological trends and developments.

Keywords: surface acoustic wave (SAW), biosensor, piezoelectric, microfluidic, phase shift

1. Introduction

Over the past three decades, the emergence of small portable lab-on-a-chip biosensors has developed into an important area in biology and medicine [1]. Lab-on-a-chip devices promise to perform all the functions of a traditional laboratory on a miniature microfluidic platform [2]. These small devices allow full automation of analysis, reduce the sample volumes, and reduce the time of analysis as well [2] SAW devices are ideally suited to provide the sensing element in the Lab-on-a-chip platform [3]. One limitation that has plagued lab-on-a-chip devices has been the lack of a miniaturized sensor that facilitates the development of high-sensitivity assays. Several technologies have been explored including Mass spectrometry field [4, 5], electrochemical sensors field [6], optical detection field [7, 8], surface plasmon resonance spectroscopy field [9], and interferometry [10, 11] but each has significant limitations in complex biological matrices. The SAW biosensor technology is based on Surface acoustic waves (SAW), a type of acoustic wave that propagates along a surface of a solid material [12–14]. Propagating SAW are impacted by mass loading and changes in viscoelastic properties of the media on the surface of the sensor and compared to a reference, as seen in **Figure 1a** and **b** [15]. These waves were first described by John William Strutt, 3rd (Lord Rayleigh), in an article on the propagation of acoustic waves in a piezoelectric material [16]. White and Voltmer introduced the concept of using interdigital transducers (IDTs) as a more efficient method of generating surface acoustic waves [17–19]. This method is still used today to generate surface acoustic waves on a piezoelectric material [20, 21]. The piezoelectric materials that are typically used for fabricating SAW devices are listed in **Table 1** [17].

To date, the primary use of SAW devices has been in the telecommunications industry, specifically as filters in cellular telephones and other smart devices [17]. SAW devices operate in the following manner: a metal IDT deposited on a piezoelectric surface is driven by a sinusoidal power source with a period specific to the IDT design [22]. This causes the electrode to vibrate, generating an acoustic wave that is perpendicular to the direction of the IDTs [23]. The penetration depth of the acoustic wave is relatively shallow. This is because the wave produces an evanescent field that cannot penetrate more than a few nanometers into the substrate from which the sensors are fabricated. If a guiding layer is used (a top layer), the acoustic wave propagation will be confined to the substrate-sample interface [24]. The confinement of the wave via a guiding layer maximizes the energy density of the acoustic wave at the substrate-sample interface.

The velocity of an acoustic wave in a piezoelectric material is an intrinsic property and varies slightly as a function of temperature [25–27] In the case of lithium tantalate, one of the more popular substrates used for the fabrication of SAW filters and devices, the wave velocity is 4200 m s^{-1} [28]. Values for the acoustic properties of commonly used piezoelectric substrates are listed in **Table 1** below. The acoustic wave velocity is approximately 10^4–10^5 times smaller than the velocity of electromagnetic waves [29]. Surface acoustic waves can be generated and detected by spatially periodic, interdigital electrodes that are deposited on the planar surface of a piezoelectric plate. Excitation

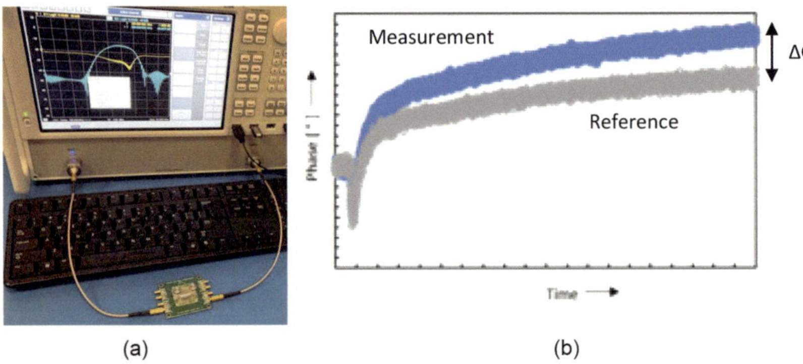

Figure 1.
Acoustic wave measurement using (a) a delay line SAW device with measurement performed via a two-port vector network analyzer (VNA). Connections are made using a customized printed circuit board with connectors to the VNA. In (b) there is a plot of the change in phase of the reference, the change in phase of the sample and the difference between the two channels.

Piezoelectric substrate	Orientation (axis)	Wave velocity (m/s)	Temperature coefficient (ppm/°C)	Coupling coefficient (%)	Wafer cost (relative cost)
Quartz	32*YX	3159	0	0.16	Low
Quartz	43*	3159	0	0.16	Low
Lithium tantalate	36°-YX	4160	5.0	28–32	Medium
Lithium tantalate	42°-YX	4022	7.6	40	Medium
Lithium niobate	128*YX	3980	75	5.5	High
Lithium niobate	64*YX	4742	70	11.3	High
Langasite	138.5*	2330	38	0.37	High

Table 1.
Properties of common piezoelectric substrates used in the fabrication of surface acoustic wave devices. Courtesy of The Roditi International Corporation Ltd, UK.

of the interdigitated electrode with a radio frequency source generates a periodic electric field, thus permitting piezoelectric coupling to a traveling surface wave. The center frequency of the acoustic wave generated by the sensor, fc, is governed by the Rayleigh wave velocity (VR). VR depends on the piezoelectric substrate and the electrode width (a) of a single finger, according to the equation fc = VR/4a [30]. The velocity for the SAW generated by the device depends on the properties of the piezoelectric substrate (crystal) that is used in the fabrication of the sensor and its crystallographic orientation. Computer models have allowed the careful sorting of numerous crystallographic orientations to enable the discovery of different types of acoustic waves. Where vs. is the SAW velocity and f_c is the center frequency of the device. The SAW velocity is an important parameter determining the center frequency. The mass sensitivity is given by Sauerbrey's equation, where:

$$\Delta f / f_0 \approx \Delta V / V_0 \tag{1}$$

and

$$f_0 = v / \lambda \tag{2}$$

Propagation loss is one of the major factors that determine the insertion loss of a device and is caused by wave scattering at crystalline defects and surface irregularities. Materials that show high electromechanical coupling factors combined with small temperature coefficients of delay are generally preferred. The free surface velocity, V_f, of the material is a function of the cut angle and propagation direction. The TCD is an indication of the frequency shift expected for a transducer due to a temperature change and is also a function of the cut angle and propagation direction. The substrate is chosen based on the device design specifications, which include operating temperature, fractional bandwidth, and insertion loss.

Indeed, the fabrication of SAW devices requires a few critical components including the physical deposition of a metal on the surface of the piezoelectric substrate, etching of that metal deposited on the surface, optional deposition of guiding, and/or sensing layer. SAW devices mainly have two kinds of structures. The first is a design that features two sets of IDTs where a sinusoidal radio frequency (*RF*) is applied to one side of the IDT structure while the other is connected to the ground. The *RF* is applied to the first set of IDTs or the input IDTs, which generates an acoustic wave, as is seen in **Figure 1a**. The wave is transmitted through a delay line and is received by the second set of output IDTs. The signal is then captured and analyzed. The second type of SAW termed a resonator, features one set of IDTs with grating reflectors that can trap the surface wave. The signal from the IDT can be amplified and then fed back to the input IDT.

There are several factors that affect the transmission of the acoustic wave in a SAW device and have to be closely monitored or controlled in order to generate repeatable results. These include temperature, pressure, humidity, and mass loading. Indeed, SAW devices can be operated as sensors for temperature, pressure, humidity and mass loading. Temperature effects are the most challenging when trying to perform sensitive acoustic-wave sensing in liquid media. This is controlled in part by including a reference delay line. The reference is functionalized with a passivating agent to minimize nonspecific binding (e.g., PEG). For biological or medical applications, the active sensing line is functionalized with capturing agents that interact specifically with the analyte being targeted. An Analyte can be quantitatively detected by monitoring changes in gas pressure, liquid pressure or from the increase mass due to binding of a biological molecule to a targeting molecule or the increase in the fluid density or mass increases due to absorption of the target. The sensitivity of SAW devices increases as the square of the frequency; therefore, higher frequencies lead to smaller, more sensitive instruments. However, the frequency also determines the depth within the sample that the device can probe; for example, for a solution placed atop a sensor, the higher frequencies will examine a shallower depth than lower frequencies. Thus, the operating frequency of the SAW must be considered when selecting targets, probes, and conjugation schemes to functionalize the active sensing region of a SAW device.

Aside from the layer of targeting molecules that is typically used to decorate a SAW device, an additional guiding layer is often deposited to enhance the sensitivity of the device. The guiding layer traps the energy of the acoustic wave near the surface of the device to increase sensitivity to surface perturbations. The SAW sensors are inherently capable of detecting analytes in solution concentrations on the order of parts-per-billion (ppb) by mass, through the use of higher frequencies >300 MHz Ideally, the guiding layer needs to have a lower density and lower acoustic velocity than the piezoelectric substrate. Materials that have been utilized in past include polymers such as poly-methyl-methacrylate and Novolac and oxides including silicon dioxide and silicon monoxide. Changes in the mass loading of the surface, if all else is kept constant, affect the acoustic wave velocity as it travels across the delay line from the input IDT to the output IDT. The time delay is a result of the interactions between any adsorbed mass, i.e. the analyte, and results in a phase shift between the applied and the detected sinusoidal wave. In the case where there is only a single IDT, the round-trip time is measured by the applied signal. In recent years, there has been an increasing demand for portable, disposable and inexpensive sensors for biological and medical applications. Due to these increasing demands for miniature sensors, SAW devices have received renewed interest for use as sensors in biochemical assays and as detectors in microfluidic biosensors, particularly since it is a label-free technique. In this review, we will outline the use of SAW biosensors in biology and medicine.

2. Principles for SAW biosensors

Surface acoustic waves are generated in a SAW device with the application of a sinusoidal *RF* to one side of the IDT patterned on the piezoelectric material, while the other side is connected to the ground. An image of a typical measurement scheme is shown in **Figure 1a** with a custom-built printed circuit board and connections with a vector network analyzer (VNA). The wavelength of the acoustic wave generated will be a function of the material properties, the shape, and layout of the IDTs, and the material deposited as the guiding layer. The main parameter utilized in data analysis is the velocity of the acoustic wave. Each piezoelectric material will allow an acoustic wave to propagate at different velocities for a given wavelength. The larger the wave velocity, the smaller time needed to have the acoustic wave travel from the input IDT to the output IDT. Another important parameter for SAW devices is the frequency that it operates. Only when the wavelength of the applied R*F* is equal to the intrinsic wavelength of the SAW, i.e. the period of the IDT, can the SAW be stimulated to produce an acoustic wave described by Eq. (2). Measurements of acoustic wave velocity is often reported as a phase shift between a reference channel and a sample channel. An image of a typical measurement is seen in **Figure 1a** while the plot of phase shift is seen in **Figure 1b**.

The IDTs can be fabricated as periodic bars with uniform lengths, widths, and gap spacing. They can be designed to give bi-directional or unidirectional acoustic wave propagation. Small IDT gap spacing and widths and thus smaller wavelengths often result in a higher frequency. In some cases, different IDT width/gap ratios can generate higher harmonic waves. The velocity of the wave that is generated can be influenced by several factors such as temperature and the analyte's concentration change. The temperature has a significant effect on the wave velocity. This effect can be described as the temperature coefficient of the frequency (TCF). TCF is described as a relative change in frequency with the temperature. Other factors that influence the device's sensitivity include humidity and pressure. Any slight fluctuations in the pressure will impact the mass loading of the device. Any change in the humidity results in changes to the electric field. The electric field strength is also impacted by charged particles that are suspended in the solution with comparatively high dipole moments (**Figure 2**).

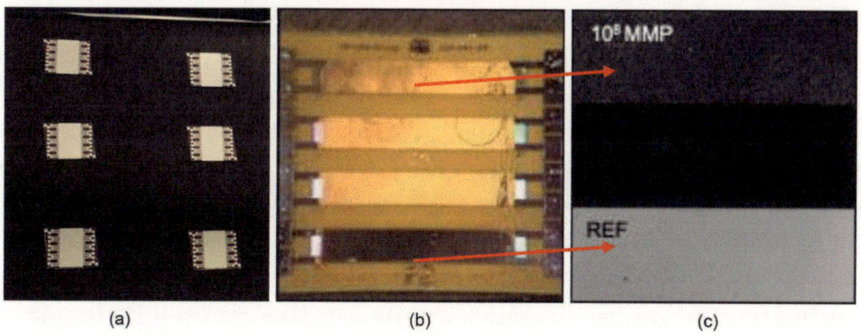

Figure 2.
Image of a surface acoustic wave biosensor where (a) is an image of new unused sensors while (b) shows an image of used sensors and (c) is a high magnification image of one of the sample channels and the reference channels from (b).

3. Biological and medical application of SAW devices

Changes in the surface mass can attenuate the wave velocity. These minute changes are measured by either measuring the changes in the resonance frequency of the piezoelectric material or by measuring the time the SAW travels from the input IDT to the output IDT. In the case when there is only a single IDT, then we measure the round-trip time.

The temperature dependence of the SAW measurements is a property that can be used in temperature sensors. Borrero et al. report a SAW resonator-based temperature sensor that was fabricated from 128° Y-X $LiNbO_3$ crystal. The device operated at a frequency of 65 MHz and was also capable of measuring pressure and impedance. The one-port SAW resonator had an IDT width of 15 μm, 20 IDT finger pairs, and an acoustic aperture of 15λ. There were also 100 electrodes on each side of the IDT pairs. A linear dynamic range was established between 50 and 200°C, while the frequency had a linear response with temperature.

Wireless temperature sensing is possible on SAW devices. This technique takes advantage of the round-trip flight time of travel. Wireless SAWs are made not to require any power supply so they can be used for remote sensing. Reindl et al. designed a delay line wireless SAW temperature sensor. The device operates by sending a VHF/UHF band RF burst delivered by a radar transceiver. The SAW then performed a measurement. Since the temperature affects the changes affect the wave velocity, measurement of the response pattern can be used to determine the temperature. The resolution of this system was ±0.2°C. This type of system could be used for biological applications in extremely isolated locations or for patients who have been isolated from the general population due to a high communicable infection.

SAW sensors can be fabricated and implanted in the body to monitor core-body temperatures in real-time. Martin and colleagues packaged a single-port resonator (single IDT) SAW temperature sensor, in a ceramic and connected it to a small antenna. In vivo tests in dogs demonstrated the capacity to perform wireless interrogation of samples. SAW devices fabricated from materials having large TCF are well suited for fabricating temperature sensors but are not well suited to fabricating other types of sensors. To perform other types of sensing, methods should be developed to compensate for the effects of TCF. One solution is to introduce a guiding layer of a material that reduces the TCF such as SiO_2. SiO_2 is often used to compensate for the negative TCF for most piezoelectric materials used to fabricate SAW devices. Zhang et al., published a report that experimentally verified that a SiO_2 layer of a thickness of 0.3λ gives a TCF of zero for $LiNbO_3$. A large electro-mechanical coupling coefficient of 7.92% was also observed when the thick SiO_2 guiding layer was used. Another method for performing temperature compensation would be to add a second SAW device and a mixer cell [1, 31]. In such a configuration, one SAW acts as a reference while the other SAW acts as a sensing unit [1, 31]. If the two SAW sensors are placed in such a manner that both devices experience the same temperature with only one sensor actually sensing changes, then any interference occurring to both systems would be canceled out after the mixer [1, 31]. The SAW velocity is strongly affected by the pressure applied to the piezoelectric material. Therefore, a SAW pressure sensor would be a device that exploits this pressure-frequency relationship [32]. To enhance the sensitivity, often a method similar to that of Grousset et al. is followed where the area below the sensing area is etched [8]. In that report, they used an AT-cut quartz film, operated at 430 MHz that was etched by Deep Reactive Ion Etching (DRIE) to expose the sensing area. The resonance frequency showed a linear relationship with the applied pressure and had a sensitivity of 25.8 kHz/bar from 0 to 4.8 bar.

SAW pressure sensors can be implanted in the human body. Liang et al. reported a blood pressure sensor where they amplified the signal from a SAW device by using a Colpitts oscillator. A static test showed a 1.75 kHz/mmHg sensitivity with a standard deviation less than 1 mmHg. Another wireless *in vivo* SAW device was reported by Murphy et al. that was designed to monitor blood pressure remotely from inside the left ventricle of the heart of a living porcine subject. A prototype of the device was able to monitor changes in blood pressure around the clock and then compared the results with a commercial catheter-tip transducer. The primary challenge to building *in vivo* SAW devices is to have a well-designed antenna to deliver the *RF* signal and to receive the data with minimal signal loss.

4. Molecular biosensors

Due to their small sizes, ability to monitor label-free, and high accuracy, SAW devices are ideally suited to function as biosensors. They can be operated remotely, they can be used as implantable devices and they facilitate real-time measurements for patients remotely. The high accuracy of the SAW supports it to use as a bacterial cell monitor, viral particle monitoring, and a DNA detection system. Cai et al. used a SAW device to detect DNA sequences and cells. As is frequently done for SAW devices, gold was deposited on the guiding layer to form a sensing layer for DNA detection. The hybridization of the target single-stranded DNA target molecules (ssDNA) with the DNA probe resulted in a frequency shift of the SAW resonator and could be recorded and measured. DNA detection using this device achieved a sensitivity of 6.7 x 10^{-16} g/cm^2 per Hz. The device was also capable of detecting a single EMT6 and 3 T3 cancer cell. Biochemical assays need to be able to monitor in liquid environments to known concentrations, however, the immersion of a traditional Rayleigh SAW tends to radiate the acoustic energy into the liquid because the displacement component is perpendicular to the surface. A type of SAW called the Love mode SAW is capable of performing analysis in liquid environments. Love-mode SAW devices guided acoustic modes which propagate in a thin layer deposited on a substrate. The acoustic energy is focused in the guiding layer where the displacement component propagates parallel to the surface. When using traditional piezoelectric substrates, SiO_2 and PMMA are frequently used as the waveguiding layer. The soft polymer poly (dimethylsiloxane) (PDMS) is often used to fabricate the channels in the device. Zhang et al. has reported a prostate-specific antigen (PSA) biosensor based on a love mode device. The sensor used $LiTaO_3$ with aluminum IDTs which were coated with a SiO_2 guiding layer and then gold forming the sensing layer. A PDMS microfluidic channel was subsequently added to the device to ensure that liquid can flow between the IDTs. The detection limit of this system was 10 mg/ml. The images and mass loading effects of a similar Love wave SAW device was used to measure the mass loading resulting from the covalent attachment of streptavidin-coated one-micron magnetic beads are shown in **Figure 3**.

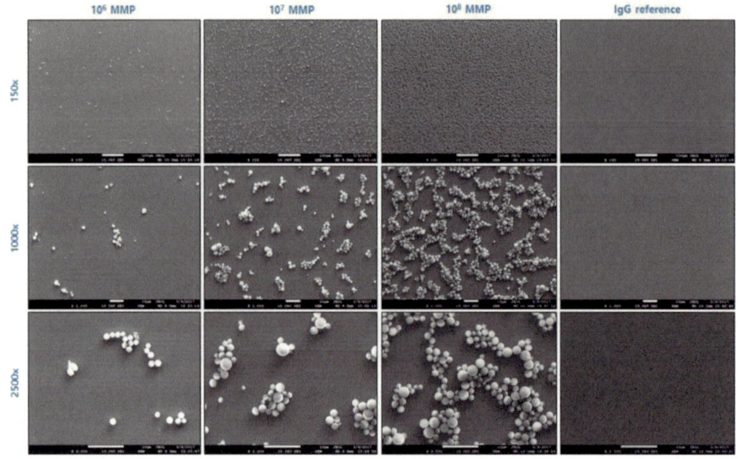

(a)

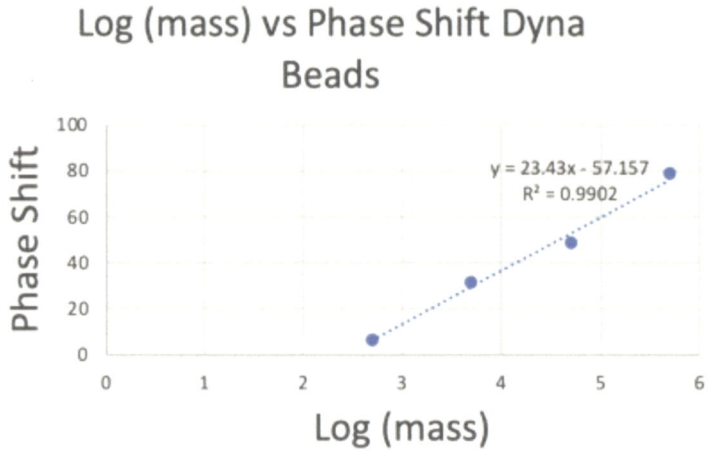

(b)

Figure 3.
Confirmation of the mass-loading correlation between magnetic nanoparticles. (a) Shows covalently bonded to the surface of the SAW sensor and (b) shows the resulting phase shifts. The semi-log plot illustrates the expected direct proportionality between mass and phase shift.

5. Pathogen detection

SAW devices have seen applications in biology and medicine in the past. Unfortunately, strong radiation losses are observed for Rayleigh surface waves and most Lamb-mode surface waves. These types of devices have surface displacement for propagation modes have displacements normal on the surface. In liquid environments, we need to use surface waves that have the particle displacement parallel to the device surface and normal to the Love-mode SAW biosensors that have also been developed for the detection of microbial species. A series of devices have been developed by Sandia National Laboratory in collaboration with the University of New Mexico's Health Science Center. Researchers Branch and Brozik at Sandia National Laboratory reported Low-level detection of endospores from *Bacillus Antracis* simulants using a love mode biosensor based on a 36° YX $LiTaO_3$ substrate. When using a polyimide guiding layer, this system was capable of detecting *Bacillus thuringiensis* B8 endospores at a level between 1 and 2 ng/cm^2. Larson and Baca from the University of New Mexico reported the benefits of using a Love-mode SAW device for viral and bacterial detection for clinical applications. **Figure 4** shows unpublished data from measurement of human cardiac troponin complex from serum samples. The values were measured on a lithium tantalate biosensor and coated with monoclonal antibodies from Hytest, Finland, as seen in **Figure 4**. In this report, they disused their findings on SAW devices that were in commercial development. In another report, Bisoffi et al. at the University of New Mexico reported using a Love-mode SAW device to detect a series of different viral particles and viral particles complex solution. In one experiment, the authors compare the detection of solutions containing sewage and other waste material. Bisoffi et al. reported developing the detection of HIV virus type 1 and type 2 using a Love-mode SAW device. In this study, three commonly occurring viral particles were detected from a complex matrix; river and sewage effluent. The SAW sensors were first treated with an organo-silane, 10% 3-glycidyloxypropyl trimethoxysilane (GPTMS), and then functionalized with an antibody. The device allowed multiplexed detection that was specific for HIV-1 and HIV-2 were introduced. The report not only confirm that the SAW could detect viral particles at a level below the standard ELISA and PCR methods but also demonstrated that the Love-mode SAW device could distinguish between HIV type 1 and type 2. Branch and Thayne reported the development of a Love-mode acoustic array biosensor platform that allowed autonomous detection of pathogenic microbes that are critical for human health and safety. Branch and Thayne reported antigen-capture of the targeted pathogens with a mass sensitivity of 7.19 ± 0.74 mm^2/ng with a detection limit of 6.7 ± 0.40 pg./mm^2. In yet another report, Baca et al. report the detection of fragmented *Ebola* antigens at the point of care without the need for added reagents, sample processing, or specialized personnel to run the test. The test could be performed by first responders. The limit of detection for this methodology was below the average level of viremia detected on the first day of symptoms by PCR. Baca and colleagues from the University of New Mexico observed a semi-log sensor response for highly fragmented Ebola viral particles with

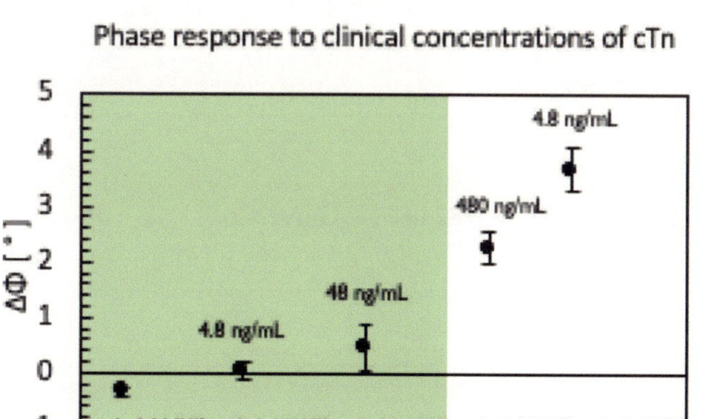

Figure 4.
The plot of injected mass versus phase shift. This investigation of rapid human cardiac troponin ITC complex (cTn-ITC) detected from human blood, which is an indication of heart muscle damage following a myocardial infarction, using a SAW biosensor. The region in green represents the clinically relevant region.

a detection limit of 1.9 x 10^4 PFU/ml. The devices used by both the researchers at Fisk University are fabricated at Sandia National Laboratory and are similar to devices used at the University of New Mexico.

6. Trends and future directions

The small size, high sensitivity, and potential low-cost nature of SAW devices make them attractive for large-scale biosensor applications. The detection is primarily focused on monitoring changes in the acoustic wave velocity due to attenuation by a surface mass loading on the surface of a piezoelectric material. The development of clinical biosensors will likely require the use of bodily fluids, which would require a primary focus will on Love-mode SAW devices that are able to operate in liquid environments. Although there are a limited number of SAW biosensors on the market, there are no commercially available devices approved by the United States Food and Drug Administration (FDA) for widespread usage. There is, however, a critical need for a portable rapid screening tool to monitor food safety and screen for infectious diseases. Therefore, point-of-care diagnostic tools are in strong demand in both biological and medical facilities. Currently, there is only one company attempting to commercialize SAW biosensors for biological and medical applications and that is TST Biomedical Company from Taiwan. This company is a subsidiary of TaiSAW.

7. Conclusion

The combination of Love-mode SAW devices with Lab-on-a-chip technology will create a new and exciting area of research. The development of SAW sensors has been welcomed by researchers working on point-of-care diagnostic tools that incorporate microfluidics for sample manipulation. These fully-integrated devices will offer tremendous capabilities since they can replace a traditional Biology or medical laboratory with highly sensitive and accurate devices that are completely portable. The added convenience of a wireless device will make monitoring remote areas or high infectious patients significantly easier.

Funding

Publication funded by NSF 181782 to Fisk University.

Author details

Marlon S. Thomas
Department of Life and Physical Sciences in the School of Natural Sciences and Mathematics, Fisk University, Nashville, Tennessee, United States

*Address all correspondence to: mthom005@gmail.com

References

[1] Lange K, Rapp BE, Rapp M. Surface acoustic wave biosensors: A review. Analytical and Bioanalytical Chemistry. 2008;**391**(5):1509-1519

[2] Luka G, Ahmadi A, Najjaran H, Alocilja E, DeRosa M, Wolthers K, et al. Microfluidics integrated biosensors: A leading technology towards lab-on-a-Chip and Sensing applications. Sensors (Basel). 2015;**15**(12):30011-30031

[3] Auroux PA, Iossifidis D, Reyes DR, Manz A. Micro total analysis systems. 2. Analytical standard operations and applications. Analytical Chemistry. 2002;**74**(12):2637-2652

[4] Oedit A, Vulto P, Ramautar R, Lindenburg PW, Hankemeier T. Lab-on-a-Chip hyphenation with mass spectrometry: Strategies for bioanalytical applications. Current Opinion in Biotechnology. 2015;**31**:79-85

[5] Arscott S. SU-8 as a material for lab-on-a-chip-based mass spectrometry. Lab on a Chip. 2014;**14**(19):3668-3689

[6] Sassa F, Biswas GC, Suzuki H. Microfabricated electrochemical sensing devices. Lab on a Chip. 2020;**20**(8):1358-1389

[7] Elsayed MY, Sherif MS, Aljaber SA, Swillam MA. Integrated lab-on-a-chip optical biosensor using ultrathin silicon waveguide SOI MMI device. Sensors (Basel). 2020;**20**(17):4955-4967

[8] Balslev S, Jorgensen AM, Bilenberg B, Mogensen KB, Snakenborg D, Geschke O, et al. Lab-on-a-chip with integrated optical transducers. Lab on a Chip. 2006;**6**(2):213-217

[9] Zhang H, Gong L, Xie FY, Zhang WH, Chen QL, Chen J. Surface enhanced spectroscopy based on lab-on-a-Chip Technology and its applications in analytical science. Guang Pu Xue Yu Guang Pu Fen Xi. 2017;**37**(2):350-355

[10] Luo J, Liu S, Chen P, Lu S, Zhang Q, Chen Y, et al. Fiber optic hydrogen sensor based on a Fabry-Perot interferometer with a fiber Bragg grating and a nanofilm. Lab on a Chip. 2021;**21**(9):1752-1758

[11] Zhu T, Zhou L, Liu M, Zhang J, Shi L. High sensitive space electric field sensing based on micro fiber interferometer with field force driven gold nanofilm. Scientific Reports. 2015;**5**:15802

[12] Hao HC, Chang HY, Wang TP, Yao DJ. Detection of cells captured with antigens on shear horizontal surface-acoustic-wave sensors. Journal of Laboratory Automation. 2013;**18**(1):69-76

[13] Josse F, Bender F, Cernose RW. Guided shear horizontal surface acoustic wave sensors for chemical and biochemical detection in liquids. Analytical Chemistry. 2001;**73**(24):5937-5944

[14] Kano K, Yatsuda H, Kondoh J. Evaluation of shear horizontal surface acoustic wave biosensors using "layer parameter" obtained from sensor responses during immunoreaction. Sensors (Basel). 2021;**21**(14):4924-4941

[15] Mandal D, Banerjee S. Surface acoustic wave (SAW) sensors: Physics, materials, and applications. Sensors (Basel). 2022;**22**(3):820-858

[16] Wells PN. Lord Rayleigh: John William Strutt, third baron Rayleigh. IEEE Transactions on Ultrasonics,

Ferroelectrics, and Frequency Control. 2007;**54**(3):591-596

[17] Hashimoto K-y. Surface Acoustic Wave Devices in Telecommunications: Modelling and Simulation. Berlin; New York: Springer; 2000. p. 330

[18] Institution of Electrical Engineers. Electronics Division. International Specialist Seminar on Component Performance and Systems Applications of Surface Acoustic Wave Devices, 25-28 September 1973 [at] Coylumbridge Hotel, Aviemore, Scotland. London: Institution of Electrical Engineers; 1974. p. vi

[19] Tsai CS. Society of Photo-Optical Instrumentation Engineers., Guided-Wave Optical and Surface Acoustic Wave Devices, Systems, and Applications: July 29-31, 1980, San Diego, California. Bellingham, Wash: Society of Photo-Optical Instrumentation Engineers; 1981. p. x

[20] Campbell C. Surface Acoustic Wave Devices for Mobile and Wireless Communications. San Diego: Academic Press; 1998. p. xxvi

[21] Datta S. Surface Acoustic Wave Devices. Englewood Cliffs, N.J: Prentice-Hall; 1986. p. 252

[22] Haofeng L, Rui J, Weilong L, Chen C, Xinyu L. Surface acoustic wave sensors of delay lines based on MEMS. Journal of Nanoscience and Nanotechnology. 2010;**10**(11):7258-7261

[23] Ward RB. Continuous-wave surface-acoustic-wave delay-difference device. IEEE Transactions on Ultrasonics, Ferroelectrics, and Frequency Control. 1989;**36**(3):300-306

[24] Djoumi L, Vanotti M, Blondeau-Patissier V. Real time cascade impactor based on surface acoustic wave delay lines for PM10 and PM2.5 mass concentration measurement. Sensors (Basel). 2018; **18**(1):255-266

[25] Huang FC, Chen YY, Wu TT. A room temperature surface acoustic wave hydrogen sensor with Pt coated ZnO nanorods. Nanotechnology. 2009;**20**(6):065501

[26] Li W, Guo Y, Tang Y, Zu X, Ma J, Wang L, et al. Room-temperature ammonia sensor based on ZnO Nanorods deposited on ST-cut quartz surface acoustic wave devices. Sensors (Basel). 2017;**17**(5):1142-1152

[27] Zellers ET, Han M. Effects of temperature and humidity on the performance of polymer-coated surface acoustic wave vapor sensor arrays. Analytical Chemistry. 1996;**68**(14):2409-2418

[28] Kadota M, Ishii Y, Tanaka S. Surface acoustic wave resonators with hetero acoustic layer (HAL) structure using lithium tantalate and quartz. IEEE Transactions on Ultrasonics, Ferroelectrics, and Frequency Control. 2021;**68**(5):1955-1964

[29] Paroni A, Henrich Bernardoni N, Savariaux C, Loevenbruck H, Calabrese P, Pellegrini T, et al. Vocal drum sounds in human beatboxing: An acoustic and articulatory exploration using electromagnetic articulography. The Journal of the Acoustical Society of America. 2021;**149**(1):191

[30] Branch DW, Huber DL, Brozik SM, Edwards TL. Shear horizontal surface acoustic wave microsensor for class A viral and bacterial detection; Sandia National Laboratories: Issued by Sandia National Laboratories, operated for the United States Department of Energy by. Sandia Corporation. 2008

[31] Rocha-Gaso MI, March-Iborra C, Montoya-Baides A,

Arnau-Vives A. Surface generated acoustic wave biosensors for the detection of pathogens: A review. Sensors (Basel). 2009;**9**(7):5740-5769

[32] Glynne-Jones P, Boltryk RJ, Hill M, Zhang F, Dong L, Wilkinson JS. Flexible acoustic particle manipulation device with integrated optical waveguide for enhanced microbead assays. Analytical Sciences. **2009;25**(2):285-291

Chapter 15

Recent Advances in Biosensing in Tissue Engineering and Regenerative Medicine

Alma T. Banigo, Chigozie A. Nnadiekwe and Emmanuel M. Beasi

Abstract

In tissue engineering and regenerative medicine, biosensors act as analytical devices that combine biological elements with electrical components to generate a measurable signal. The application of biosensing in the nearest future may need high performance, incorporation of biosensors into feedback-based devices, advanced diagnostics as well as detection of toxins. These functionalities will aid the biosensors with increased sensitivity, specificity, and the ability to detect multiple analytes. With the newly improved strategies in fabrication, sensors may develop high spatial sensitivity and draw us near actualizing capable devices. Although biosensors have been produced in past years, there are still pending challenges such as scale-up process and long-term stability of commercial products that should be addressed. This review will also involve the application of additive manufacturing techniques such as 3D bioprinting to produce world-recognized biosensors. We will focus on some bioprinting techniques including laser direct-write and also consider microfluidic tissue engineering which can sense biomolecules in the miniaturized tissue constructs in real time at quite low concentration through different sensing systems. We also review its advances in mobile Health (mhealth) technologies for detection and monitoring as biosensors are produced with living cells encapsulated in 3D microenvironments. These advances and many more will, however, grow the community of biosensors and their availability in tissue engineering and regenerative medicine.

Keywords: Biosensor, biofabrication, challenges, application, tissue engineering, 3D bioprinting, regenerative medicine

1. Introduction

The biosensor is an analytical device or probe that combines biological elements (enzymes or antibodies) with an electronic component to produce signals that can easily be measured. It can also be defined as an integrated single device with the capacity to provide results by recognizing a biological element that is in direct contact with a transducer [1]. This electronic device identifies, processes, and communicates data about the physiological changes of an analyte and the presence of various chemical or biological materials in the environment.

All these biosensors are produced in a variety of sizes and shapes. They can detect and measure even low levels of infections, harmful chemicals, and pH values. On the other hand, biosensing is the act of measuring or detecting the presence of particular chemicals in a physiological activity with the aid of a biosensor device. The major components of the biosensor including the transducer are displayed in **Figure 1**, and they are briefly defined in the following section.

Analyte: This biosensor component is the biochemical substance of interest to be identified by the biosensor. A typical example of an analyte in blood glucose can be detected by the glucometer (biosensor) [2].

Bioreceptor: This is a biological molecule that recognizes the analytes. Some examples include enzymes, cells, aptamers, deoxyribonucleic acid (DNA), and antibodies. The biological receptor generates a signal in the form of light, heat, pH, charge, or mass change when it interacts with a target analyte in the process known as biorecognition [2].

Transducer: This component converts the biochemical signal received from the biological receptor into a measurable and quantifiable signal in a process known as signalization [2].

Electronics: This part processes the transduced signals and prepares them for display. Its electronic circuitry is complex, and it also performs signal conditioning such as amplification and conversion of an analog signal into a digital form [2].

Display: The display unit consists of a user interpretation system such as the liquid crystal display (LCD) of a computer or a direct printer that generates numbers or curves understandable by the user. It usually consists of a combination of hardware and software that generates results of the biosensor in a user-friendly manner. The output signal on the display can be numeric, graphic, tabular, or an image, depending on the end user's requirements [2].

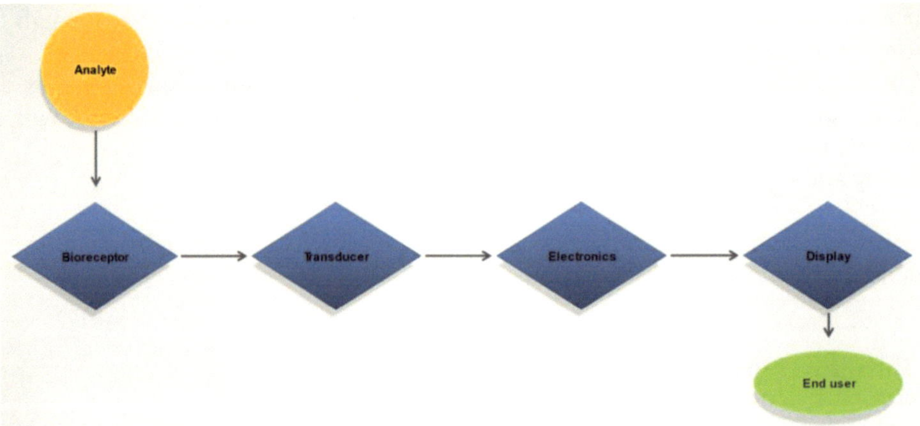

Figure 1.
The main components of a biosensor arranged in chronological order. It begins with the analyte and ends with the end user.

1.1 History of biosensors

The concept of biosensors has gone through a series of evolution in terms of what is referred to as a "biosensor." Accordingly, biosensing devices have metamorphosed into complex systems since their first invention.

The premier reported idea of biosensing rather than its "term" began in 1906 by M. Cremer. He emphasized that the concentration of an acid suspended in an aqueous solution is equal to the electric potential produced between sections of the solution when separated by a glass membrane [2]. Cremer's discovery led to the introduction of pH by Soren Peder Lauritz Sorensen in 1909. After the invention of an electrode to measure the pH was achieved by Hughes in 1922, 34 years later, an oxygen probe was developed by Leland C. Clark who eventually became the father of biosensors after building what is described as a "real biosensor" in 1959 [3]. Based on this study, he described how "to make electrochemical sensors (pH, polarographic, potentiometric, or conductometric) more intelligent 'by incorporating' enzyme transducers as membrane-enclosed sandwiches" at a conference in New York in 1962 [4].

The term "enzyme electrode" which was originally used to describe the first biosensor was adopted by Updike and Hicks to describe a similar device in 1967 [5]. Guilbault & Montalvo [6] used glass electrodes coupled with urease to measure urea concentration by potentiometric measurement instead of the amperometric method.

In the electrochemical community during that period, the research on ion ion-selective electrodes (ISEs) was very active, and the idea of extending the range of sensors to non-electrochemical active compounds had been widely accepted, even for nonionic substances like glucose [5, 7]. Since then, great strides have been made in developing highly sensitive and selective biosensing devices where biological elements are combined with electrochemical sensors [5, 8]. Some of these changes are listed as follows:

- The first change took place by Clemen's team where they developed a "bedside artificial pancreas" that included an electrochemical glucose biosensor. This was performed in 1976 and was sold by Miles (Elkhart) as the Biostator Glucose-Controlled Insulin Infusion System shortly after [5].

- The second change that occurred was performed by Pharmacia researchers. They began collaborating with physics and biochemistry academics at Linkoping University in 1982 to develop a novel bioanalytical device capable of monitoring biomolecule interactions. Pharmacia biosensor was founded in 1984 and in 1990, the business launched BIA core, a new instrument [5].

- In 1984, Cass and his colleagues published a scientific paper demonstrating the use of ferrocene and its derivatives as mediators for amperometric biosensors. A few years later, the Medisense Exac Tech Glucose Meter was launched on the market and became the world's bestselling biosensor product. The initial product was a pen-shaped meter with a disposable screen-printed electrode [5].

- From 1999 till the present, research in biosensing has led to the development of a nanoelectromechanical biosensor (BioNMES), quantum dots, nanoparticles, nanocantilever, nanowire, and nanotube. The biosensor's "driving force" exploits the selectivity of the biological element [4, 7].

1.2 Features of a biosensor: the basic features of a biosensor are as follows

1.2.1 Selectivity

This is usually the most important feature of a biosensor. A bioreceptor detects a specific analyte in a sample containing other admixtures and contaminants. The interaction of an antigen with the antibody depicts an example of this selectivity of a biosensor. Antibodies act as bioreceptors and are immobilized on the surface of the transducer. A solution (usually a buffer containing salts) containing the antigen is then exposed to the transducer where antibodies interact only with the antigens [2].

1.2.2 Reproducibility

This is the ability of the biosensor to produce identical results in different experimental setups. Reproducibility is characterized by the precision and accuracy of the transducer and electronics in a biosensor. Precision is the ability of the sensor to provide reproducible results every time a sample is measured and accuracy indicates the sensor's capacity to provide a mean value close to the true value when a sample is measured more than once [2]. Reproducible signals provide high reliability and robustness to the inference made on the response of a biosensor.

1.2.3 Stability

This is the degree of susceptibility to ambient disturbances in and around the biosensing system [2]. These disturbances can cause a drift in the output signals of a biosensor under measurement. An error can occur in the measured concentration and can affect the precision and accuracy of the biosensor, and stability is the most crucial feature in applications where a biosensor requires long incubation steps or continuous monitoring [2]. The response of transducers and electronics can be temperature-sensitive, and this may likely influence the stability of a biosensor. Therefore, appropriate tuning of electronics is required to ensure a stable response of the sensor. Another factor that can affect the stability is the affinity of the bioreceptor, which is the degree to which the analyte binds to the bioreceptor. Bioreceptors with high affinities encourage either strong electrostatic bonding or covalent linkage of the analyte that fortifies the stability of a biosensor. Also, the degradation of the bioreceptor over some time is another factor that affects the stability of measurement [2].

1.2.4 Sensitivity

The minimum amount of analyte that can be detected by a biosensor defines its limit of detection (LOD) or sensitivity. In several medical and environmental monitoring applications, a biosensor is required to detect analyte concentrations as low as nanogram/milliliter (ng/ml) or even femtogram/milliliter (fg/ml) to confirm the presence of traces of analytes in a sample [2]. For instance, a prostate-specific antigen (PSA) concentration of 4 ng/ml in the blood is associated with prostate cancer for which doctors suggest biopsy tests. Hence, sensitivity is considered to be an important property of a biosensor [2].

1.2.5 Linearity

Linearity is the feature that shows the accuracy of the measured response (for a set of measurements with different concentrations of the analyte) to a straight line, mathematically represented as y = mc, where c is the concentration of the analyte, y is the output signal, and m is the sensitivity of the biosensor [2]. Linearity of the biosensor can be associated with the resolution of the biosensor and the range of analyte concentrations under test. The resolution of the biosensor is defined as the smallest change in the concentration of an analyte that is required to bring a change in the response of the biosensor. Depending on the application, a good resolution is required as most biosensor applications require not only analyte detection but also the measurement of concentrations of the analyte over a wide working range. Another term associated with linearity is a linear range, which is defined as the range of analyte concentrations for which the biosensor response changes linearly with the concentration [2]. These features are essential for the biosensors' proper functioning, which can be used for various applications.

1.3 Applications of biosensors

The use of biosensors aims to improve the quality of life, for environmental monitoring, disease detection, food safety, defense, drug discovery, and many more. One of the main applications of biosensors is the detection of biomolecules that are either indicators of a disease or targets of a drug. For example, electrochemical biosensing techniques can be used as clinical tools to detect protein cancer biomarkers [9, 10].

Biosensors can also be used as platforms for monitoring food traceability, quality, safety, and nutritional value [11, 12]. Furthermore, an application such as pollution monitoring [12, 13] requires a biosensor to function from a few hours to several days. Such biosensors can be termed as "long-term monitoring" analysis tools. Long-term monitoring biosensors find their use as technologically advanced devices both in resource-limited settings and sophisticated medical setups. Some examples are as follows:

- Applications in drug discovery [14, 15];
- For the detection of several chemical and biological agents that are considered to be toxic materials of defense interest [16];
- For use in artificial implantable devices such as pacemakers [17];
- Used in prosthetic devices [18];
- Sewage epidemiology [19].

A range of electrochemical, optical, and acoustic sensing techniques have been utilized, along with their integration into analytical devices for various applications. **Figure 2** depicts the various applications of biosensors. This book chapter will focus on tissue engineering, regenerative medicine, and mobile health (mHealth) technologies.

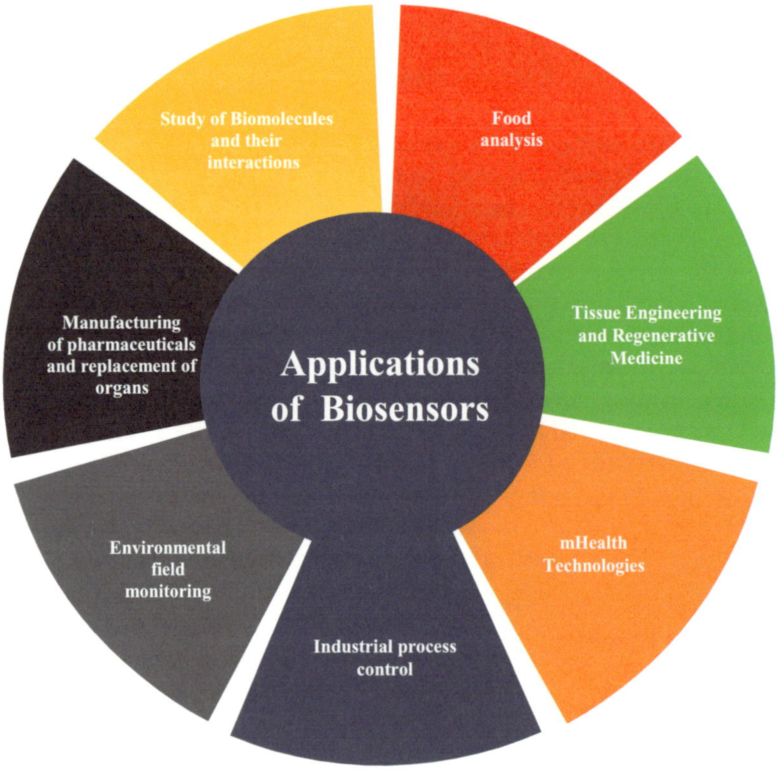

Figure 2.
Applications of Biosensors in different areas of specialization.

1.4 Types of biosensors

Biosensors are grouped based on the type of transducer deployed. They are as follows:-

- Electrochemical biosensors;
- Calorimetric/thermal detection biosensors;
- Optical biosensors;
- Piezoelectric biosensors.

1.4.1 Electrochemical biosensors

Electrochemical biosensors are simple devices that use bioelectrodes to measure electric current, ionic, or conductance changes. These biosensors have different types according to the transducer deployed and also based on the measurements of electrical parameters including potentiometric, amperometric, and voltammetric biosensors. The electrochemical biosensor has three electrodes namely reference, working, and counter electrodes [1]. A typical example of the electrochemical biosensor is shown in **Figure 3**.

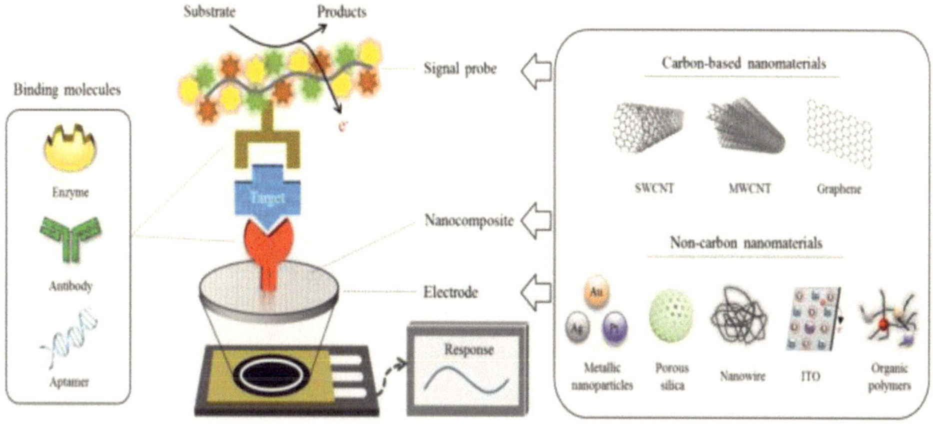

Figure 3.
A schematic representation of an electrochemical biosensor illustrating its application in enzyme, antibody, or aptamer measurements [20].

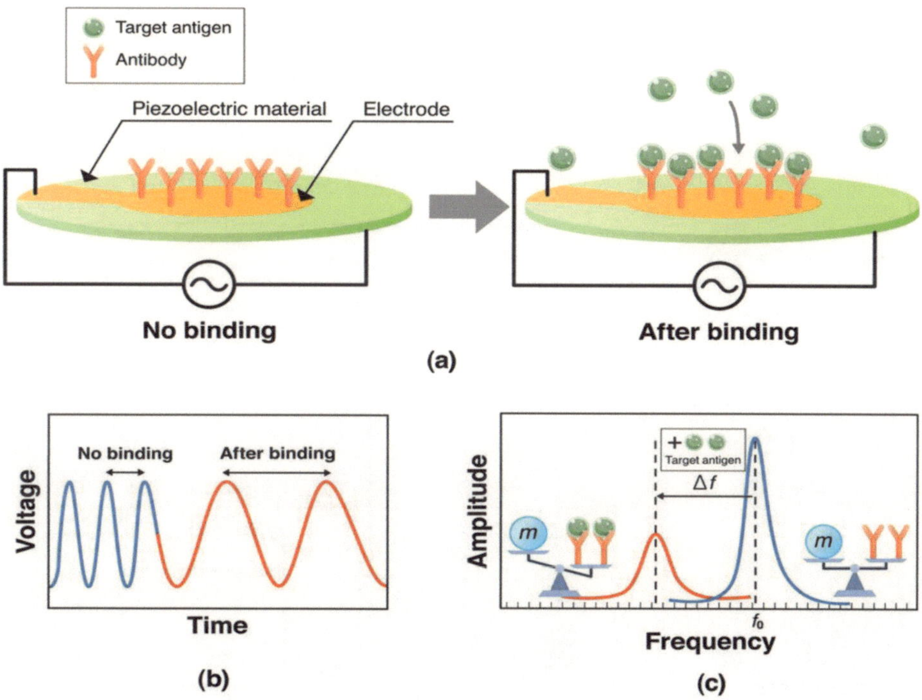

Figure 4.
A schematic representation of a piezoelectric sensor. (a) Target antigen and antibody on a piezoelectric material before and after binding, (b) voltage-time curve before and after binding in a piezoelectric sensor and (c) amplitude of a piezoelectric sensor before and after binding concerning frequency [21].

1.4.2 Piezoelectric biosensors

They produce an electrical signal based on the principle of acoustics (sound vibrations) when mechanical force is applied. Quartz crystals are a common piezoelectric material used in biosensors. **Figure 4** displays a commonly used piezoelectric biosensor.

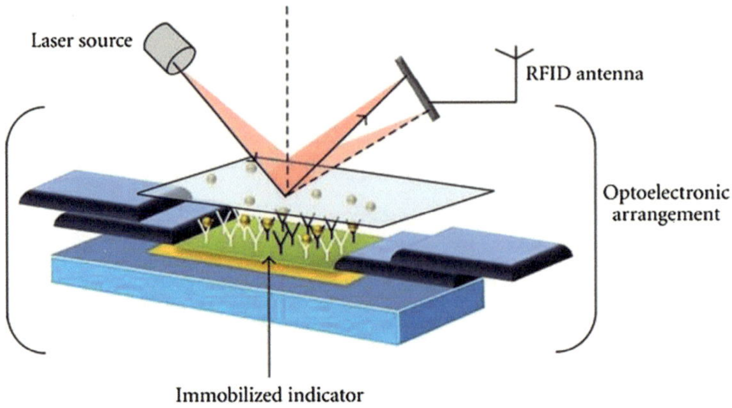

Figure 5.
A schematic representation of an optoelectrical arrangement of an optical biosensor [24].

1.4.3 Optical biosensors

Optical biosensors are used for analyte detection by absorption, fluorescence, or light scattering. They can also detect microscopic changes when cells bind to receptors immobilized on the transducer surface. They utilize the changes that occur in mass, concentration, or several molecules to direct changes in the characteristics of light [22, 23]. Here,

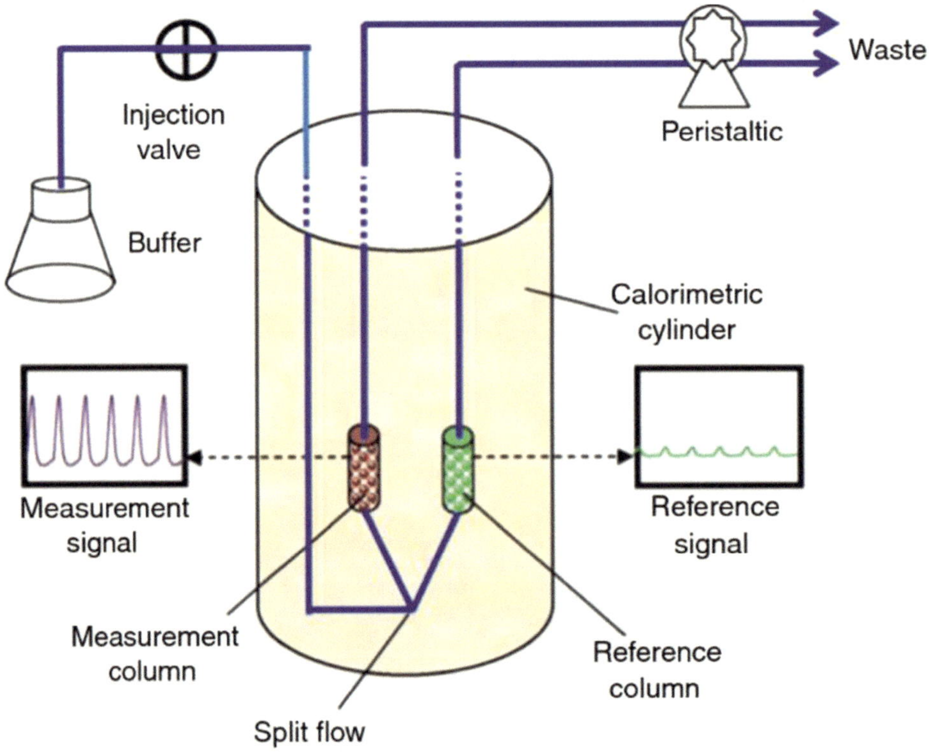

Figure 6.
A schematic diagram of an optical biosensor showing its components [25].

S/N	Types of biosensors		Some applications	References
1	Electrochemical biosensors	Potentiometric biosensor	Detection of urea in blood serum	[26]
		Amperometric biosensor	Detection of ethanol, glucose, and lactate	[27]
		Impedimetric biosensor	Detection, identification, and quantification of bacteria in the field of microbiology	[28]
		Immuno-sensor	Detection of several pathogens such as viruses like COVID-19 and influenza.	[29]
		Voltammetric biosensor	It can be used for analyzing paracetamol	[30]
2	Piezoelectric biosensor Example is micromembrane biosensor		They are able to detect the presence of cells and their masses, used in the rapid detection of HIV in biological fluids	[31, 32]
3	Thermal biosensor Examples are micro-electromechanical systems (MEMSs) biosensors		Low-cost integration of miniaturized devices, allow-cost batch fabrication, and measurement of multiple samples in parallel. It is used to measure enzyme activity, clinical monitoring, environmental monitoring, etc.	[33, 34]
4	Optical biosensor Examples are evanescent wave fluorescence biosensors and bioluminescent optical fiber biosensors		For the rapid, sensitive, and highly selective detection of 17β-estradiol, an endocrine-disrupting compound is frequently detected in environmental water samples. It enables the multi-detection of genotoxins and is used in the study of transferrin-binding proteins, lipooligosaccharide (LOS)-antibody interactions, and serum responses to experimental vaccines	[35–37]

Table 1.
The various types of biosensors, some of their applications, and references.

both catalytic and affinity reactions can both be assessed. **Figure 5** depicts a type of optical biosensor.

1.4.4 Thermometric biosensors

They are made up of a heat-insulated box with a heat exchanger (calorimetric cylinder), and the reaction takes place in a tiny enzyme-packed bed reactor. The substrate is transformed into a product and heat is created as it enters the bed. **Figure 6** shows a typical example of an optical biosensor.

A summary of types of biosensors and some of their applications that can be used in tissue engineering, regenerative medicine, or mhealth technology are shown in **Table 1**.

2. Design and fabrication of a biosensor

There are many types of biosensors including electrochemical biosensors (potentiometric biosensors, amperometric biosensors, and conductometric biosensors). These biosensors are uniquely designed and fabricated based on their applications. This book chapter will explore the design and fabrication of two biosensors such as an amperometric electrochemical biosensor and a surface plasmon resonance (SPR) optical biosensor used for glucose level detection or measurement and bioprinting, respectively.

2.1 Amperometric electrochemical biosensor

The design of the electrodes and chip is a crucial aspect in the development of an amperometric electrochemical biosensor. In general, designing electrochemical biosensor electrodes necessitate a thorough understanding of fluid flow, particularly its behavior in microscales. Furthermore, it also requires a detailed understanding of mass transport phenomena and microflow mass transport foundations.

Biosensors have been improved using a variety of designs. The design of electrodes in a microfluidic system is a crucial pillar for improved performance. Electrode design necessitates a thorough understanding of electron diffusion phenomena. In most current flows, electron diffusion is the limiting step. Diffusion is generally hampered by crucial parameters such as the electrode surface and the number of active sites available for the target. When a device with a microchannel is utilized as an analytical platform, the analyte is injected into the channel using two alternative methods namely pressure-driven flow and electrokinetic flow [38]. A pressure gradient induces flow in pressure-driven flow, and the nature of the flow is influenced by the channel geometry and flow rates. The Reynolds number is commonly used to express the ratio of inertial and viscous forces:

$$R_e = \frac{\rho V D}{\mu}$$

where R_e is the Reynolds number, V is the characteristic velocity for the flow, D is the characteristic distance, ρ is the density of the fluid, and μ is the fluid viscosity. Laminar flow occurs at Reynolds numbers below 2300 [38]. Flow in the microchannel is laminar because of the micron-scale size of microchannels, and the low velocity requires fluids to move across the channels. For laminar flow, fluid travels in a steady and time-independent manner at each location. The flow profile is parabolic, in which the velocity of the flow is negligible at the wall surfaces.

Materials used in the design of amperometric electrochemical biosensors are classified as: (1) materials for the electrode and supporting substrate; (2) materials for the immobilization of biological recognition elements; (3) materials for the fabrication of the outer membrane; and (4) biological elements, such as enzymes, antibodies, antigens, mediators, and cofactors.

Solid electrode systems and supporting substrates are frequently constructed with metals and carbon. Due to their superior electrical and mechanical qualities, metals such as platinum, gold, silver, and stainless steel have long been employed as electrochemical electrodes [39]. **Figure** 7 depicts the various techniques used for the production of conductive supporting substrates.

The basic elements of biosensors are the bioelement and the sensing element. Any organic organism that can detect specific analytes from the medium of interest while remaining unresponsive to any other potentially inquisitive/interfering species is referred to as a bioelement. The signal transducing section of the biosensor is known as the sensing element, and it can take the shape of any magnetic, optical, electrical, or electrochemical transducing mechanism [40].

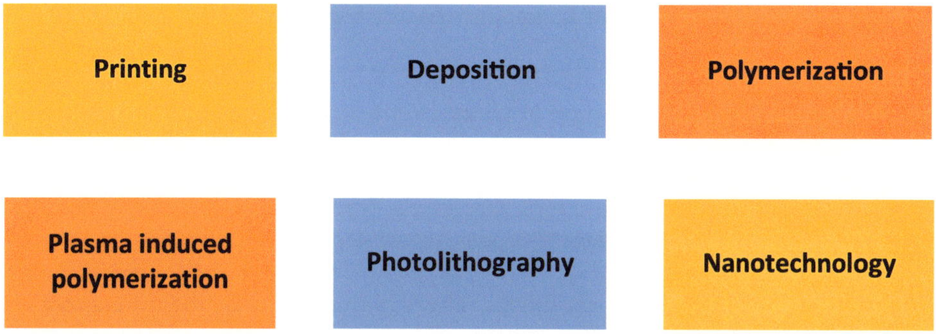

Figure 7.
A schematic diagram of the techniques used for the production of the conductive supporting substrate.

2.2 Design and fabrication of a surface plasmon resonance (SPR) biosensor

A surface plasmon resonance biosensor can be designed and manufactured using a variety of periodic structural patterns. One of the structural patterns employed in the design and fabrication of a surface plasmon resonance biosensor is the nanohole creation procedure using thermal nanoimprint lithography which is discussed in this book chapter.

The stamps for the nanohole array are made by thermal nanoimprint lithography, residual layer etching, (titanium/gold) Ti/Au deposition, and lift-off procedures. For example, if a 10-cm thick glass wafer is utilized for the imprinting process and is coated with a 100-nm thermoplastic polymer layer, it has to be spin-coated at 3000 rpm for 30s to obtain this layer. A hot embossing system can be used to perform nanoimprint lithography. The leftover layer is then etched with oxygen (O_2) plasma [41].

The polymer is etched uniformly in this procedure until the residual layer is completely removed and the pattern is transferred to the substrate. A metallic titanium (Ti) (adhesion layer, 5 nm)/gold (Au) (50 nm) layer is deposited using electron beam evaporation. Finally, the resist lift-off operation is carried out in an ultrasonic hot acetone bath to obtain the nanohole array structure [42].

2.2.1 Design and fabrication considerations for biosensors

Studying the target analyte and identifying how it reacts with biological molecules is the first phase in constructing a biosensing device.

Other phases include are as follows:

2.2.1.1 Biological receptor selection

The sensitivity and selectivity of a biosensor to the analyte of interest are decided by the biological receptor used. As a result, a receptor with a high affinity for the analyte is suggested. It is critical to understand the benefits and drawbacks of various biological receptors in diverse biosensor applications when selecting an appropriate receptor [41, 43, 44].

2.2.1.2 Selection of an appropriate immobilization method

Biological molecule must be attached to the surface of a transducer to function consistently as a biological receptor. Immobilization is the term for this procedure. This goal has been accomplished using a variety of techniques including adsorption, entrapment, covalent attachment, microencapsulation, and crosslinking [45, 46].

2.2.1.3 Transducer element selection

The efficiency of the biosensor device is heavily influenced by the transducer element. The use of an effective transducer will result in a device with greater efficiency, whereas the use of an ineffective transducer will result in a device with reduced efficiency [45, 47].

2.3 Recent advances in biosensing

2.3.1 Tissue engineering

Biosensors are particularly useful in tissue engineering applications, such as maintaining three-dimensional (3D)-printed cell cultures [48] and developing "organs-on-chips" models, where biomolecule concentrations such as glucose, adenosines, and hydrogen peroxide levels play a key role in determining the fate of cells and tissues. Changes in oxygen consumption, pH, membrane potentials, ion concentrations, and the release of numerous metabolic chemicals and proteins are all well-known physical and chemical signals that living cells communicate [49]. Monitoring these analytes in real time can provide insight into cellular activity.

2.3.1.1 Application of biosensors in tissue engineering

2.3.1.1.1 3D-bioprinted sensing devices

The deposition of a bioink (living cells and biomaterials) onto a printing surface is described as bioprinting, and it is a new approach for fabricating tissues and organs by accurately controlling the periodic arrangement of diverse biological materials, such as biomolecules and biocells. It has a wide range of characteristics that can be used in biosensing applications, such as fast deposition and patterning of proteins and other biomolecules [50]. A typical illustration of a 3D-printed tissue construct can be seen in **Figure 8**.

There are a variety of bioprinting technologies that can be used to make biosensors, and they are basically grouped into two methods, namely contact-based and noncontact-based printing. Both biomaterials and bioinks are essential for biological signal transduction. For advanced extrusion-based bioprinting such as coaxial or triaxial, optimization of the bioink viscosity is a major consideration to prevent clogging. Other properties including pore size and cellular behavior may influence biosensing [52]. Using an electric field, some printing processes, such as electrodeposition, may be able to transfer thin films of metal nanoparticles [50] or nanowires [53] to a substrate. Creating circuits that could be an intrinsic part of a biosensor, as well as some immunoassays or microarrays, can be done by printing thin metal sheets [54, 55]. Even thin films of biological material, such as proteins, enzymes, nucleic acids, polysaccharides, and bacterial cells, have been printed using electrodeposition

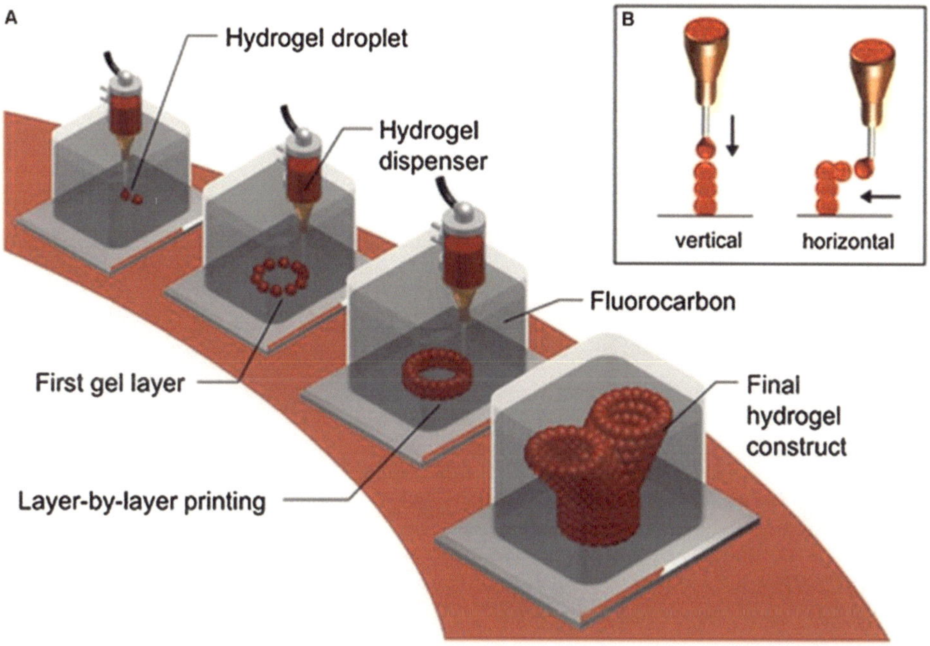

Figure 8.
Stages in submerged bioprinting of a 3D tissue construct. A) The cell-laden hydrogel bioink is printed in droplets, layer by layer following the provided model. The printing nozzle is submerged in high-density perfluorocarbons that are immiscible in water and oil. Perfluorocarbons are suitable for submerged cells due to the presence of oxygen and carbon dioxide transport capability. B) The hydrogel droplets are printed in a vertical or lateral dimension to produce branching constructs without solid support [51].

[56–58]. More work needs to be done on bioprinting techniques that may be utilized to deposit a wide range of biologics and mammalian cells in precise spatial positions, rather than thin films, which have been used for biosensing applications.

2.3.1.1.2 Biosensors for diabetes

Diabetes is a serious chronic metabolic illness that affects over 400 million people globally. Uncontrolled chronic hyperglycemia damages and destroys various organs, resulting in significant morbidity and mortality [59]. Blood glucose control can help to reduce the frequency and severity of these problems [60]. By putting the glucose oxidase enzyme on an oxygen electrode, Clark and Lyons created the first biosensor for monitoring glucose levels in 1962 [61]. The care of diabetic patients was transformed when the first self-monitoring blood glucose (SMBG) gadget based on the glucose dehydrogenase enzyme was introduced in 1987 [62]. SMBG in **Figure 9** is now widely used in the treatment of diabetes, particularly type I [64, 65].

2.3.1.1.3 Biosensors for wound healing

Wound healing is a multistep process that necessitates the collaboration of numerous tissues and biochemical pathways [66]. Chronic wounds result from the failure of these processes to proceed in a timely and organized manner, possibly putting a huge financial strain on healthcare systems [67]. Uncontrolled inflammatory processes, bacterial infections, alterations in the acidic pH of the skin, oxygen levels, and matrix

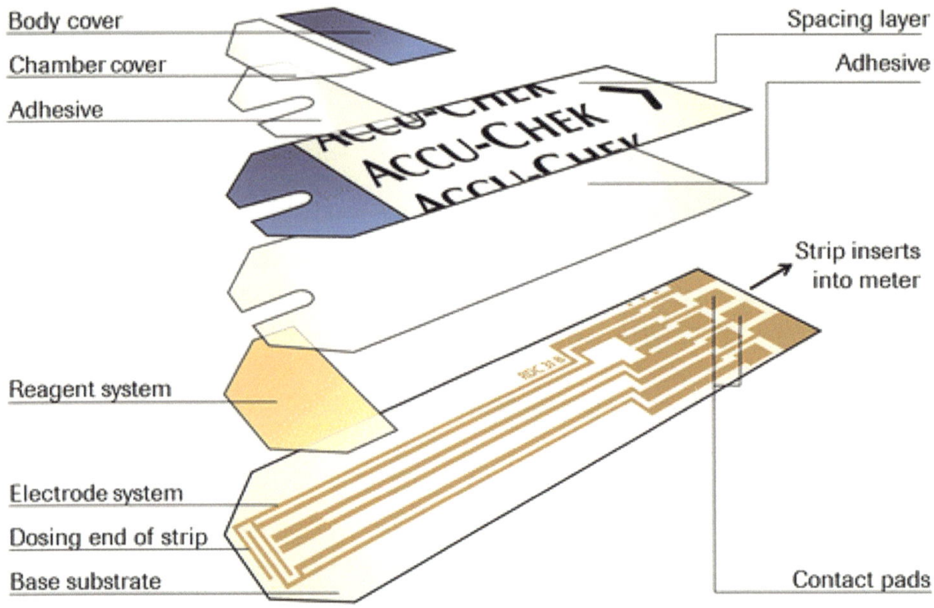

Figure 9.
Various parts of an electrochemical glucose biosensor for diabetes care [63].

metalloproteinases (MMPs) are all involved in such failures [67, 68]. Biosensors are being researched to allow doctors to closely monitor the healing process, as regular monitoring is crucial in chronic wound management [67]. Screen-printing electrodes with Ag/AgCl-conductive ink were used to create a wearable pH sensor [69]. Wearable sensors for biomarkers detection for wound infections can be shown in **Figure 10**.

2.3.1.1.4 Biosensors for cancer applications

The use of biosensors in cancer diagnostics has a lot of promise. Cancer is the second biggest cause of mortality [71], and because biomarker concentrations in the early stages of tumor formation are relatively low, biosensor sensitivities or their LODs are critical for early diagnosis [72]. Early diagnosis of malignant cells before they spread has been shown to improve treatment outcomes and save lives. As a result, specialized, accurate, and rapid-response biosensors are in high demand in oncology, some of which can be seen in **Figure 11**. Recent biosensor advancements have greatly improved breast cancer diagnosis [74]. Breast cancer is the second most frequent cancer in women in the United States, after skin cancer, and the second most lethal, after lung cancer [75]. Traditional breast cancer diagnostic methods such as mammography, magnetic resonance imaging, and enzyme-linked immunosorbent assays (ELISAs) have produced impressive results; however, many false-negative or false-positive results continue to occur, and the adverse effects of some invasive techniques necessitate the development of new highly sensitive, reliable, and noninvasive methods for detection and prognosis [74].

2.3.1.1.5 Biosensors for cardiovascular applications

Cardiovascular illnesses are the leading cause of death worldwide, and early identification could save tens of thousands of lives each year. Biosensors are being

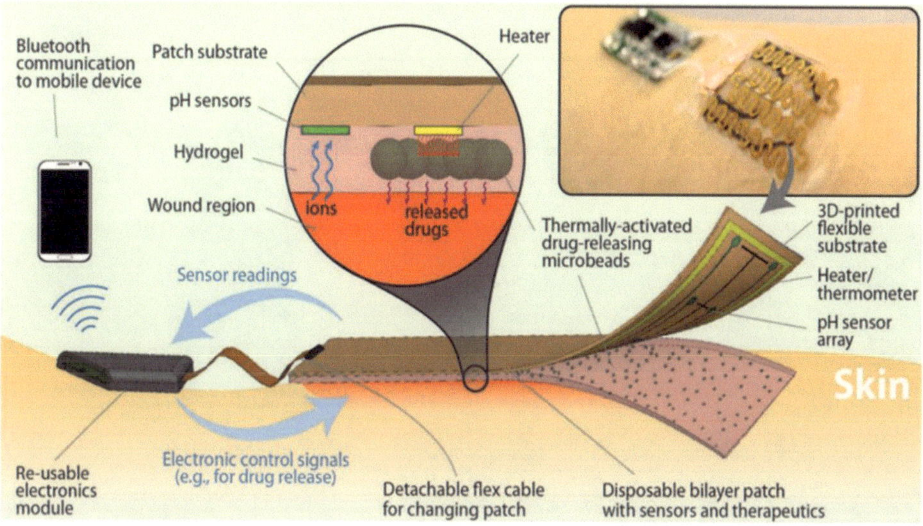

Figure 10.
Wearable Sensors for the detection of biomarkers for wound infection [70].

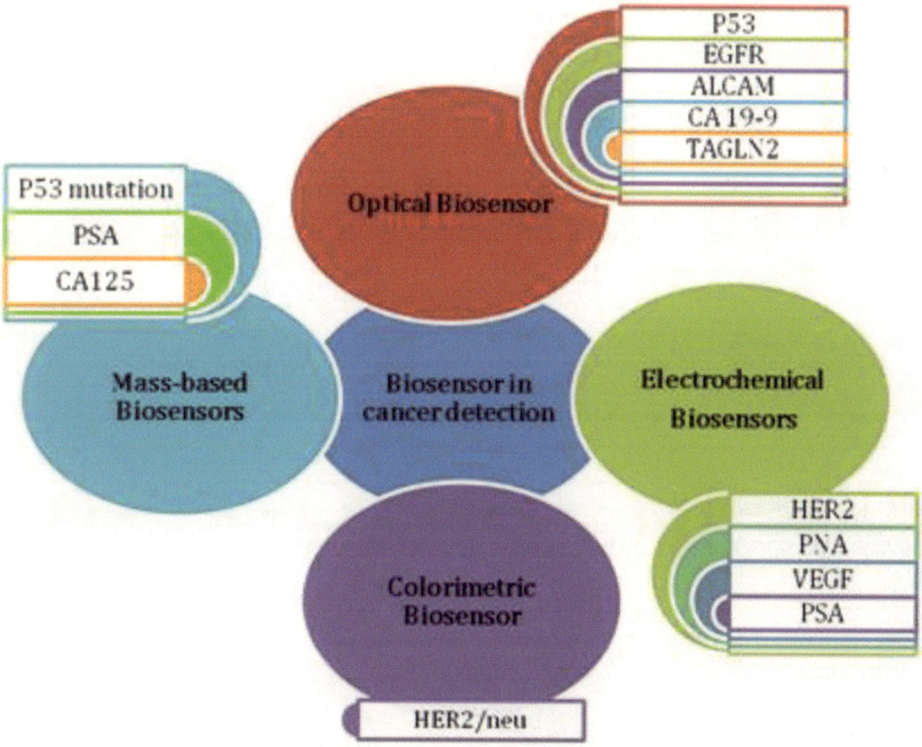

Figure 11.
Common biosensors and biomarkers used in the detection of cancer [73].

utilized to measure cardiac troponin (both T and I), C-reactive protein (CRP), creatine kinase (CK), myoglobin, and other cardiac indicators. One of the most significant indicators for detecting myocardial infarction is cardiac troponin [76].

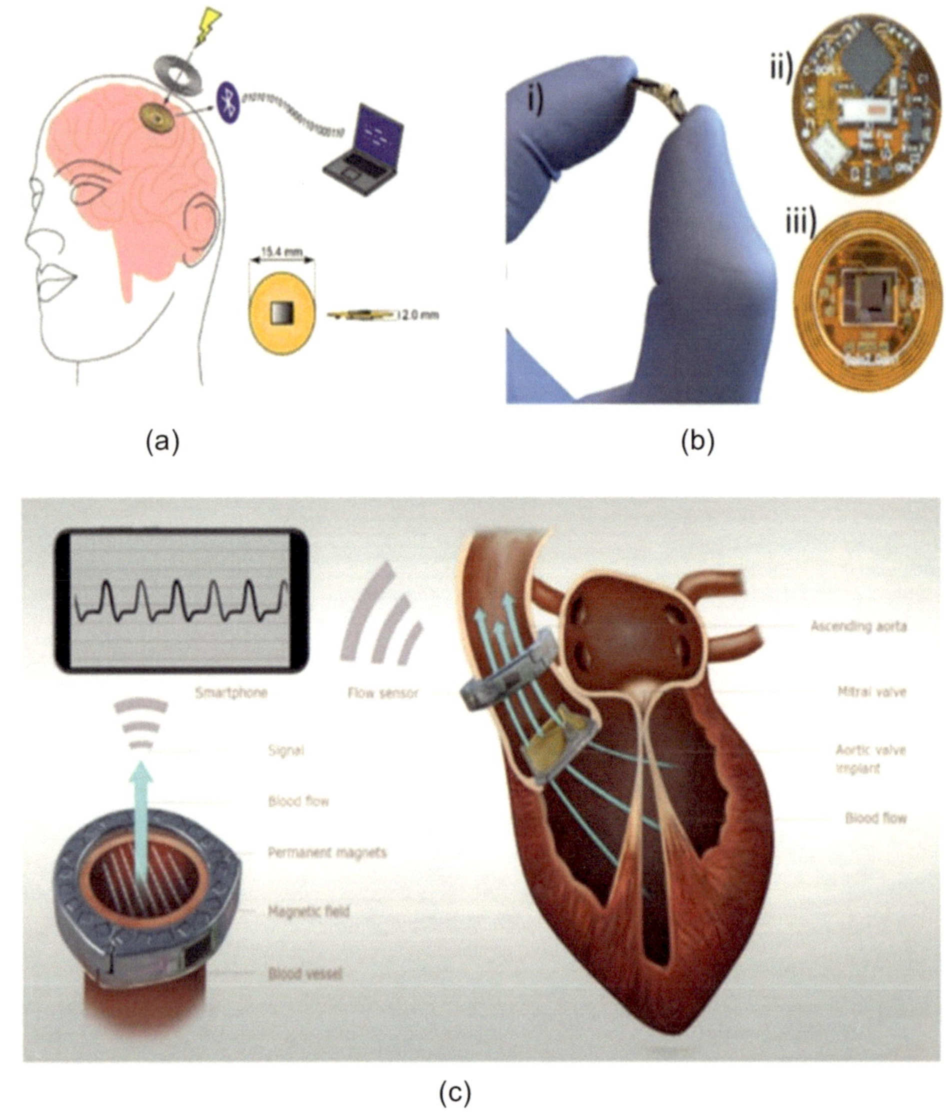

Figure 12.
Implantable biosensor: (a) head implant (in vivo); (b) head implant (in vitro); and (c) heart implant for recording electrocardiogram [77].

Some implantable biosensors can be used for cardiovascular applications. A typical example can be seen in **Figure 12**.

2.3.1.1.6 Biosensors in artificial limbs (prostheses)

The potential of prostheses to restore human skin's sensory capabilities would provide users of mechanical limbs with a more natural feeling [78]. The use of a pressure sensor on an artificial hand, for example, might change the amount of force applied by the fingers when gripping objects. This could protect the object from falling due to an underapplied force or breaking due to an overapplied force. A system with sensors for electromyography, temperature, and strain incorporated into stimulation electrodes was developed [79], and its practical use for prosthesis control with sensory input as well as electrical muscle stimulation was reported [80].

2.3.2 Regenerative medicine

Biosensors serve as a control platform for other technologies, allowing for real-time monitoring of system behavior for improved efficiency. Biosensing technologies are used in regenerative medicine for a variety of purposes, including biomanufacturing (for example, product release requirements), organ-on-a-chip technologies, and therapeutic efficacy indicators.

2.3.2.1 Application of biosensors in regenerative medicine

2.3.2.1.1 Biomanufacturing

Biomanufacturing is a relatively recent industrial strategy to produce economically relevant biological goods such as human tissues by leveraging biological systems. Industrial-scale bioproducts are made using additive manufacturing techniques such as 3D printing and other biofabrication technologies **Figure 13** [81]. shows DNA biosensing with 3D printing technology.

Biomanufacturing facilities may also use altered cells to manufacture chemical or molecular products, as well as mass culture cells for organ fabrication. Biomanufacturing may be used in a variety of industries, including healthcare, food production, and even agriculture. Controlling the quality and condition of the biological structure is crucial for producing trustworthy goods, and biosensing technologies can help with this. Electrochemical enzyme-based biosensors, for example, have been utilized to monitor metabolites in cell culture medium in real time [81].

2.3.2.1.2 Organ-on-a-chip technologies

Using microfluidic technology and organoids, organ-on-a-chip technologies have opened up a new biomedical research field. Organoids are tiny cell clusters of a certain tissue type that can mimic the behavior of regular tissues and organs more accurately. Organ-on-a-chip technology is utilized for a variety of purposes, including evaluating the response of organoids to medications and other external stimuli [83]. The use of biosensors for real-time monitoring of the behavior of microtissues and organoids has progressed the technique significantly. Damage to cardiac organoids was monitored using a new microfluidic aptamer-based electrochemical biosensor **Figure 14** [84]. shows the use of biosensors to develop organs-on-a-chip technology.

2.3.2.1.3 As indicators for therapeutic efficacy

Given that most outcomes are observed visually (e.g. a regenerated tissue or a healed wound) or functionally (e.g. improved sensory ability), biosensors for detecting the efficacy of regenerative medicine-related therapies remain relatively unexplored. Biosensors, on the other hand, may play an increasingly essential role in therapeutic evaluation in the future. For example, with glucose sensors, patients undergoing treatment can make use of biosensors to self-monitor the efficacy of the

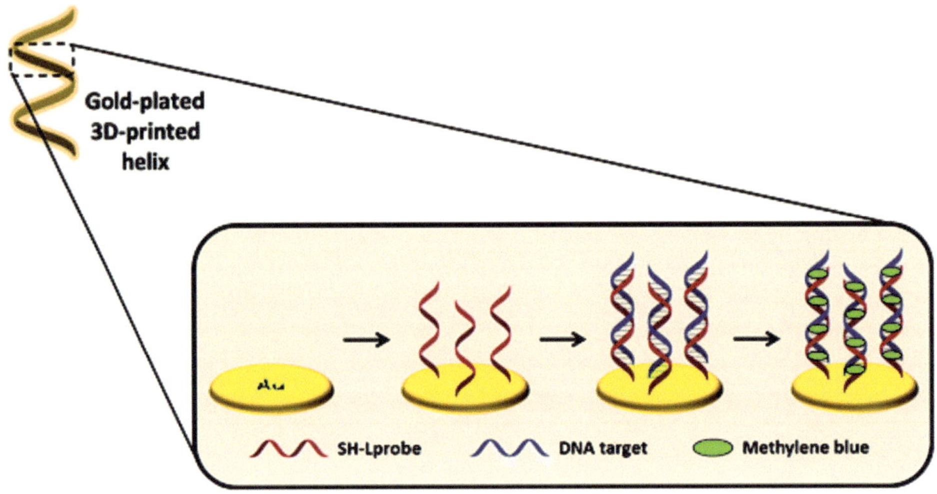

Figure 13.
DNA biosensing with 3D printing technology [82].

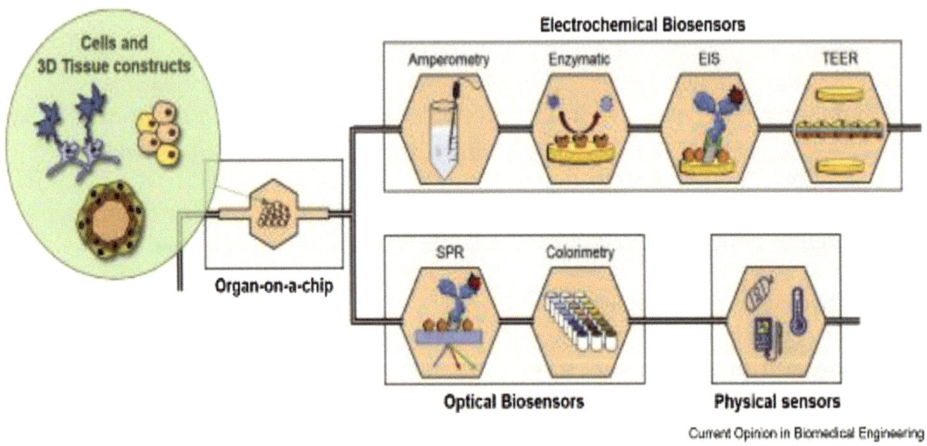

Figure 14.
Diagram showing the use of biosensors in organ-on-a-chip integration [85].

treatment (for instance, the presence of the required growth factors in their bloodstream after undergoing treatment).

Also, biosensors that monitor stem cell differentiation status before transplantation for therapeutic purposes can be made with nanotechnology [86]. Small cellular surface proteins and neurotransmitters, for example, can be measured to validate the differentiation of stem cells into dopamine-producing brain cells before their implantation into Parkinson's disease patients [87].

Future applications of biosensing can be seen in the monitoring of regenerative medicine therapies in patients, such as biosynthesized tissue preparation and posttreatment self-monitoring. With the advancement of technology and stem cell-related applications, physicians and patients will be able to use biosensors in new ways.

2.3.3 Mobile health (mHealth)

The pathbreaking spread of mobile technologies together with innovative application advancements has brought up deliberate attempts to address health-related matters using mobile devices. This has led to the evolution of a new pathway of electronic health (eHealth), known as mHealth. According to the International Telecommunication Union, there are about 5 billion mobile phone subscriptions in the world, with over 85% of the world's population now covered by a commercial wireless signal [88]. Mobile phones have penetrated most low-income countries more than other infrastructures such as paved roads and electricity. The increasing quality of these networks which involves providing higher speeds of data transmission alongside cheaper and more powerful handsets is transforming the way health services and information are accessed, delivered, and managed. With increased accessibility comes a greater possibility of personalization and adoption in healthcare delivery [89].

The term "mobile" in mHealth connotes a sense of freedom and flexibility to function anywhere and at any time [90]. There is no one generally accepted definition for the term – mobile health, and how it is defined keeps changing with time, and as you move from one field to the other. However, World Health Organization Global Observatory for eHealth (WHO, GOe) has defined mHealth as a subdivision of eHealth (electronic health). This subdivision is referred to as medical and public health practice supported by mobile devices. The mobile devices include the following:

- Mobile phones
- Patient monitoring devices
- Personal digital assistants (PDAs)
- Other wireless devices

mHealth capitalizes on a mobile phone's core utility of voice and short messaging service (SMS) as well as more complex functionalities and applications including general packet radio service (GPRS), third- and fourth-generation mobile telecommunications (3G and 4G systems), a global positioning system (GPS), and Bluetooth technology [89].

On the other hand, [91] it has described mHealth as wireless devices and sensors (which include mobile phones) which are meant to be carried or accessed by an individual throughout regular activities that are performed daily. This definition tells us that an important component of mHealth is the sensor that can monitor and measure physiological data; hence, the sensors can be used for various applications including monitoring and measuring physiological data in mHealth.

2.3.3.1 Application of biosensors in mHealth

There are many types of biosensors employed in mHealth for telecare. For biosensors to fit into mobile devices, they have to be of high quality and miniaturized, and consume low power. This has been better achieved through innovation in materials and instrumentation [92–95]. As biosensors gain more and more attachments with smart devices for mHealth, they become necessary for researchers to design biosensors with suitable functionalities and specifications to work flawlessly with accompanying hardware and software [96].

Two features will remain immutable with mHealth devices: a sensing technology for sensing health parameters and processing software to transform the sensor data into useful information. Hence, biosensors will remain invaluable components of mHealth. In designing a biosensor for mHealth, the biosensor can be built as a distinct microfluidic chip to communicate with the smartphone via wired or wireless connectivity. Alternatively, the biosensing chip with computing features can be incorporated directly into the design of smartphones, and this will eliminate additional hardware, thereby improving portability and possibly bringing about overall cost reduction [97].

Regarding smartphone-based mHealth, recent smartphones lack some key health sensor modalities. An integrated smartphone biosensor has limitations in the types of health data it can collect. Yet, the presence of connectivity technology such as USB, Bluetooth, and WiFi that enable them to interface with a large number of external biosensors to expand their range of signal acquisition is a great advantage. In mHealth, data processing can either be local processing (on the smartphone or a standalone biosensing accessory) or server processing (taking place on the cloud or on a nearby computer that communicates with the smartphone or a standalone biosensing accessory) [97].

Smartphones are not very suitable for data processing that requires high computing power as they may take a long time to process the data into useful information. However, smartphones can take advantage of their built-in connectivity features to transfer sensor data to a more powerful server. After the processing is completed, the server can transmit the results back to the smartphone to be accessible to the user.

2.3.3.1.1 Some of the specific applications of biosensors in mHealth

2.3.3.1.1.1 Detection of melanoma

The biosensor has been employed in the detection of melanoma using a fully integrated smartphone application [98]. A 10x detachable lens is used to capture the image of the target site of the skin, and the image is then passed through a series of processing steps such as preprocessing, segmentation, and feature extraction. A support vector machine classifier is then used to determine whether the image is an indication of a malignant or benign lesion [98].

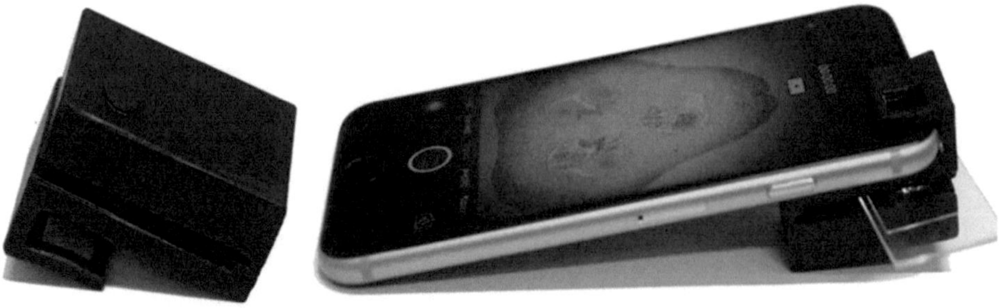

Figure 15.
Dual-mode microscope attachment (left) designed for the smartphone [99].

2.3.3.1.1.2 Phone microscopy

Orth et al. developed a dual-mode smartphone microscope. The system uses a camera flash or ambient light for brightfield and darkfield imaging [99]. They devised a clip-on 3D-printed attachment that easily attaches to the smartphone as shown in **Figure 15**. A cell nuclei imaging of unlabeled cells, cattle sperm, and zooplankton were demonstrated with this system. Another phone microscopy device called MoleScope is a commercially available smartphone attachment for dermoscopy that allows the user to obtain magnified images of the skin with controlled lighting. The images can be stored and viewed on a computer using a web platform and can be shared with a dermatologist, thereby facilitating teledermatology [97].

2.3.3.1.1.3 Semen analysis

Kanakasabapathy et al. developed a smartphone-based semen analyzer for point-of-care (POC) male infertility screening as shown in **Figure 16**. The system is composed of a disposable microfluidic device that handles the semen samples and an optical attachment for the smartphone that enhances image magnification and device alignment [100].

2.3.3.1.1.4 Lung function test

An acoustic-based diagnostic biosensor used for lung function tests has been developed by researchers as shown in **Figure 17**. It uses the audio signal from the in-built microphone of the smartphone with a mouthpiece attachment. The mechanism is based on a variable frequency complex demodulation using lung function parameter estimation [101].

2.3.3.1.1.5 Enzyme-linked immunosorbent assays at the point of care

Ozcan and the group developed a smartphone-based microplate reader for performing enzyme-linked immunosorbent assays at the point of care [102]. The system

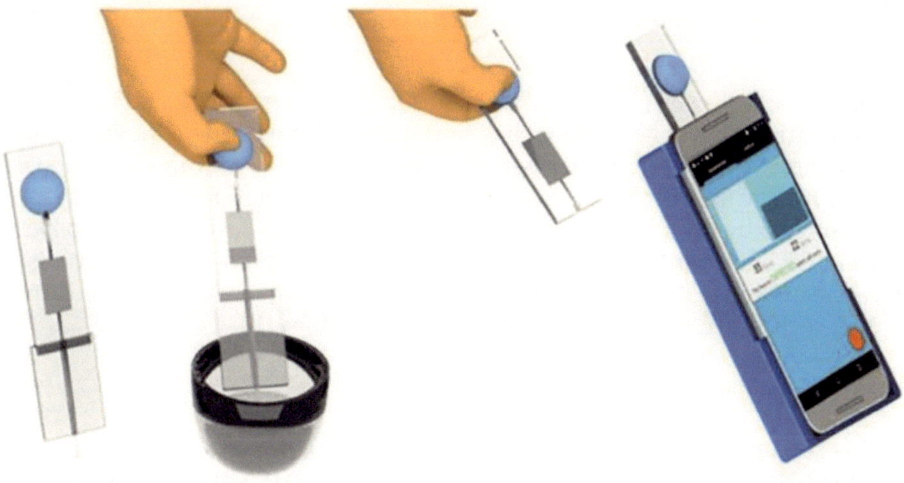

Figure 16.
Semen analyzer for point-of-care male fertility screening [100].

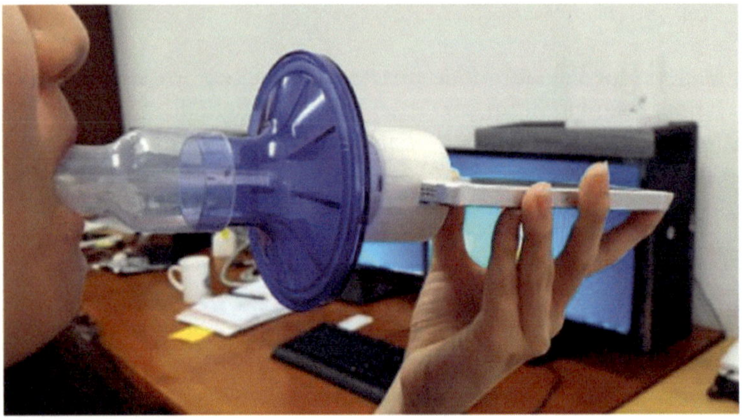

Figure 17.
Smartphone device with mouthpiece attachment for lung function testing [101].

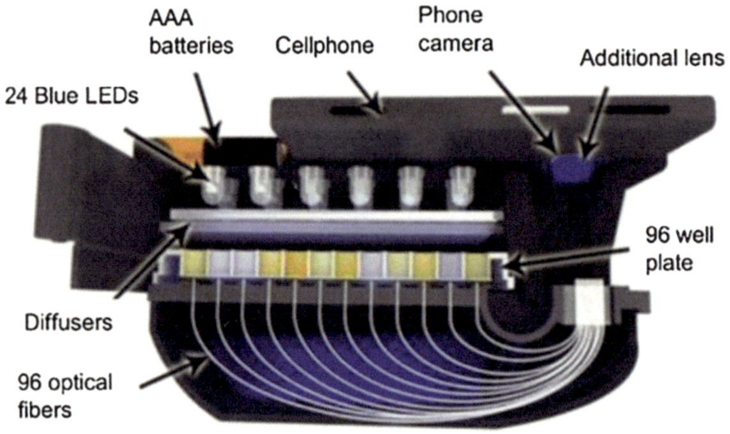

Figure 18.
Smartphone-based microplate reader for point-of-care enzyme-linked immunosorbent assays [102].

is composed of a 96-well plate held by a 3D-printed attachment and an LED array for the illumination of the plate. The smartphone camera is mounted on the same attachment, connected with the optical fibers that carry the light to the camera as shown in **Figure 18**. The image taken is sent to online servers for analysis, and the results are sent back to the phone in about 1-minute time. [103] also developed injectable dermal tattoo biosensors for measuring pH, glucose, and albumin concentrations. The biosensors undergo a colorimetric change upon exposure to varying levels of these analytes, such as pH, glucose, and albumin concentrations [103].

2.3.3.1.1.6 Amperometric electrochemical analysis

Guo devised a system for measuring blood ketones in order to detect diabetic ketoacidosis early. The concentration of blood ketone is detected using disposable test strips from fingerstick whole blood analysis on a smartphone-powered electrochemical analyzer. The -hydroxybutyrate dehydrogenase integrated with the test strip

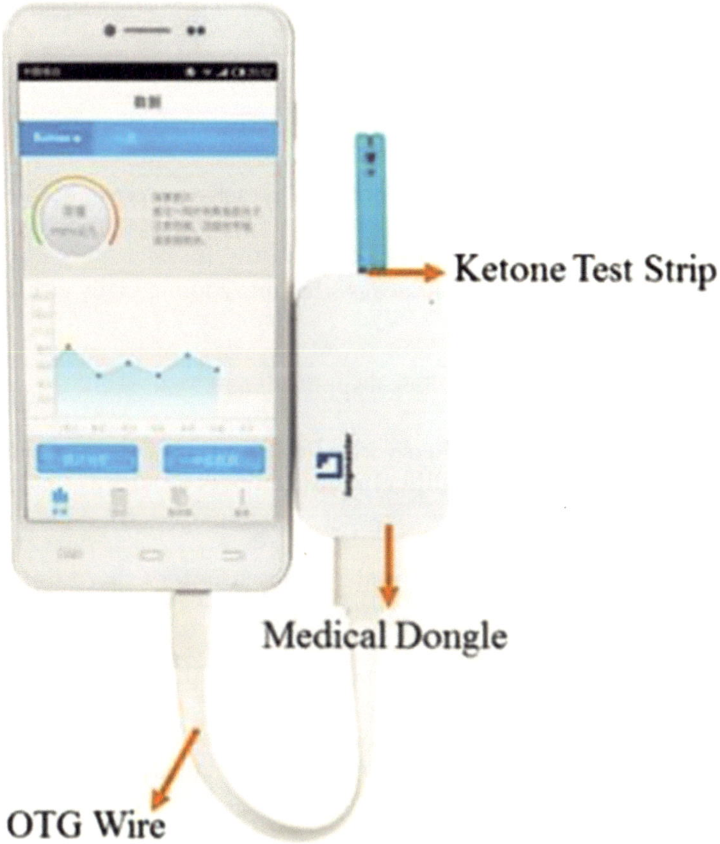

Figure 19.
Amperometric-based system for blood ketone monitoring [104].

converts -hydroxybutyrate to acetyl acetic acid after a drop of whole blood is added. The oxidation of NADH into NAD+ is then triggered by this cascade, which may be monitored amperometrically using an electrochemical analyzer. The results of mapping the current produced to the concentration of hydroxybutyrate are then sent to the smartphone through USB as shown in **Figure 19** [104].

3. Advantages of biosensing in tissue engineering and regenerative medicine

- It can be used in real-time monitoring of bioanalytes [52, 81].
- Development of "organs-on-chips" models in which concentrations of biomolecules such as glucose, adenosines, and hydrogen peroxide levels play important roles in determining the fate of the cells and tissues [48].
- Biosensing can be employed for the early detection of cancer biomarkers from blood samples in a noninvasive manner. Surface plasmon resonance (SPR) and electrochemical biosensors have been successfully used for the detection

of carcinoembryonic antigen (CEA) biomarkers in the early diagnosis of lung cancer in serum [105–107].

4. Challenges

There are many challenges researchers face in biosensing research. These include the following:

- Difficulties in translating academic research into commercially viable prototypes by industries.
- Complex regulatory issues in clinical applications.
- Difficulties in finding researchers with a background in biosensor technology or engaging researchers from different disciplines of science and engineering to work together.
- Identifying a market that is interested in a biosensor for a specific analyte of interest.
- Clear-cut advantages over existing methods for the analysis of that analyte.
- Testing the performance of the biosensor both in use and after storage. Response of a biosensor after 6 months of storage is the absolute minimum for any practical commercial application.
- Stability, costs, and ease of manufacturing of each component of the biosensor; hazards and ethics associated with the use of the developed biosensor [2].

5. Conclusion and future perspectives

The application of biosensing in tissue engineering, regenerative medicine, and mHealth has been fast growing. However, the growth has been limited even though some sensors including piezoelectric sensors have been described in previous research works and are already present in the market depicting high sensitivity and sensibility. The popularly known and successful ones among all are the electrochemical and mHealth, whereas some others cannot be used practically.

In tissue engineering and regenerative medicine, real-time monitoring of analytes is still at its early stage, and further research can bring enormous possibilities in the field. Future studies should focus on overcoming the challenges of miniaturization and integration of biosensors in microfluidic systems. Microfluidic technology with automated, sensitive, and real-time monitoring capabilities will play significant roles in translating to clinics. The use of microfluidic technology and many other mentioned technologies (methods) for global biosensing applications will need the utmost high standard of the systems and the whole process.

Incorporating biofabrication techniques into biosensing fields is important. For multiplexing signals and evaluating cellular responses in 2D and 3D, high-quality transducers could be used to separate and quantify analytes of interest. Future studies could be carried out by joining the recent biofabrication techniques (contact-based and noncontact-based), to yield better advances in biosensing technology, more particularly, in advanced extrusion-based bioprinting (noncontact-based printing method), to print living biosensing structures (as implantable therapeutics) with the use of coaxial and triaxial nozzles for various healthcare-related issues. The synergy of biofabrication and sensing will generate the next generation of biosensors possessing a high degree of sensitivity, throughput, and dynamic range in one sensor. In the end, the synergetic effect will yield a great impact on future sensing, monitoring of diseases, research, diagnostics, and therapeutic applications.

Acknowledgements

The authors would like to thank Mr. Ekwebelem George and Ms. Nwaigwe Ogochukwu for their great contributions to the areas of design and fabrication of a biosensor, and recent advances in biosensing.

Authors' contributions

This book chapter was written by all authors. All authors have approved the final version of the book chapter. A.T.B (corresponding author): conceptualization, writing, editing, supervision, and review. C.A.N: co-ordination, writing, and editing. E.M.B: conceptualization and writing.

Conflict of interest

The authors declare no conflict of interest.

Author details

Alma T. Banigo[1*], Chigozie A. Nnadiekwe[2] and Emmanuel M. Beasi[2]

1 Department of Developmental BioEngineering, University of Twente, The Netherlands

2 Department of Biomedical Engineering, Federal University of Technology, Owerri, Imo State, Nigeria

*Address all correspondence to: a.tamunonengioforibanigo@utwente.nl

References

[1] Hasan A, Nurunnabi M, Morshed M, Paul A, Polini A, Kuila T, et al. Recent advances in application of biosensors in tissue engineering. BioMed Research International. 2014;**2014**:1-18. DOI: 10.1155/2014/307519

[2] Bhalla N, Jolly P, Formisano N, Estrela P. Introduction to biosensors. Essays in Biochemistry. 2016;**60**:1-8. DOI: 10.1042/EBC20150001

[3] Tetyana P, Shumbula PM, Njengele-Tetyana Z. Biosensors: Design, development and applications. In: Ameen S, Akhtar MS, Shin H-S, editors. Nanopores. London: IntechOpen; 2021. pp. 1-172. DOI: 10.5772/intechopen.97576

[4] Palchetti I, Mascini M. Biosensor technology: A brief history. In: Malcovati P, Baschirotto A, d'Amico A, Natale C, editors. Sensors and Microsystems. Lecture Notes in Electrical Engineering. Dordrecht: Springer; 2010. pp. 15-23. DOI: 10.1007/978-90-481-3606-3_2

[5] Mascini M, Giardi MT, Piletska E. A brief story of biosensor technology. In: Giardi MT, Piletska EV, editors. Biotechnological Applications of Photosynthetic Proteins: Biochips, Biosensors and Biodevices. Florence: Landes Bioscience; 2007. pp. 4-10. DOI: 10.1007/978-0-387-36672-2_2

[6] Guilbault GG, Montalvo JG. Urea-specific enzyme electrode. Journal of the American Chemical Society. 1969;**91**:2164-2165. DOI: 10.1021/ja01036a083

[7] Javed H, Niazi KM. Overview, History & Types of Biosensors. Biosensors [Internet]; 2009. Available from: http://myweb.sabanciuniv.edu/javed/files/2009/10/JHNiazi_Introductory-Week-Overview-history-types-of-biosensors.pdf [Accessed: 2022-03-09]

[8] Li Y-CE, Lee IC. The current trends of biosensors in tissue engineering. Biosensors. 2020;**10**:1-22. DOI: 10.3390/bios10080088

[9] Jolly P, Formisano N, Estrela P. DNA aptamer-based detection of prostate cancer. Chemical Papers. 2015;**69**:77-89. DOI: 10.1515/chempap-2015-0025

[10] Formisano N, Jolly P, Bhalla N, Cromhout M, Flanagan SP, Fogel R, et al. Optimization of an electrochemical impedance spectroscopy aptasensor by exploiting quartz crystal microbalance with dissipation signals. Sensors & Actuators, B: Chemical. 2015;**220**:369-375. DOI: 10.1016/j.snb.2015.05.049

[11] Sharma TK, Ramanathan R, Rakwal R, Agrawal GK, Bansal V. Moving forward in plant food safety and security through nanobiosensors: adopt or adapt biomedical technologies? Proteomics. 2015;**15**:1680-1692. DOI: 10.1002/pmic.201400503

[12] Van Dorst B, Mehta J, Bekaert K, Rouah-Martin E, De Coen W, Dubruel P, et al. Recent advances in recognition elements of food and environmental biosensors: A review. Biosensors & Bioelectronics. 2010;**26**:1178-1194. DOI: 10.1016/j.bios.2010.07.033

[13] Gavrilescu M, Demnerová K, Aamand J, Agathos S, Fava F. Emerging pollutants in the environment: present and future challenges in biomonitoring, ecological risks and bioremediation. New Biotechnology. 2015;**32**:147-156. DOI: 10.1016/j.nbt.2014.01.001

[14] Bhalla N, Di Lorenzo M, Pula G, Estrela P. Protein phosphorylation analysis based on proton release detection: potential tools for drug discovery. Biosensors & Bioelectronics. 2014;**54**:109-114. DOI: 10.1016/j.bios.2013.10.037

[15] Bhalla N, Formisano N, Miodek A, Jain A, Di Lorenzo M, Pula G, et al. Plasmonic ruler on field-effect devices for kinase drug discovery applications. Biosensors & Bioelectronics. 2015;**71**:121-128. DOI: 10.1016/j.bios.2015.04.020

[16] Paddle BM. Biosensors for chemical and biological agents of defence interest. Biosensors & Bioelectronics. 1996;**11**:1079-1113. DOI: 10.1016/0956-5663(96)82333-5

[17] Grayson ACR, Shawgo RS, Johnson AM, Flynn NT, Li Y, Cima MJ, et al. A BioMEMS review: MEMS technology for physiologically integrated devices. Proceedings of the IEEE. 2004;**92**:6-21. DOI: 10.1109/JPROC.2003.820534

[18] Porous Electro Active Hydrogels and Uses Thereof. 8,999,378 B2. U.S. Pat. 2015 [Internet]. 2009. Available from: https://patentimages.storage.googleapis.com/51/4e/0d/756fbf2287a759/WO2010036800A1.pdf [Accessed on 2022-04-01]

[19] Yang Z, Kasprzyk-Hordern B, Frost CG, Estrela P, Thomas KV. Community sewage sensors for monitoring public health. Environmental Science & Technology. 2015;**49**:5845-5846. DOI: 10.1021/acs.est.5b01434

[20] Cho IH, Kim DH, Park S. Electrochemical biosensors: Perspective on functional nanomaterials for on-site analysis. Biomaterials Research. 2020;**24**:1-12. DOI: 10.1186/s40824-019-0181-y

[21] Narita F, Wang Z, Kurita H, Li Z, Shi Y, Jia Y, et al. A review of piezoelectric and magnetostrictive biosensor materials for detection of COVID-19 and other viruses. Advanced Materials. 2021;**33**:2005448 (1-24). DOI: 10.1002/adma.202005448

[22] Lazcka O, Del Campo FJ, Muñoz FX. Pathogen detection: A perspective of traditional methods and biosensors. Biosensors & Bioelectronics. 2007;**22**:1205-1217. DOI: 10.1016/j.bios.2006.06.036

[23] Watts HJ, Lowe CR, Pollard-Knight DV. Optical biosensor for monitoring microbial cells. Analytical Chemistry. 1994;**66**:2465-2470. DOI: 10.1021/ac00087a010

[24] Dey D, Goswami T. Optical biosensors: A revolution towards quantum nanoscale electronic device fabrication. Journal of Biomedicine & Biotechnology. 2011;**2011**:348218. DOI: 10.1155/2011/348218

[25] Adlerberth J, Meng Q, Mecklenburg M, Tian Z, Zhou Y, Bülow L, et al. Thermometric analysis of blood metabolites in ICU patients. Journal of Thermal Analysis and Calorimetry. 2020;**140**:763-771. Available from. DOI: 10.1007/s10973-019-08873-7

[26] Marchenkoa SV, Kucherenkoa IS, Hereshkob AN, Panasiuk I, Soldatkin O, El'skaya, Soldatkin A. Application of potentiometric biosensor based on recombinant urease for urea determination in blood serum and hemodialyzate. Sensors and Actuators, B: Chemical. 2015;**207**:981-986. DOI: 10.1016/j.snb.2014.06.136

[27] Goriushkina TB, Soldatkin AP, Dzyadevych SV. Application of amperometric biosensors for analysis of ethanol, glucose, and lactate in

wine. Journal of Agricultural and Food Chemistry. 2009;**57**:6528-6535. DOI: 10.1021/jf9009087

[28] Guana JG, Miao YQ, Zhang QJ. Impedimetric biosensors. Journal of Bioscience and Bioengineering. 2004;**97**:219-226. DOI: 10.1016/S1389-1723(04)70195-4

[29] Aizawa M. Immunosensors for clinical analysis. Advances in Clinical Chemistry. 1994;**31**:247-275. DOI: 10.1016/s0065-2423(08)60337-6

[30] Goyal RN, Gupta VK, Chatterjee S. Voltametric biosensors for the determination of paracetamol at carbon nanotube modified pyrolytic graphite electrode. Sensors & Actuators, B: Chemical. 2010;**149**:252-258. DOI: 10.1016/j.snb.2010.05.019

[31] Woolley AT, Cheung CL, Hafner JH, Lieber CM. Structural biology with carbon nanotube AFM probes. Chemistry and Biology. 2000;**7**:R193-R204. DOI: 10.1016/s1074-5521(00)00037-5

[32] Pohanka M. The piezoelectric biosensors: principles and applications, A review. International Journal of Electrochemical Science. 2016;**12**:496-506. DOI: 10.20964/2017.01.44

[33] Vasuki S, Varsha V, Mithra ARD, Abinaya S, Deva RD, Sivarajasekar N. Thermal biosensors and applications. In: Proceeding of the American International Journal of Research in Science, Technology, Engineering & Mathematics, Special issue of National Conference on Innovations in Bio. Tamil Nadu. India: Chemical and Food Technology (IBCFT '19): February 02, 2019; pp. 262-264

[34] Ramanathan K, Danielsson B. Principles and applications of thermal biosensors. Biosensors & Bioelectronics. 2001;**16**:417-423. DOI: 10.1016/S0956-5663(01)00124-5

[35] Yildirim N, Long F, Gao C, He M, Shi HC, Gu AZ. Aptamer-based optical biosensor for rapid and sensitive detection of 17beta-estradiol in water samples. Environmental Science & Technology. 2012;**46**:3288-3294. DOI: 10.1021/es203624w

[36] Biran I, Rissin DM, Ron EZ, Walt DR. Optical imaging fiber-based live bacterial cell array biosensor. Analytical Biochemistry. 2003;**315**:106-113. DOI: 10.1016/S0003-2697(02)00700-5

[37] Suker J, Charalambous BM. Application of optical biosensor techniques to the characterization of PorA-antibody binding kinetics. Methods in Molecular Medicine. 2001;**66**:129-143. DOI: 10.1385/1-59259-148-5:129

[38] Beebe D, Mensing GA, Walker GM. Physics and application of microfluidics in biology. In Yarmush, editor. Annual Review of Biomedical Engineering. 2002;**4**:261-286. DOI: 10.1146/annurev.bioeng.4.112601.125916

[39] Ce'spedes F, Alegret S. New materials for electrochemical sensing: glucose biosensors based on rigid carbon-polymer biocomposites. Food Technology and Biotechnology. 1996;**34**:143-146. Available from: https://www.ftb.com.hr/images/pdfarticles/1996/December-October/34-4-4.pdf

[40] Vidal JC. Electrochemical affinity biosensors for detection of mycotoxins: A review. Biosensors and Bioelectronics. 2013;**49**:146-158. DOI: 10.1016/j.bios.2013.05.008

[41] Grieshaber D, MacKenzie R, Voros J, Reimhult E. Electrochemical biosensors - sensor principles and

architectures. Sensors. 2008;**8**:1400-1458. DOI: 10.3390/s80314000

[42] Akhtar KL. Design of Surface Plasmon Resonance Devices for Biosensing [thesis]. Barcelona: Universitat de Barcelona; 2021

[43] Chaubey A, Malhotra BD. Mediated biosensors. Biosensors & Bioelectronics. 2002;**17**:441-456. DOI: 10.1016/S0956-5663 (01)00313-X

[44] Saha K, Agasti SS, Kim C, Li X, Rotello VM. Gold nanoparticles in chemical and biological sensing. Chemical Reviews. 2012;**112**:2739-2779. DOI: 10.1021/cr2001178

[45] Morales MA, Halpern JM. Guide to selecting a biorecognition element for biosensors. Bioconjugate Chemistry. 2018;**29**:3231-3239. DOI: 10.1021/acs.bioconjchem.8b00592

[46] Korotkaya EV. Biosensors: Design, classification, and applications in the food industry. Foods and Raw Materials. 2014;**2**:161-171. DOI: 10.12737/5476

[47] Sassolas A, Blum LJ, Leca-Bouvier BD. Immobilization strategies to develop enzymatic biosensors. Biotechnology Advances. 2012;**30**:489-511. DOI: 10.1016/j.biotechadv.2011.09.00

[48] Wheeldon I, Farhadi A, Bick AG, Jabbari E, Khademhosseini A. Nanoscale tissue engineering: Spatial control over cell-materials interactions. Nanotechnology. 2011;**22**:212001. DOI: 10.1088/0957-4484/22/21/212001

[49] Wang Y, Chen Q, Zeng X. Potentiometric biosensor for studying hydroquinone cytotoxicity in vitro. Biosensors and Bioelectronics. 2010;**25**:1356-1362. DOI: 10.1016/j.bios.2009.10.027

[50] Salimi A, Noorbakhsh A, Rafiee-Pour H-A, Ghourchian H. Direct voltammetry of copper, zinc-superoxide dismutase immobilized onto electrodeposited nickel oxide nanoparticles: Fabrication of amperometric superoxide biosensor. Electroanalysis. 2011;**23**:683-691 Available from: https://www.chemeurope.com/en/publications/83510/direct-voltammetry-of-copper-zincsuperoxide-dismutase-immobilized-onto-electrodeposited-nickel-oxide-nanoparticles-fabrication-of-amperometric-superoxide-biosensor.html

[51] Hanaphy P. South African Researchers Identify Solutions for Challenges in Using Bioinks to 3d Print Tissue Constructs [Internet]. 2020. Available from: https://3dprintingindustry.com/news/south-african-researchers-identify-solutions-for-challenges-in-using-bioinks-to-3d-print-tissue-constructs-172589/ [Accessed: 2022-03-21]

[52] Dias AD, Kingsley DM, Corr DT. Recent advances in bioprinting and applications for biosensing. Biosensors (Basel). 2014;**4**:111-136. DOI: 10.3390/bios4020111

[53] Xiang C, Kung S, Taggart DK, Yang F, Thompson MA, Gu AG, et al. Lithographically patterned nanowire patterning electrically continuous metal nanowires on dielectrics. ACS Nano. 2008;**2**:1939-1949. DOI: 10.1021/nn800394k

[54] Peng S, Zhang X. Electrodeposition of CdSe quantum dots and its application to an electrochemiluminescence immunoassay for α-fetoprotein. Microchimica Acta. 2012;**178**:323-330. DOI: 10.1007/s00604-012-0844-z

[55] Loget G, Wood JB, Cho K, Halpern AR, Corn RM. Electrodeposition of polydopamine thin films for DNA

patterning and microarrays. Analytical Chemistry. 2013;**85**:9991-9995. DOI: 10.1021/ac4022743

[56] Novak S, Maver U, Peternel Š, Venturini P, Bele M, Gaberšček M. Electrophoretic deposition as a tool for separation of protein inclusion bodies from host bacteria in suspension. Colloids and Surfaces A: Physicochemical and Engineering Aspects. 2009;**340**:155-160. DOI: 10.1016/j.colsurfa.2009.03.023

[57] Ammam M, Fransaer J. Two-enzyme lactose biosensor based on β-galactosidase and glucose oxidase deposited by AC-electrophoresis: Characteristics and performance for lactose determination in milk. Sensors & Actuators, B: Chemical. 2010;**148**:583-589. DOI: 10.1016/j.snb.2010.05.027

[58] Poortinga AT, Bos R, Busscher HJ. Controlled electrophoretic deposition of bacteria to surfaces for the design of biofilms. Biotechnology and Bioengineering. 2000;**67**:117-120. DOI: 10.1002/(SICI)1097-0290(20000105)67:1<117::AID-BIT14>3.0.CO;2-6

[59] WHO. World Health Organization: Global report on diabetes [Internet]. 2016. Available from: https://www.who.int/publications/i/item/9789241565257 [Accessed: 2022-03-21]

[60] Holman RR, Paul SK, Bethel MA, Matthews DR, Neil HAW. 10- year follow-up of intensive glucose control in type 2 diabetes. The New England Journal of Medicine. 2008;**359**:1577-1589. DOI: 10.1056/nejmoa0806470

[61] Clark LC, Lyons C. Electrode systems for continuous monitoring in cardiovascular surgery. Annals of the New York Academy of Sciences. 1962;**102**:29-45. DOI: 10.1111/j.1749-6632.1962.tb13623

[62] Matthews DR, Holman RR, Bown E, Steemson J, Watson A, Hughes S, et al. Pen-sized digital 30-second blood glucose meter. Lancet. 1987;**1**:778. DOI: 10.1016/s0140-6736(87)92802-9

[63] Ocvirk G, Buck H, DuVall SH. Electrochemical glucose biosensors for diabetes care. Bioanalytical Reviews. 2017;**6**:1-101. Available from: https://www.springerprofessional.de/en/electrochemical-glucose-biosensors-for-diabetes-care/11029372 Retrieved: 2022-03-22

[64] Murata GH, Shah JH, Hoffman RM, Wendel CS, Adam KD, Solvas PA, et al. Intensified blood glucose monitoring improves glycemic control in stable, insulin-treated veterans with type 2 diabetes. Diabetes Care. 2003;**26**:1759-1763. DOI: 10.2337/diacare.26.6.1759

[65] Poolsup N, Suksomboon N, Rattanasookchit S. Meta-analysis of the benefits of self-monitoring of blood glucose on glycemic control in type 2 diabetes patients: An update. Diabetes Technology & Therapeutics. 2009;**11**:775-784. DOI: 10.1089/dia.2009.0091

[66] Martin P. Wound healing—aiming for perfect skin regeneration. Science. 1997;**276**:75-81. DOI: 10.1126/science.276.5309.75

[67] Schreml S, Szeimies RM, Prantl L, Karrer S, Landthaler M, Babilas P. Oxygen in acute and chronic wound healing. The British Journal of Dermatology. 2010;**163**:257-268. DOI: 10.1111/j.1365-2133.2010.09804.x

[68] Werdin F, Tenenhaus M, Rennekampff H-O. Chronic wound care. Lancet. 2008;**372**:1860-1862. DOI: 10.1016/s0140-6736(08)61793-6

[69] Guinovart T, Valdés-Ramírez G, Windmiller JR, Andrade FJ, Wang J.

Bandage-based wearable potentiometric sensor for monitoring wound pH. Electroanalysis. 2014;**26**:1345-1353. DOI: 10.1002/elan.201300558

[70] Pusta A, Tertiș M, Cristea C, Mirel S. Wearable sensors for the detection of biomarkers for wound infection. Biosensors. 2021;**12**:1-20. DOI: 10.3390/bios12010001

[71] Bohunicky B, Mousa SA. Biosensors: The new wave in cancer diagnosis. Nanotechnology, Science and Applications. 2010;**4**:1-10. DOI: 10.2147/nsa.s13465

[72] Wang H, Wang X, Wang J, Fu W, Yao C. An SPR biosensor based on signal amplification using antibody-QD conjugates for the quantitative determination of multiple tumor markers. Scientific Reports. 2016;**6**:33140. DOI: 10.1038/srep33140

[73] Patel P, Patel J. Biosensors and biomarkers: Promising tools for cancer diagnosis. International Journal of Biosensors & Bioelectronics. 2017;**3**:313-316. DOI: 10.15406/ijbsbe.2017.03.00072

[74] Mittal S, Kaur H, Gautam N, Mantha AK. Biosensors for breast cancer diagnosis: A review of bioreceptors, biotransducers, and signal amplification strategies. Biosensors & Bioelectronics. 2017;**88**:217-231. DOI: 10.1016/j.bios.2016.08.028

[75] DeSantis C, Ma J, Bryan L, Jemal A. Breast cancer statistics, 2013. CA: A Cancer Journal for Clinicians. 2014;**64**:52-62. DOI: 10.3322/caac.21203

[76] Aldous SJ. Cardiac biomarkers in acute myocardial infarction. International Journal of Cardiology. 2013;**164**:282-294. DOI: 10.1016/j.ijcard.2012.01.081

[77] Rodrigues D, Barbosa AI, Rebelo R, Kwon IK, Reis RL, Correlo VM. Skin-integrated wearable systems and implantable biosensors: A comprehensive review. Biosensors. 2020;**10**:79. DOI: 10.3390/bios10070079

[78] Anders O. Restoring touch. Nature Materials. 2016;**15**:919. DOI: 10.1038/nmat4748

[79] Xu B, Akhtar A, Liu Y, Chen H, Yeo W-H, Park SI, et al. An epidermal stimulation and sensing platform for sensorimotor prosthetic control, management of lower back exertion, and electrical muscle activation. Advanced Materials. 2015;**28**:4462-4471. DOI: 10.1002/adma.201504155

[80] Merrill DR, Lockhart J, Troyk PR, Weir RF, Hankin DL. Development of an implantable myoelectric sensor for advanced prosthesis control. Artificial Organs. 2011;**35**:249-252. DOI: 10.1111/j.1525-1594.2011.01219.x

[81] Boero C, Casulli MA, Olivo J, Foglia L, Orso E, Mazza M, et al. Design, development, and validation of an in-situ biosensor array for metabolite monitoring of cell cultures. Biosensors & Bioelectronics. 2014;**61**:251-259. DOI: 10.1016/j.bios.2014.05.030

[82] Loo AH, Chua CK, Pumera M. DNA biosensing with 3D printing technology. Analyst. 2017;**142**:279-283. DOI: 10.1039/c6an02038k

[83] Shafiee A, Atala A. Tissue engineering: Toward a new era of medicine. Annual Review of Medicine. 2017;**68**:29-40. DOI: 10.1146/annurev-med-102715-092331

[84] Shin SR, Zhang YS, Kim DJ, Manbohi A, Avci H, Silvestri A, et al. Aptamer-based microfluidic electrochemical biosensor for monitoring cell-secreted trace cardiac

biomarkers. Analytical Chemistry. 2016;**88**:10019-10027. DOI: 10.1021/acs.analchem.6b02028

[85] Zhu Y, Mandal K, Hernandez AL, Kawakita S, Huang W, Bandaru P, et al. State of the art in integrated biosensors for organ-on-a-chip applications. Current Opinion in Biomedical Engineering. 2021;**19**:100309. DOI: 10.1016/j.cobme.2021.100309

[86] Lee J-H, Lee T, Choi J-W. Nano-biosensor for monitoring the neural differentiation of stem cells. Nano. 2016;**6**:224. DOI: 10.3390/nano6120224

[87] Yea C-H, Kim T-H, Yin PT-T, Conley B, Dardir K, Pak Y, et al. Large-scale nanoelectrode arrays to monitor the dopaminergic differentiation of human neural stem cells. Advanced Materials. 2015;**27**:6356-6362. DOI: 10.1002/adma.201502489

[88] Resolution WHA. 58.28. eHealth. In: Fifty-eighth World Health Assembly. 2005. Available from: http://apps.who.int/gb/ebwha/pdf_files/WHA58/WHA58_28-en.pdf Accessed 2022-03-08

[89] Ryu S. Book Review: mHealth: New horizons for health through mobile technologies: Second global survey on eHealth. Global Observatory for eHealth Series. 2012;**18**:231-233. DOI: 10.4258/hir.2012.18.3.231

[90] Sulley AM. Mobile health technology & mHealth [thesis]. Health Information Science Program, Faculty of Information & Media Studies, The University of Western Ontario; 2016. DOI:10.13140/RG.2.2.30652.44165

[91] Carlos DAO, Magalhães TO, Filho JEV, da Silva RM, Brasil CCP. Design and evaluation of mHealth technology for vocal health promotion. RISTI - Revista Iberica de Sistemas e Tecnologias de Informacao. 2016;**19**:46-60. DOI: 10.17013/risti.19.46-60

[92] Wood CS, Thomas MR, Budd J, Mashamba-Thompson TP, Herbst K, Pillay D, et al. Taking connected mobile-health diagnostics of infectious diseases to the field. Nature. 2019;**566**:467-474. DOI: 10.1038/s41586-019-0956-2

[93] Sackmann EK, Fulton AL, Beebe DJ. The present and future role of microfluidics in biomedical research. Nature. 2014;**507**:181-189. DOI: 10.1038/nature13118

[94] Nayak S, Blumenfeld NR, Laksanasopin T, Sia SK. Point-of-care diagnostics: Recent developments in a connected age. Analytical Chemistry. 2017;**89**:102-123. DOI: 10.1021/acs.analchem.6b04630

[95] Thuau D, Ducrot PH, Poulin P, Dufour I, Ayela C. Integrated electromechanical transduction schemes for polymer MEMS sensors. Micromachines (Basel). 2018;**9**:197. DOI: 10.3390/mi9050197

[96] Arumugam S, Colburn DAM, Sia SK. Biosensors for personal mobile health: A system architecture perspective. Advanced Materials Technologies. 2020;**5**:1900720. DOI: 10.1002/admt.201900720

[97] Sun AC, Hall AD. Point-of-care smartphone-based electrochemical biosensing. Electroanalysis. 2019;**31**:2. DOI: 10.1002/elan.201800474

[98] Kalwa U, Legner C, Kong T, Pandey S. Skin cancer diagnostics with an all-inclusive smartphone application. Symmetry. 2019;**11**:790. DOI: 10.3390/sym11060790

[99] Orth A, Wilson ER, Thompson JG, Gibson BC. A dual-mode mobile phone

microscope using the onboard camera fash and ambient light. Scientific Reports. 2018;**8**:3298. DOI: 10.1038/s41598-018-21543-2

[100] Kanakasabapathy MK, Sadasivam M, Singh A, Preston C, Thirumalaraju P, Venkataraman M, et al. An automated smartphone-based diagnostic assay for point-of-care semen analysis. Science Translational Medicine. 2017;**9**:1-14. DOI: 10.1126/scitranslmed.aai7863

[101] Thap T, Chung H, Jeong C, Hwang KE, Kim HR, Yoon KH, et al. High-resolution time-frequency spectrum-based lung function test from a smartphone microphone sensors. Baseline. 2016;**16**:1305. DOI: 10.3390/s16081305

[102] Berg B, Cortazar B, Tseng D, Ozkan H, Feng S, Wei QS, et al. Cellphone-based hand-held microplate reader for point-of-care testing of enzyme-linked immunosorbent assays. ACS Nano. 2015;**9**:7857. DOI: 10.1021/acsnano.5b03203

[103] Yetisen AK, Moreddu R, Seifi S, Jiang N, Vega K, Dong XC, et al. Dermal tattoo biosensors for colorimetric metabolite detection. Angewandte Chemie International. 2019;**58**:10506-10513. DOI: 10.1002/anie.201904416

[104] Guo J. Smartphone-powered electrochemical dongle for point-of-care monitoring of blood β-ketone. Analytical Chemistry. 2017;**89**:8609-8613. DOI: 10.1021/acs.analchem.7b02531

[105] Shevchenko Y, Camci-Unal G, Cuttica DF, Dokmeci MR, Albert J, Khademhosseini A. Surface plasmon resonance fiber sensor for real-time and label-free monitoring of cellular behavior. Biosensors and Bioelectronics. 2014;**56**:359-367. DOI: 10.1016/j.bios.2014.01.018

[106] Altintas Z, Kallempudi SS, Sezerman U, Gurbuz Y. A novel magnetic particle-modified electrochemical sensor for immunosensor applications. Sensors and Actuators, B: Chemical. 2012;**174**:187-194. DOI: 10.1016/j.snb.2012.08.052

[107] Ladd J, Lu H, Taylor AD, Goodell V, Disis ML, Jiang S. Direct detection of carcinoembryonic antigen autoantibodies in clinical human serum samples using a surface plasmon resonance sensor. Colloids and Surfaces B: Biointerfaces. 2009;**70**:1-6. DOI: 10.1016/j.colsurfb.2008.11.032

Chapter 16

NanoBioSensors: From Electrochemical Sensors Improvement to Theranostic Applications

Anielle C.A. Silva, Eliete A. Alvin, Lais S. de Jesus, Caio C.L. de França, Marílya P.G. da Silva, Samaysa L. Lins, Diógenes Meneses, Marcela R. Lemes, Rhanoica O. Guerra, Marcos V. da Silva, Carlo J.F. de Oliveira, Virmondes Rodrigues Junior, Renata M. Etchebehere, Fabiane C. de Abreu, Bruno G. Lucca, Sanívia A.L. Pereira, Rodrigo C. Rosa and Noelio O. Dantas

Abstract

This chapter comments on the advantages of nanobiosensors using nanocrystals in improving electrochemical sensors' response and their use as theragnostic tools in biomedical applications. The use of nanomaterials to modify electrochemical sensors' surfaces to increase these devices' sensitivity and their bio-functionality enables high-quality nanotechnological platforms. Thus, graphene nanostructures and CdSe/CdS magic-sized quantum dots (MSQDs) were shown to improve biosensor's sensitivity. In addition, the use of CdSe/CdS MSQDs and cobalt ferrite nanocrystals (NCs) as potential tools for drug delivery systems and biocompatible titanium dioxide NCs in osseointegration processes and their bio-location are also demonstrated. So, this chapter shows some impressive results on which the group has been working regarding the applications of nanocrystals to electrochemical sensors and theranostic applications.

Keywords: nanocrystals, luminescence, magnetic nanocrystals, magic-sized quantum dots, drug delivery systems, biosensors, biomaterials, theranostic applications

1. Introduction

Nanotechnology allows the development of nanomaterials with controllable physical, chemical, and biological properties [1–4]. These properties are controlled according to the nanomaterials' size and shape, enabling the development of new innovative technologies, from new device development to tools in the health field [4–9]. In this context, nanobiotechnology is a recent field emerging from science, which establishes an interface between biology and nanotechnology, evaluating and assigning new functionalized nano biosystems [8]. Thus, this multidisciplinary research field has great potential in developing improved medical engineering [1, 10].

Nanoparticles can be amorphous or crystalline (nanocrystals), and this difference reflects directly on the physical, chemical, and biological properties. Spanó et al. demonstrated that zinc oxide (ZnO) nanocrystals are more biocompatible when compared to amorphous nanoparticles [11]. Amorphous nanoparticles have a long-range disorder of their atoms and are more reactive [12]. On the other hand, nanocrystals show the periodicity of atoms forming crystalline arrangements and consequently fewer defects and less reactivity [13–15].

Nanocrystals (NCs) are often and successfully applied in several sensors, such as colorimetric, fluorescence, surface plasmon resonance, and electrochemical [16]. Regarding electroanalytical chemistry, conductive nanostructured crystals are interesting for application in electrochemical sensing due to their well-known ability to improve the catalytic activity, the electron transfer speed, and the conductivity of the sensors. Furthermore, the deposition of nanocrystals over electronic surfaces can increase the superficial area and amplify the analytical signal, enhancing the sensitivity regarding the detection of target analytes [17]. Nowadays, nanocrystal-based sensors have been widely explored in various applications and attracted the attention of several researchers [18].

Nanoparticle drug delivery can be used to target the tissue, promote the slow-release, protect against degradation, and diminish toxicity [19, 20]. The pharmacokinetic properties of a compound of biological activity are, among other factors, related to its solubility. The low solubility will result in problems from absorption until elimination. So, it is essential to search for alternatives, and they can increase the solubility of drugs without interfering in their pharmacological activity. Several active compounds are usually poorly soluble in aqueous media [21, 22]. A vast literature reports the possibility of complexation between lipophilic organic molecules appropriately sized, inorganic ions, and other species, with cyclodextrin, dendrimers, and liposomes. Whether for the drug's application for pharmaceutical use, the nanocrystal compounds are essential on the medical and economic side [23, 24].

The development of biomaterials arouses tremendous scientific and clinical interest, given the possibility of replacing, in part or whole, human bones and/or favoring bone regeneration, both in the craniofacial complex and in other parts of the skeleton. Therefore, it is expected that the materials have osteoconductive properties (materials that function as a support surface for adhesion and proliferation of osteoblastic cells, which promote the formation of mineralized bone tissue), osteoinduction (materials that contain inductive proteins present in the matrix bone tissue and are capable of inducing differentiation of undifferentiated mesenchymal cells into chondroblasts or osteoblasts), osteogenesis (materials that have viable osteoblasts, capable of determining the formation of the new bone when grafted into the host tissue) and/or osteopromotion (materials that constitute physical barriers for the anatomical isolation of the site under repair, aiming at the selection of cells that promote the restoration, while excluding competing for inhibitory cells) [25]. This chapter book will comment specifically on titanium dioxide nanocrystals in dental and orthopedic applications.

Therefore, this chapter shows the innovative results obtained by the group of carbon-based, semiconductor, and magnetic nanocrystals that can be used in biosensors and biomedical applications, further strengthening the development of new tools.

2. NanoBioSensors and applications

This section shows nanocrystals' results in improved electrochemical sensors and their use as theranostic tools in biomedical applications. We will demonstrate how graphene nanostructures and CdSe/CdS MSQDs can improve sensors sensitivity. In the biomedical applications, we will show CdSe/CdS MSQDs and cobalt ferrite ($CoFe_2O_4$) NCs to drug deliveries and biocompatible titanium dioxide (TiO_2) NCs in osseointegration processes and their bio-location.

2.1 Nanocrystals to biosensors improvement

Graphene has been the nanostructured material most utilized in electroanalytical applications due to its unique features [26]. Graphene consists of a single layer of carbon atoms in the sp^2 hybridization organized in a honeycomb structure with six-membered rings, yielding 2D nanocrystals [27]. Some advantages of using graphene in electrochemical sensors are enhanced conductivity, decreased overpotentials, increased electroactive areas, and enhanced charge transfer rate [28]. Graphene is usually synthesized by the chemical reduction of graphene oxide [29, 30].

In this field, the advantages of using graphene-based nanocrystals in electroanalytical sensing have been previously demonstrated by several researchers and our research group [31]. We have reported the modification of a glassy carbon rod electrode (GCRE) with reduced graphene oxide doped with copper nanoparticles (RGO-CuNP). The synthesis of the RGO used in this work was carried out by the modified Hummers' method [32]. This GCRE modified with RGO-CuNP was coupled, for the first time, to a paper-based electrochemical platform and applied in the electroanalysis of analytes of clinical interest, as illustrated in **Figure 1**.

The modified sensor was thoroughly studied, optimized, and characterized. The results showed that the modification with RGO-CuNP significantly improved the electrochemical properties of the working electrode. In comparison with the unmodified GCRE, the RGO-CuNP sensor presented lower peak potentials, better sensitivity (ca. two-fold higher), lower electron transfer resistance (857 vs. 21,497 Ω), and larger electroactive area (0.067 vs. 0.040 cm^2). These improvements are directly related to the modification with RGO-Cu nanocrystals, which are responsible for enhancing the conductivity and increasing the superficial area of the GCRE. As proof of concept, this modified sensor was employed to determine paracetamol and caffeine in real urine samples simultaneously. These two analytes were successfully quantified in low levels without matrix interferences, and the results showed excellent concordance with high-performance liquid chromatography used to validate the method. So, it evidences some of the advantages of using graphene-based nanocrystal in sensing platforms.

In this context, quantum dots (QDs) are among the most explored nanomaterials nowadays. The synthesis and practical application of QDs are among the main focuses in the development directions of nanotechnology [33]. QDs are semiconductor nanocrystals with optical and electrical properties that are widely employed in sensing

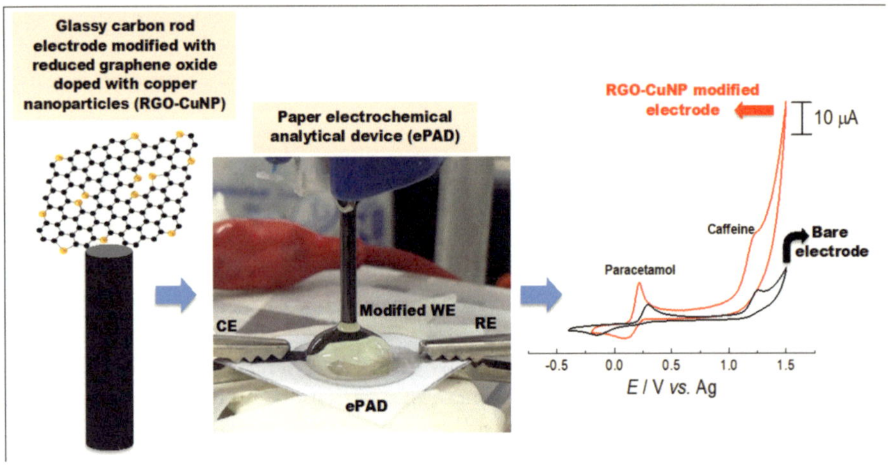

Figure 1.
Representation of the modification of the GCRE with RGO-CuNP, coupling of the modified sensor to the paper-based electrochemical platform such as used in work, and voltammetric responses of unmodified and modified electrodes in the simultaneous electroanalysis of paracetamol and caffeine.

applications. Another exciting feature of QDs is that properties such as size, shape, composition, and structure can be controlled and tuned. It allows obtaining QDs with unique properties according to the desired application [34, 35].

Although, promising, conventional QDs have some drawbacks that include moderate stability, limited luminescence spectra, and large size to some applications. At this point, the magic-sized quantum dots (MSQDs) are a class of nanocrystals that show smaller particle sizes, broader spectra, and more excellent stability than conventional QDs [36]. Among other applications, the MSQDs are a promising nanomaterial for electrochemical sensing use. The small size (in nanometric scale) and the electrical properties of these nanocrystals can significantly increase the surface area and the conductivity of the sensors.

Our research group recently explored, for the first time, the application of MSQDs for the modification of electrochemical sensors [37]. This pioneering work proposed a simple and inexpensive paper electrochemical device (PED) whose carbon-based working electrode was modified with CdSe/CdS MSQDs. The three-electrode setup (working, counter, and pseudo-reference) was fabricated on the paper substrate by a simple pencil-drawing method. At the same time, the CdSe/CdS MSQDs were synthesized according to the method described by Silva et al. [36, 38, 39]. This PED was modified with CdSe/CdS MSQDs to demonstrate the analytical feasibility and applied for clinical quantification of dopamine in biological samples, as represented in **Figure 2**.

Electrochemical and morphological techniques investigated the miniaturized CdSe/CdS MSQDs-based PED. This modified PED presented improved analytical signal (ca. 46% higher), lower charge transfer resistance (32 vs. 169 Ω), and larger superficial area (0.28 vs. 0.14 cm^2) in comparison with the unmodified PED. It can be attributed to CdSe/CdS nanocrystals in the sensor, which was also confirmed by microscopy analysis. The electroanalysis of dopamine in real human blood serum samples was successfully carried out, and the limit of detection obtained was lower than other recent reports that utilize more complex electrochemical platforms for detecting the same analyte. In this way, MSQDs have been shown as a promising nanomaterial to be explored in electrochemical sensing.

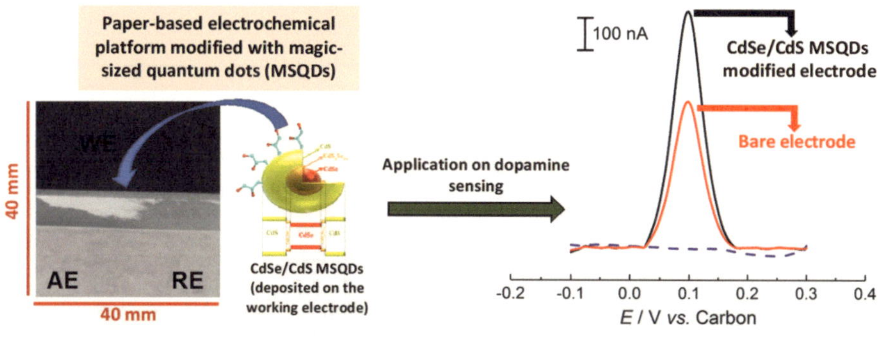

Figure 2.
Picture of the paper electrochemical device containing the pencil-drawn carbon electrodes used in work, representing a modification of the working electrode with CdSe/CdS MSQDs, and the voltammetric dopamine response regarding the unmodified and modified electrodes.

2.2 Nanocrystals to biomedical applications

In the last decade, several nanostructured systems for the delivery of chemotherapeutic agents have been developed to eliminate tumor cells. However, most of these systems cannot reach specific tumor cells without adequate control of these drug release processes, resulting in serious side effects [40, 41]. It is necessary to direct efforts to improve ideal drug distribution systems to release stimuli and selectively target cancer cells. Thus, quantum dots, liposomes, magnetic nanoparticles, and TiO2 nanocrystals have enormous potential.

Quantum dots have been the subject of extensive investigations in different science and technology areas in the past years [42, 43]. There are few studies of MSQDs, even though they exhibit features such as tiny size, higher fluorescence quantum efficiency, molar absorptivity greater than traditional QDs, and highly stable luminescence in theranostic, which refers to the simultaneous integration of diagnosis and therapy [36, 39, 44, 45].

Our group investigated the first study about the core-shell MSQDs by analyzing the electrochemical behavior of CdSe/CdS MSQDs immobilized on a gold electrode modified with a self-assembled cyclodextrin monolayer using cyclic voltammetry and electrochemical impedance spectroscopy techniques [46]. The work showed a good interaction between the thiol group from thiolated cyclodextrin and CdSe/CdS MSQDs (**Figure 3a**). The proposed method was successfully applied to encapsulation studies of Mangiferin, a natural antioxidant compound, and cyclodextrin associated with the CdSe/CdS MSQDs, and the response was compared with that of the modified electrode without MSQDs. The fluorescence study revealed that CdSe/CdS MSQDs emit blue light when excited by an optical source of the wavelength of 350 nm, and a significant increase in fluorescence and absorbance intensity is observed from the core-shell CdSe/CdS MSQDs when quantities of Mangiferin are added to the solution containing thiolated cyclodextrin. CdSe/CdS MSQDs are optically and electrochemically sensitive and can be used to detect and interact with compounds encapsulated in cyclodextrin and can be applied in theranostic.

Because of their reduced size, lipophilic nanoparticles of less than 100 nm can cross the brain-blood barrier by diffusion, allowing the drug delivery directly to the Central Nervous System (CNS) [47]. Neurodegenerative diseases (ND) such as Alzheimer's, Parkinson's, strokes, glioblastoma, Huntington's, amyotrophic lateral

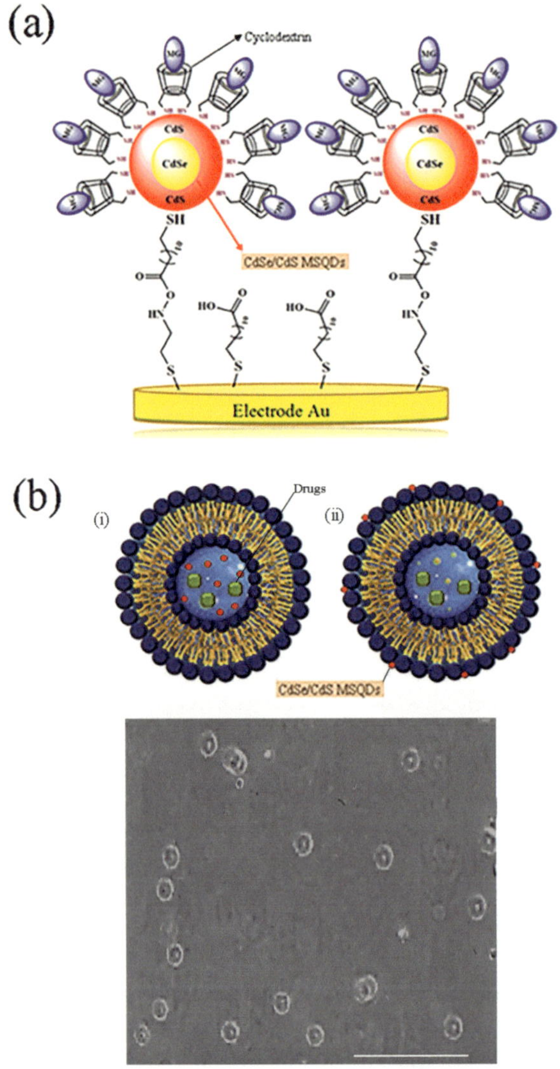

Figure 3.
(a) CdSe/CdS MSQDs immobilized on a gold electrode modified with a self-assembled cyclodextrin to encapsulation studies of Mangiferin, and (b) illustration of liposome with MSQDs (top panel) when MSQDs are (i) inside or (ii) outside and optical image the scale bar is 1 mm (bottom panel).

sclerosis may be treated differently with this approach [19]. Just like liposomes, polymeric nanoparticles may be environmentally sensitive to drug release, such as temperature change, pH change, among others. These systems may be combined therapy, delivering two or more drugs, allowing different therapy combinations.

The group has also been developing liposomes containing CdSe/CdS MSQDs aiming at a new luminescent tool for drug delivery. **Figure 3b** shows the illustration of liposomes with MSQDs (top panel); when MSQDs are (i) inside or (ii) outside and optical image, the scale bar is 1 mm (bottom panel). Therefore, we demonstrate that CdSe/CdS MSQDs can be used in drug delivery systems, which serve as photostable fluorescent reporters. A combination of MSQDs with liposomes is a powerful theranostic tool since it is possible to monitor their location via luminescence in addition to drug delivery.

Since the 1990's Liposomal Amphotericin B has been available in the market, being one of the oldest and most clinical used nanoparticle formulations in the treatment of leishmaniasis. In 1978, Alvin et al. proved that the use of liposomal leishmanicidal drugs could enhance 700 times the efficacy [48]. Liposome functionalization is another advance that can enhance circulation time and release drugs according to temperature change and pH change; magnetic prepared liposomes can be target-directed by applying a magnetic field, and ligands in the lipidic bilayer can actively target cellular types [49]. Thus, the group has been working to develop drug systems containing liposomes and nanocrystals.

The study of bioactive substances by electrochemical and UV-visible spectroscopic methods is already very conceptual. The association of magnetic nanoparticles has emerged as a new bias of these techniques. We group reported the interaction between the molecule LQM10, a derivative of guanylhydrazone, with the $CoFe_2O_4$ NCs coated with polyamidoamine dendrimer (PAMAM), generating a nanocarrier to benefit LQM10 (**Figure 4**). The PAMAM dendrimer has empty spaces that change according to its generation. In these places, as well as cyclodextrins, "guest-host" interactions can occur, where the hydrophobic molecule can interact with dendrimers by hydrogen bonds, ionic bonding, or hydrophobic interactions, being possible interaction with LQM10 due to the tert-butyl group attached to its ring, which gives it a hydrophobic character, as well as with $CoFe_2O_4$ NCs. In addition to this type of interaction. PAMAM can make covalent and non-covalent bonds through its primary and tertiary amine groups, which would also be possible by observing the structure of LQM10. Both interactions can occur in an isolated or simultaneous way, making it possible for a single molecule of PAMAM to interact with several other substances, which enables its association with $CoFe_2O_4$ NCs, producing a better nanocarrier for LQM10 [50].

The magnetic properties of $CoFe_2O_4$ NCs and each nanocarrier were confirmed by a vibrating sample magnetometer and field-effect calorimetry. LQM10 showed good interaction corroborating with the results of UV-visible and electrochemistry data.

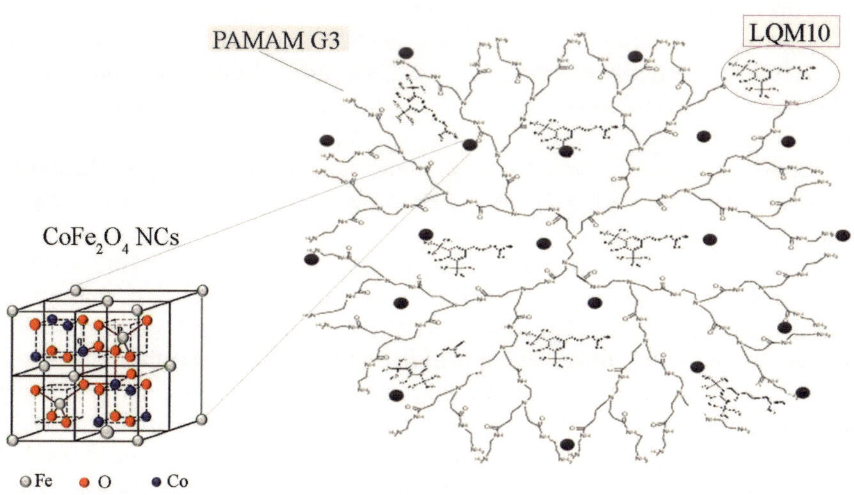

Figure 4.
Illustrative scheme of the nanocarrier composed by the PAMAN molecule, the black spheres represent the $CoFe_2O_4$ NCs and the LQM10 molecule.

The heat generation by magnetic hyperthermia of $CoFe_2O_4$ NCs in the presence of PAMAM G3 and LQM10 was observed, demonstrating the association of promising nanocarriers (PAMAM G3 and $CoFe_2O_4$ NCs) with anticancer substances and their applicability as magnetic hyperthermia [50].

The implantation of material inside biological tissues must meet a minimum requirement, called biocompatibility, defined as a biomaterial's ability to perform the desired therapeutic function without triggering any undesirable local or systemic effect, generating the most cellular or tissue response. Therefore, optimizing clinical therapeutic performance should be as beneficial as possible [51]. After application, an interaction occurs between the host's immune system and the implanted biomaterial, leading to a specific cellular reaction to the biomaterial [52]. Proteins play a crucial role in the interaction between biomaterials and cells or tissues. Thus, the absorption of proteins on the material surface is the first event of this interaction, which is decisive for the subsequent cell growth processes, differentiation, and extracellular matrix formation [53].

The deliberate, accidental implantation of any foreign material into living tissues causes a response, and it is not the response itself but the extent, intensity, and duration that define biocompatibility. The ideal response of biological tissues to a biomaterial is when the initial inflammatory response resulting from the surgical procedure is quickly resolved, without the presence of a chronic inflammatory infiltrate or the development of an immune response. Thus, the biomaterial must be biocompatible and have characteristics that include predictability, clinical applicability, absence of transoperative risks and minimal postoperative sequelae, and acceptance by the patient. It is also expected that this biomaterial is not carcinogenic, that it presents adequate chemical and biological stability, mechanical and elastic resistance, and has low cost [54].

The biomaterial is a natural or synthetic material intended to interact with biological systems to assess, treat, augment, or replace an organism's organ, tissue, or function [51]. The primary function of biomaterials is to replace damaged tissue and passively assume its function, selection, and manufacture, based on the imitation of the chemical and physical properties of natural tissue, causing minimal response as a foreign body [53].

Since the early 1970s, various synthetic bone substitutes have been developed to minimize the difficulties inherent in using autogenous bone grafts and homogeneous and heterogeneous bone implants [25]. The main advantages of grafts created from synthetic materials through bioengineering are biocompatibility and good reabsorption [55]. The alloplastic materials most commonly used in the medical-dental field are metals or metal alloys, ceramics, polymers, composites, and bioactive glasses [25]. Despite the wide variety of organic and synthetic materials capable of replacing bone tissue or stimulating reparational osteogenesis, there is still no material that meets all the desired requirements.

Titanium dioxide (TiO_2) is a semiconductor that absorbs and emits in the ultraviolet region with numerous applications in biomedical fields such as cosmetics, medicines, and pharmaceutical products [56–58]. This material has three crystalline phases: anatase, brookite, rutile, and physical and biological properties [59]. The anatase phase is more electroactive than the rutile phase, having greater genotoxicity and photocatalytic effects [60–63]. The TiO_2 NCs have shown great potential for use in implants due to their excellent physical, chemical, and biological properties, such as high specific surface area, ability to provoke positive cellular response and stability in body fluids, is suitable for the propagation, proliferation, and differentiation of osteoblast cells [56, 64]. Thus, will show exciting results obtained by the group using TiO_2 nanocrystals as well as their luminescence bio-location.

The porous structure of TiO_2 nanotubes increases bone regeneration and repair, presenting good osteointegration, being used as a graft and biological fixation element for implants [57, 65–70]. In an experimental study carried out by our research group using TiO_2 NCs, adequate osteointegration in bone failure in the calvary of rats was evidenced, with the presence of a large amount of newly formed tissue, suggesting effective osteoinductive action, as can be seen in **Figure 5**.

Despite the promising findings with TiO_2 NCs, it is essential to report that there may be a high contamination rate and post-surgical infection since, currently, the spread of antibiotic-resistant bacteria is a worrying threat to human health.

In this context, it is essential to establish new antimicrobial strategies, in which the idea of coating device surfaces with active antimicrobial metals is considered one of the essential strategies. Therefore, bimetallic corrosion is inevitable, in which TiO_2 photocatalytic nanomaterials, in the anatase form, offer more significant advantages for antimicrobial purposes [71]. Still, the photocatalytic activity of TiO_2 under exposure to ultraviolet radiation results in disinfectant properties, mainly related to the generation of reactive oxygen species [72].

In this perspective, the sensitive and accurate detection of biological analytes in low concentrations is another application of TiO_2 nanostructures that is beneficial for biomedical research and clinical diagnosis. There has been significant interest in applying TiO_2 detection in biosensors [57, 67]. Therefore, those reported in the literature point out that TiO_2 nanocrystals are inert and safe structures when exposed to the human organism, thus contributing to new promising nanotechnologies with the biomedical application.

Luminescence is related to some materials' ability to light emissions. This excitation energy (absorbed energy) can be obtained from different sources: photons usually in the ultraviolet region of the electromagnetic spectrum (emission called photoluminescence), electrical energy (electroluminescence), electron beam (cathodoluminescence), physical impact (gives rise to triboluminescence) and heating the luminophore (results in thermoluminescence) [73, 74]. Photoluminescent materials are often called phosphors or luminophores [73]. Efficient luminophore requirements are efficient absorption of light in a suitable spectral region; chemical stability of the excited electronic state populated after light absorption; high conversion efficiency to the excited luminescent state; a long lifetime of excited state luminescence; high luminescent efficiency [75].

Photoluminescent materials require a host crystalline matrix, such as TiO2, as well as an activating ion, such as lanthanides. Lanthanide ions are known to have

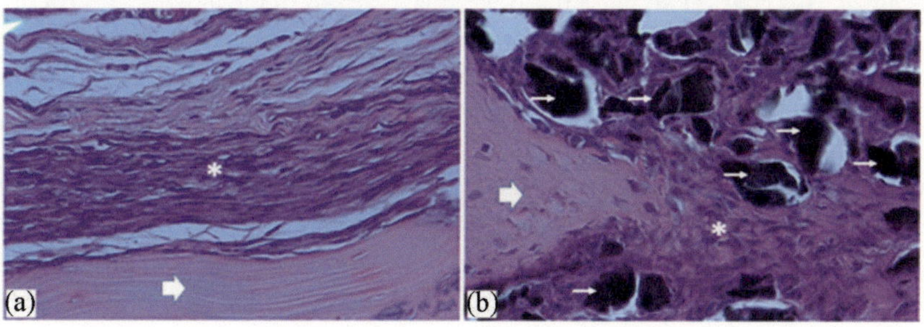

Figure 5.
Histological section of rats' calvaria: (a) fibrous connective tissue (asterisk); bone tissue (arrow); and (b) TiO_2 NCs (arrows), bone tissue (arrow), and neoformed fibrous connective tissue (asterisk) (hematoxylin and eosin staining, 400×).

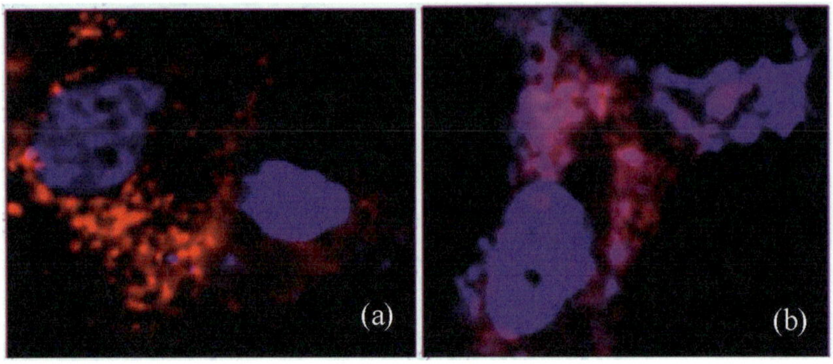

Figure 6.
Fluorescence microscopy of mesenchymal stem cells treated with europium doped TiO_2 NCs: (a) culture medium with 50 μg of mesenchymal stem cells; and (b) culture medium with 100 μg of mesenchymal stem cells.

characteristic luminescence (high color purity). Among lanthanides, the europium ion (Eu^{3+}) is one of the most used for biomarking due to its intrinsic electronic spectroscopic properties in the visible region under excitation in the ultraviolet region [76, 77].

Compounds with trivalent europium ions emit red light, with emission spectra of thin bands of approximately 614 nm. Therefore, it has been applied to investigate the properties and functions of biochemical systems and the determination of biologically active substances. In this context, we find reports of its application mainly as spectroscopic probes in the study of biomolecules [78]; in biological tracers to follow the path taken by medicines in the human organism and animals; as markers in immunology (fluoroimmunoassays) [79], as well as contrast agents in non-invasive diagnosis of pathologies in tissues by nuclear magnetic resonance imaging [80].

In a study carried out by our research group with TiO_2 NCs doped with Eu^{3+}, in the culture of mesenchymal stem cells, isolated from bone marrow cells, the presence of these nanocrystals was observed in the cytoplasm of the cells after 24 hours of incubation, not being found in the cell nucleus, suggesting the absence of cytotoxicity and genotoxicity (**Figure 6**).

3. Conclusion

Therefore, this chapter showed nanocrystals inserted in biosensors and their use in drug delivery tools or biomaterials. Graphene and magic-sized quantum dots into biosensors enable an increase in sensitivity and specificity, making the development of nanotechnological platforms in biological diagnosis possible. In theranostic applications, magic-sized quantum dots, magnetic nanoparticles, and TiO_2 nanocrystals can be innovative drug delivery tools and dental and orthopedic applications. Thus, the fabrication of nanomaterials with interesting properties makes it possible to generate several potential tools to improve electrochemical sensors and in theranostic applications.

Acknowledgements

This work was supported by CNPq, CAPES, FAPEAL, and FAPEMIG.

Conflict of interest

The authors declare no conflict of interest.

Author details

Anielle C.A. Silva[1,2*], Eliete A. Alvin[1,2], Lais S. de Jesus[1], Caio C.L. de França[3], Marílya P.G. da Silva[3], Samaysa L. Lins[3], Diógenes Meneses[3], Marcela R. Lemes[4], Rhanoica O. Guerra[4], Marcos V. da Silva[4], Carlo J.F. de Oliveira[4], Virmondes Rodrigues Junior[4], Renata M. Etchebehere[5], Fabiane C. de Abreu[3], Bruno G. Lucca[6], Sanívia A.L. Pereira[7,8], Rodrigo C. Rosa[9] and Noelio O. Dantas[1]

1 Laboratory of New Nanostructured and Functional Materials, Physics Institute, Federal University of Alagoas, Maceió, AL, Brazil

2 Programa de Pós-Graduação da Rede Nordeste de Biotecnologia (RENORBIO), Federal University of Alagoas, Maceió, AL, Brazil

3 LEMAN, Institute of Chemistry and Biotechnology, Federal University of Alagoas Maceió, Maceió, AL, Brazil

4 Department of Microbiology, Immunology, and Parasitology, Institute of Biological and Natural Sciences, Federal University of Triângulo Mineiro, Uberaba, MG, Brazil

5 Clinics Hospital, Service of Surgical Patology, Federal University of Triângulo Mineiro, Uberaba, MG, Brazil

6 Institute of Chemistry, Federal University of Mato Grosso do Sul, Campo Grande, MS, Brazil

7 Laboratory of Cell and Molecular Biology, University de Uberaba (UNIUBE), Uberaba, MG, Brazil

8 Professional Education Center, Federal University of Triângulo Mineiro, Uberaba, MG, Brazil

9 Department of Structural Biology, Institute of Biological and Natural Sciences, Federal University of Triângulo Mineiro, Uberaba, MG, Brazil

*Address all correspondence to: acalmeida@fis.ufal.br

References

[1] Darvishi MH, Nomani A, Hashemzadeh H, Amini M, Shokrgozar MA, Dinarvand R. Targeted DNA delivery to cancer cells using a biotinylated chitosan carrier. Biotechnology and Applied Biochemistry. 2017;**64**:423-432. DOI: 10.1002/bab.1497

[2] Razavi H, Janfaza S. Ethosome: A nanocarrier for transdermal drug delivery. Archives of Advances in Biosciences. 2015;**6**:38-43. DOI: 10.22037/jps.v6i2.8856

[3] Hashemzadeh H, Allahverdi A, Sedghi M, Vaezi Z, Moghadam TT, Rothbauer M, et al. PDMS nano-modified scaffolds for improvement of stem cells proliferation and differentiation in microfluidic platform. Nanomaterials. 2020;**10**:668. DOI: 10.3390/nano10040668

[4] Esfandyari J, Shojaedin-Givi B, Hashemzadeh H, Mozafari-Nia M, Vaezi Z, Naderi-Manesh H. Capture and detection of rare cancer cells in blood by intrinsic fluorescence of a novel functionalized diatom. Photodiagnosis and Photodynamic Therapy. 2020;**30**:101753. DOI: 10.1016/j.pdpdt.2020.101753

[5] Garimella R, Eltorai AEM. Nanotechnology in orthopedics. Journal of Orthopaedics. 2017;**14**:30-33. DOI: 10.1016/j.jor.2016.10.026

[6] Janfaza S, Banan Nojavani M, Nikkhah M, Alizadeh T, Esfandiar A, Ganjali MR. A selective chemiresistive sensor for the cancer-related volatile organic compound hexanal by using molecularly imprinted polymers and multiwalled carbon nanotubes. Microchimica Acta. 2019;**186**:137. DOI: 10.1007/s00604-019-3241-z

[7] Razavi H, Darvishi MH, Janfaza S. Silver sulfadiazine encapsulated in lipid-based nanocarriers for burn treatment. Journal of Burn Care & Research. 2018;**39**:319-325. DOI: 10.1097/BCR.0000000000000602

[8] Hashemzadeh H, Allahverdi A, Ghorbani M, Soleymani H, Kocsis Á, Fischer MB, et al. Gold nanowires/fibrin nanostructure as microfluidics platforms for enhancing stem cell differentiation: Bio-AFM study. Micromachines. 2020;**11**:50. DOI: 10.3390/mi11010050

[9] Hashemzadeh H, Javadi H, Darvishi MH. Study of structural stability and formation mechanisms in DSPC and DPSM liposomes: A coarse-grained molecular dynamics simulation. Scientific Reports. 2020;**10**:1-10. DOI: 10.1038/s41598-020-58730-z

[10] Jha RK, Jha PK, Chaudhury K, Rana SVS, Guha SK. An emerging interface between life science and nanotechnology: Present status and prospects of reproductive healthcare aided by nano-biotechnology. Nano Reviews. 2014;**5**:22762. DOI: 10.3402/nano.v5.22762

[11] de Reis ÉM, de Rezende AAA, Santos DV, de Oliveria PF, Nicolella HD, Tavares DC, et al. Assessment of the genotoxic potential of two zinc oxide sources (amorphous and nanoparticles) using the in vitro micronucleus test and the in vivo wing somatic mutation and recombination test. Food and Chemical Toxicology. 2015;**84**:55-63. DOI: 10.1016/j.fct.2015.07.008

[12] Hoang V, Ganguli D. Amorphous nanoparticles—Experiments and computer simulations. Physics Reports. 2012;**518**:81-140. DOI: 10.1016/j.physrep.2012.07.004

[13] Chen Y, Lai Z, Zhang X, Fan Z, He Q, Tan C, et al. Phase engineering of nanomaterials. Nature Reviews Chemistry. 2020;**4**:243-256. DOI: 10.1038/s41570-020-0173-4

[14] Jiang J, Oberdörster G, Elder A, Gelein R, Mercer P, Biswas P. Does nanoparticle activity depend upon size and crystal phase? Nanotoxicology. 2008;**2**:33-42. DOI: 10.1080/17435390701882478

[15] Moreau LM, Ha DH, Zhang H, Hovden R, Muller DA, Robinson RD. Defining crystalline/amorphous phases of nanoparticles through X-ray absorption spectroscopy and X-ray diffraction: The case of nickel phosphide. Chemistry of Materials. 2013;**25**:2394-2403. DOI: 10.1021/cm303490y

[16] Geetha Bai R, Muthoosamy K, Zhou M, Ashokkumar M, Huang NM, Manickam S. Sonochemical and sustainable synthesis of graphene-gold (G-Au) nanocomposites for enzymeless and selective electrochemical detection of nitric oxide. Biosensors & Bioelectronics. 2017;**87**:622-629. DOI: 10.1016/j.bios.2016.09.003

[17] Song BB, Zhen YF, Yin HY, Song XC. Electrochemical sensor based on platinum nanoparticles modified graphite-like carbon nitride for detection of phenol. Journal of Nanoscience and Nanotechnology. 2019;**19**:4020-4025. DOI: 10.1166/jnn.2019.16297

[18] Yin HY, Zheng YF, Wang L. Au/CeO 2/g-C 3 N 4 nanocomposite modified electrode as electrochemical sensor for the determination of phenol. Journal of Nanoscience and Nanotechnology. 2020;**20**:5539-5545. DOI: 10.1166/jnn.2020.17857

[19] Gondim BLC, da Silva Catarino J, de Sousa MAD, de Oliveira Silva M, Lemes MR, de Carvalho-Costa TM, et al. Nanoparticle-mediated drug delivery: Blood-brain barrier as the main obstacle to treating infectious diseases in CNS. Current Pharmaceutical Design. 2019;**25**:3983-3996. DOI: 10.2174/1381612825666191014171354

[20] Téllez J, Echeverry MC, Romero I, Guatibonza A, Santos Ramos G, Borges De Oliveira AC, et al. Use of liposomal nanoformulations in antileishmania therapy: Challenges and perspectives. Journal of Liposome Research. 2020;**31**:169-176. DOI: 10.1080/08982104.2020.1749067

[21] Feitosa RC, Geraldes DC, Beraldo-de-Araújo VL, Costa JSR, Oliveira-Nascimento L. Pharmacokinetic aspects of nanoparticle-in-matrix drug delivery systems for oral/buccal delivery. Frontiers in Pharmacology. 2019;**10**:1057. DOI: 10.3389/fphar.2019.01057

[22] Raza K, Kumar P, Kumar N, Malik R. Pharmacokinetics and biodistribution of the nanoparticles. In: Advances in Nanomedicine for the Delivery of Therapeutic Nucleic Acids. Amsterdam, Netherlands: Elsevier Inc; 2017. pp. 166-186

[23] Abdifetah O, Na-Bangchang K. Pharmacokinetic studies of nanoparticles as a delivery system for conventional drugs and herb-derived compounds for cancer therapy: A systematic review. International journal of Nanomedicine. 2019;**14**:5659-5677. DOI: 10.2147/IJN.S213229

[24] Rodallec A, Benzekry S, Lacarelle B, Ciccolini J, Fanciullino R, Benzekry S. Pharmacokinetics variability: Why nanoparticles are not magic bullets in oncology. Critical Reviews in Oncology/Hematology. 2018;**129**:1-12. DOI: 10.1016/j.critrevonc.2018.06.008ï

[25] Moore WR, Graves SE, Bain GI. Synthetic bone graft substitutes. ANZ Journal of Surgery. 2001;**71**:354-361. DOI: 10.1046/j.1440-1622.2001.02128.x

[26] Hong J, Wang Y, Zhu L, Jiang L. An electrochemical sensor based on gold-nanocluster-modified graphene screen-printed electrodes for the detection of β-lactoglobulin in milk. Sensors. 2020;**20**:3956. DOI: 10.3390/s20143956

[27] Chen D, Tang L, Reviews JL-CS. undefined graphene-based materials in electrochemistry. Chemical Society Reviews. 2010;**8**:3157-3180. DOI: 10.1039/b923596e

[28] Zhang X, Wang KP, Zhang LN, Zhang YC, Shen L. Phosphorus-doped graphene-based electrochemical sensor for sensitive detection of acetaminophen. Analytica Chimica Acta. 2018;**1036**:26-32. DOI: 10.1016/j.aca.2018.06.079

[29] Wang X, Sun G, Routh P, Kim DH, Huang W, Chen P. Heteroatom-doped graphene materials: Syntheses, properties and applications. Chemical Society Reviews. 2014;**43**:7067-7098. DOI: 10.1039/c4cs00141a

[30] Yu X, Feng L, Park HS. Highly flexible pseudocapacitors of phosphorus-incorporated porous reduced graphene oxide films. Journal of Power Sources. 2018;**390**:93-99. DOI: 10.1016/j.jpowsour.2018.04.032

[31] Petroni JM, Lucca BG, da Silva Júnior LC, Barbosa Alves DC, Souza Ferreira V. Paper-based electrochemical devices coupled to external graphene-Cu nanoparticles modified solid electrode through meniscus configuration and their use in biological analysis. Electroanalysis. 2017;**29**:2628-2637. DOI: 10.1002/elan.201700398

[32] Hummers WS, Offeman RE. Preparation of graphitic oxide. Journal of the American Chemical Society. 1958;**80**:1339. DOI: 10.1021/ja01539a017

[33] Saquib Q, Faisal M, Al-Khedhairy AA, Alatar AA, editors. Cellular and Molecular Toxicology of Nanoparticles. Vol. 1048. Cham: Springer International Publishing; 2018

[34] Rezaei B, Jamei HR, Ensafi AA. Lysozyme aptasensor based on a glassy carbon electrode modified with a nanocomposite consisting of multi-walled carbon nanotubes, poly(diallyl dimethyl ammonium chloride) and carbon quantum dots. Microchimica Acta. 2018;**185**:1-10. DOI: 10.1007/s00604-017-2656-7

[35] Jasieniak J, Smith L, Van Embden J, Mulvaney P, Califano M. Re-examination of the size-dependent absorption properties of CdSe quantum dots. Journal of Physical Chemistry C. 2009;**113**:19468-19474. DOI: 10.1021/jp906827m

[36] Silva ACA, de Deus SLV, Silva MJB, Dantas NO. Highly stable luminescence of CdSe magic-sized quantum dots in HeLa cells. Sensors and Actuators B: Chemical. 2014;**191**:108-114. DOI: 10.1016/j.snb.2013.09.063

[37] de França CCL, Meneses D, Silva ACA, Dantas NO, de Abreu FC, Petroni JM, et al. Development of novel paper-based electrochemical device modified with CdSe/CdS magic-sized quantum dots and application for the sensing of dopamine. Electrochimica Acta. 2021;**367**:137486. DOI: 10.1016/j.electacta.2020.137486

[38] Silva ACA, Da Silva SW, Morais PC, Dantas NO. Shell thickness modulation in ultrasmall CdSe/CdSxSe 1-x/CdS core/shell quantum dots via 1-thioglycerol.

ACS Nano. 2014:8, 1913-1922. DOI: 10.1021/nn406478f

[39] Almeida Silva A, Silva MJ, da Luz FA, Silva D, de Deus S, Dantas N. Controlling the cytotoxicity of CdSe magic-sized quantum dots as a function of surface defect density. Nano Letters;**14**:5452-5457. DOI: 10.1021/nl5028028

[40] Lammers T, Subr V, Ulbrich K, Hennink WE, Storm G, Kiessling F. Polymeric nanomedicines for image-guided drug delivery and tumor-targeted combination therapy. Nano Today. 2010;**5**:197-212. DOI: 10.1016/j.nantod.2010.05.001

[41] Zahednezhad F, Zakeri-Milani P, Shahbazi Mojarrad J, Valizadeh H. The latest advances of cisplatin liposomal formulations: Essentials for preparation and analysis. Expert Opinion on Drug Delivery. 2020;**17**:523-541. DOI: 10.1080/17425247.2020.1737672

[42] Kargozar S, Hoseini SJ, Milan PB, Hooshmand S, Kim HW, Mozafari M. Quantum dots: A review from concept to clinic. Biotechnology Journal. 2020;**15**:e2000117. DOI: 10.1002/biot.202000117

[43] Wagner AM, Knipe JM, Orive G, Peppas NA. Quantum dots in biomedical applications. Acta Biomaterialia. 2019;**94**:44-63. DOI: 10.1016/j.actbio.2019.05.022

[44] Silva ACA, Correia LIV, Silva MJB, Zóia MAP, Azevedo FVPV, Rodrigues JP, et al. Biocompatible magic sized quantum dots: Luminescent markers and probes. In: State of the Art in Nano-Bioimaging. Vol. 1. 2017. pp. 95-104

[45] Silva ACA, Azevedo FVPV, Zóia MAP, Rodrigues JP, Dantas NO, Melo VRÁ, et al. Magic sized quantum dots as a theranostic tool for breast cancer. In: Recent Studies & Advances in Breast Cancer. Wilmington: Open Access eBooks; 2017. pp. 1-10

[46] de Lima França CC, da Silva Terto EG, Dias-Vermelho MV, Silva ACA, Dantas NO, de Abreu FC. The electrochemical behavior of core-shell CdSe/CdS magic-sized quantum dots linked to cyclodextrin for studies of the encapsulation of bioactive compounds. Journal of Solid State Electrochemistry. 2016;**20**:2533-2540. DOI: 10.1007/s10008-016-3221-8

[47] Mansoor KR, Sima KR, Soheila KR. Advancement of polymer–based nanoparticles as smart drug delivery systems in neurodegenerative medicine. Journal of Nanomedicine Reseasrch. 2019;**8**:277-280. DOI: 10.15406/jnmr.2019.08.00198

[48] Alving CR, Steck EA, Chapman WL, Waits VB, Hendricks LD, Swartz GM, et al. Therapy of leishmaniasis: Superior efficacies of liposome encapsulated drugs. Proceedings of the National Academy of Sciences of the United States of America. 1978;**75**:2959-2963. DOI: 10.1073/pnas.75.6.2959

[49] Cheng R, Liu L, Xiang Y, Lu Y, Deng L, Zhang H, et al. Advanced liposome-loaded scaffolds for therapeutic and tissue engineering applications. Biomaterials. 2020;**232**:119706. DOI: 10.1016/j.biomaterials.2019.119706

[50] da Silva MPG, Candido ACL, de Araújo-Júnior JX, Silva ACA, Dantas NO, de Aquino TM, et al. Evaluation of the interaction of a guanylhydrazone derivative with cobalt ferrite nanoparticles and PAMAM electrochemical and UV/visible spectroscopic techniques. Journal of Solid State Electrochemistry. 2020;**25**:743-752. DOI: 10.1007/s10008-020-04848-z

[51] Williams DF. On the mechanisms of biocompatibility. Biomaterials. 2008;**29**:2941-2953. DOI: 10.1016/j.biomaterials.2008.04.023

[52] Al-Maawi S, Orlowska A, Sader R, James Kirkpatrick C, Ghanaati S. In vivo cellular reactions to different biomaterials—Physiological and pathological aspects and their consequences. Seminars in Immunology. 2017;**29**:49-61. DOI: 10.1016/j.smim.2017.06.001

[53] Othman Z, Cillero Pastor B, van Rijt S, Habibovic P. Understanding interactions between biomaterials and biological systems using proteomics. Biomaterials. 2018;**167**:191-204. DOI: 10.1016/j.biomaterials.2018.03.020

[54] Boss JH, Shajrawi I, Aunullah J, Mendes DG. The relativity of biocompatibility. A critique of the concept of biocompatibility. Israel Journal of Medical Sciences. 1995;**31**:203-209

[55] Karalashvili L, Kakabadze A, Uhryn M, Vyshnevska H, Ediberidze K, Kakabadze Z. Bone grafts for reconstruction of bone defects (review). Georgian Medical News. 2018;**282**:44-49

[56] Hasanzadeh Kafshgari M, Goldmann WH. Insights into Theranostic Properties of Titanium Dioxide for Nanomedicine. Nano-Micro Letters. 2020;**12**:1-35. DOI: 10.1007/s40820-019-0362-1

[57] Molaeirad A, Janfaza S, Karimi-Fard A, Mahyad B. Photocurrent generation by adsorption of two main pigments of halobacterium salinarum on TiO2 nanostructured electrode. Biotechnology and Applied Biochemistry. 2015;**62**:121-125. DOI: 10.1002/bab.1244

[58] Naseri N, Janfaza S, Irani R. Visible light switchable bR/TiO2 nanostructured photoanodes for bio-inspired solar energy conversion. RSC Advances. 2015;**5**:18642-18646. DOI: 10.1039/c4ra16188b

[59] Chen X, Selloni A. Introduction: Titanium dioxide (TiO2) nanomaterials. Chemical Reviews. 2014;**114**:9281-9282. DOI: 10.1021/cr500422r

[60] de Melo Reis É, de Rezende AAA, de Oliveira PF, Nicolella HD, Tavares DC, Silva ACA, et al. Evaluation of titanium dioxide nanocrystal-induced genotoxicity by the cytokinesis-block micronucleus assay and the Drosophila wing spot test. Food and Chemical Toxicology. 2016;**96**:309-319. DOI: 10.1016/j.fct.2016.08.023

[61] Carvalho Naves MP, de Morais CR, Silva ACA, Dantas NO, Spanó MA, de Rezende AAA. Assessment of mutagenic, recombinogenic and carcinogenic potential of titanium dioxide nanocristals in somatic cells of drosophila melanogaster. Food and Chemical Toxicology. 2018;**112**:273-228. DOI: 10.1016/j.fct.2017.12.040

[62] Abdel Moniem SM, Ali MEM, Gad-Allah TA, Khalil ASG, Ulbricht M, El-Shahat MF, et al. Detoxification of hexavalent chromium in wastewater containing organic substances using simonkolleite-TiO2photocatalyst. Process Safety and Environment Protection. 2015;**95**:247-254. DOI: 10.1016/j.psep.2015.03.010

[63] Bakbolat B, Daulbayev C, Sultanov F, Beissenov R, Umirzakov A, Mereke A, et al. Recent developments of TiO2-based photocatalysis in the hydrogen evolution and photodegradation: A review. Nanomaterials. 2020;**10**:1-16. DOI: 10.3390/nano10091790

[64] Bezerra Neta IA, Mota MF, Lira HL, Neves GA, Menezes RR. Nanostructured titanium dioxide for use in bone implants: A short review. Cerâmica. 2020;**66**:440-450. DOI: 10.1590/0366-69132020663802905

[65] Weetall HH. Biosensor technology what? where? when? and why? Biosensors and Bioelectronics. 1996;**11**: i-iv. DOI: 10.1016/0956-5663(96)83729-8

[66] Razavi H, Janfaza S. Medical nanobiosensors: A tutorial review. Nanomedicine Journal. 2015;**2**:74-87

[67] Abdullah M, Kamarudin SK. Titanium dioxide nanotubes (TNT) in energy and environmental applications: An overview. Renewable and Sustainable Energy Reviews. 2017;**76**:212-225. DOI: 10.1016/j.rser.2017.01.057

[68] Viter R, Tereshchenko A, Smyntyna V, Ogorodniichuk J, Starodub N, Yakimova R, et al. Toward development of optical biosensors based on photoluminescence of TiO2 nanoparticles for the detection of Salmonella. Sensors and Actuators B: Chemical. 2017;**252**:95-102. DOI: 10.1016/j.snb.2017.05.139

[69] Wang T, Jiang H, Wan L, Zhao Q, Jiang T, Wang B, et al. Potential application of functional porous TiO2 nanoparticles in light-controlled drug release and targeted drug delivery. Acta Biomaterialia. 2015;**13**:354-363. DOI: 10.1016/j.actbio.2014.11.010

[70] Zhao L, Mei S, Chu PK, Zhang Y, Wu Z. The influence of hierarchical hybrid micro/nano-textured titanium surface with titania nanotubes on osteoblast functions. Biomaterials. 2010;**31**:5072-5082. DOI: 10.1016/j.biomaterials.2010.03.014

[71] Chung CJ, Lin HI, Tsou HK, Shi ZY, He JL. An antimicrobial TiO2 coating for reducing hospital-acquired infection. Journal of Biomedical Materials Research Part B: Applied Biomaterials: An Official Journal of The Society for Biomaterials, The Japanese Society for Biomaterials, and The Australian Society for Biomaterials and the Korean Society for Biomaterials. 2008;**85**:220-224. DOI: 10.1002/jbm.b.30939

[72] Foster HA, Ditta IB, Varghese S, Steele A. Photocatalytic disinfection using titanium dioxide: Spectrum and mechanism of antimicrobial activity. Applied Microbiology and Biotechnology. 2011;**90**:1847-1868. DOI: 10.1007/s00253-011-3213-7

[73] Parker D. Luminescent lanthanide sensors for pH, p O2 and selected anions. Coordination Chemistry Reviews. 2000;**205**:109-130. DOI: 10.1016/s0010-8545(00)00241-1

[74] Barth A, Haris P. Advances in biomedical spectroscopy. In: Biological and Biomedical Infrared Spectroscopy. Vol. 2. Amsterdam, Netherlands: IOS Press; 2009

[75] Lima FF, Andrade CT. Synthesis and characterization of aba-type copolymers for encapsulation of bovine hemoglobin. Quimica Nova. 2012;**35**:956-961. DOI: 10.1590/s0100-40422012000500017

[76] Trotochaud L, Boettcher SW. Synthesis of rutile-phase SnxTi1-xO2 solid-solution and (SnO2)x/(TiO2)1-x core/shell nanoparticles with tunable lattice constants and controlled morphologies. Chemistry of Materials. 2011;**23**:4920-4930. DOI: 10.1021/cm201737x

[77] Rodrigues LCV, Stefani R, Brito HF, Felinto MCFC, Hls J, Lastusaari M, et al.

Thermoluminescence and synchrotron radiation studies on the persistent luminescence of BaAl2O4:Eu2,Dy3. Journal of Solid State Chemistry. 2010;**183**:2365-2371. DOI: 10.1016/j.jssc.2010.07.044

[78] Richardson FS. Terbium(III) and europium(III) ions as luminescent probes and stains for biomolecular systems. Chemical Reviews. 1982;**82**:541-552. DOI: 10.1021/cr00051a004

[79] Kodaira CA, Brito HF, Malta OL, Serra OA. Luminescence and energy transfer of the europium (III) tungstate obtained via the Pechini method. Journal of Luminescence. 2003;**101**:11-21. DOI: 10.1016/S0022-2313(02)00384-8

[80] Silva HRM, Fonseca MG, Espínola JGP, Brito HF, Faustino WM, Teotonio EES. Luminescent Eu^{III} complexes immobilized on a vermiculite clay surface. European Journal of Inorganic Chemistry. 2014;**2014**: 1914-1921. DOI: 10.1002/ejic.201301494